August 1998

Cancer

Cancer
A Comprehensive
Clinical Guide

Edited by

David Morris
Professor of Surgery, The St. George Hospital
Kogarah, Australia

John Kearsley
Professor of Radiation Oncology, The St. George Hospital
Kogarah, Australia

and

Chris Williams
Co-ordinator — Cochrane Cancer Network
Institute of Health Sciences, Oxford, UK

h⚫ap **harwood academic publishers**
Australia • Canada • China • France • Germany • India • Japan • Luxembourg
Malaysia • The Netherlands • Russia • Singapore • Switzerland

Copyright © 1998 OPA (Overseas Publishers Association) N.V. Published by license under the Harwood Academic Publishers imprint, part of The Gordon and Breach Publishing Group.

Amsteldijk 166
1st Floor
1079 LH Amsterdam
The Netherlands

British Library Cataloguing in Publication Data

A catalogue record for this book is available from the British Library.

ISBN: 90-5702-215-X (hardcover)

Contents

Preface

The aim of this book is to provide a simple, comprehensive and structured medical text on cancer. It is truly multidisciplinary, as is the reality of cancer care. We felt that there was a considerable need for such a book. It is principally aimed at helping senior medical students and early graduates, oncology nurses and scientists with an interest in clinical aspects of cancer care. A large number of very eminent people from all over the world have kindly made great contributions to it and the publisher has provided enthusiastic support.

We hope that it will improve the training of cancer carers and ultimately improve care for this increasingly important cause of morbidity and death.

List of Contributors

Nicholas Armitage
Department of Surgery
University Hospital
Queen's Medical Centre
Nottingham
UK

Michael Baum
Professor of Surgery
University College Hospital
London
UK

Patrick Boland
Orthopaedic Surgery
Memorial Sloan-Kettering Cancer Center
New York
USA

Michael Boyer
Medical Oncologist
Royal Prince Alfred Hospital
Camperdown NSW
Australia

Michael Brada
Senior Lecturer and Consultant
Radiotherapy and Oncology
The Institute of Cancer Research and The Royal
  Marsden NHS Trust
Sutton
Surrey
UK

Frank J. Branicki
Professor and Head of Department of Surgery
University of Queensland
Clinical Sciences Building
Royal Brisbane Hospital
Herston QLD
Australia

Michael Burgess
Bristol Royal Hospital for Sick Children
St. Michael's Hill
Bristol
UK

T.J. Christmas
Consultant
Department of Urology
Charing Cross Hospital
London
UK

Philip R. Clingan
410 Crown Street
Wollongong NSW
Australia

Marylon Coates
Biostatistician
NSW Central Cancer Registry
Cancer Epidemiology Research Unit
NSW Cancer Council
Woolloomooloo NSW
Australia

Helen Collins
Department of Medical Oncology
Stanford University School of Medicine
Palo Alto CA
USA

Carol L. Davis
Macmillan Senior Lecturer in Palliative Medicine
Countess Mountbatten House
Moorgreen Hospital
Southampton
UK

David Goldstein
Senior Staff Specialist in Medical Oncology
Prince of Wales Hospital
Randwick, Sydney
Australia

David Gotley
Senior Lecturer in Surgery
Department of Surgery
University of Queensland
Clinical Sciences Building
Royal Brisbane Hospital
Herston QLD
Australia

Sandra J. Horning, MD
Department of Medical Oncology
Stanford University School of Medicine
Palo Alto CA
USA

C.W. Imrie
PancreatoBiliary Surgical Unit
Royal Infirmary
Glasgow
UK

J. Jorgensen
8/40-42 Montgomery Street
Kogarah NSW
Australia

John Kearsley
Professor of Radiation Oncology
The St. George Hospital
Kogarah
Australia

Denis W. King
Director — Division of Surgery
The St. George Hospital
Kogarah
Australia

Laurence Klotz
Toronto-Sunnybrook Regional Cancer Centre
University of Toronto
Ontario
Canada

Simon Law
Department of Surgery
University of Hong Kong Medical Centre
Queen Mary Hospital
Hong Kong

C. Soon Lee
Staff Specialist and Head of Teaching and
    Research, Hunter Area Pathology Service
Head of Anatomical Pathology
University of Newcastle
Callaghan
Australia

Joanne Lester
6360 Rising Sun Road
Grove City OH
USA

Peter Maguire
Honorary Consultant Psychiatrist and Director
Christie CRC Research Centre
University of Manchester
Withington
UK

Jo Marsden
Professor of Surgery
Institute of Cancer Research
The Royal Marsden Hospital NHS Trust
London
UK

W.H. McCarthy
Sydney Melanoma Unit
Royal Prince Alfred Hospital
Camperdown NSW
Australia

Margaret McCredie
Chief Epidemiologist
NSW Central Cancer Registry
Cancer Epidemiology Research Unit
NSW Cancer Council
Woolloomooloo NSW
Australia

David L. Morris
Professor of Surgery
The St. George Hospital
Kogarah
Australia

Martin Mott
Bristol Royal Hospital for Sick Children
St. Michael's Hill
Bristol
UK

John E. deB. Norman
Clinical Professor, University of Sydney
St. George Private Medical Centre
Kogarah
Australia

Mark Noss
Toronto-Sunnybrook Regional Cancer Centre
University of Toronto
Ontario
Canada

Michael Poulsen
Queensland Radium Institute
Herston, Queensland
Australia

Tom S. Reeve
Executive Officer, Australian Cancer Network
Emeritus Professor of Surgery
University of Sydney at Royal
North Shore Hospital
Sydney NSW
Australia

William B. Ross
Director, Department of Surgery
St. George Hospital
Kogarah
Australia

Geoffrey Sharpe
Senior Clinical Research Fellow
Academic Unit of Radiotherapy
The Royal Marsden NHS Trust
Sutton
Surrey
UK

Martin H.N. Tattersall
Department of Cancer Medicine
Royal Prince Alfred Hospital
Camperdown NSW
Australia

N.A. Watkin
Specialist Registrar
Department of Urology
Charing Cross Hospital
London
UK

Maurice J. Webb
Professor, Obstetrics & Gynecology
Head — Section of Gynecologic Surgery
Mayo Clinic
Rochester MN
USA

Chris Williams
Co-ordinator, Cochrane Cancer Network
Institute of Health Sciences
Oxford
UK

H.R. Withers
St. George Hospital
Kogarah
Australia

John Wong
Professor of Surgery
University of Hong Kong Medical Centre
Department of Surgery
Queen Mary Hospital
Hong Kong

1. Epidemiology of Cancer

MARGARET McCREDIE and MARYLON COATES

NSW Central Cancer Registry, Cancer Epidemiology Research Unit, NSW Cancer Council, Australia

Epidemiology is the study of the distribution and "determinants" of disease in human populations. In the context of cancer, this involves examination of differences in rates according to age, sex, race and place of residence, and how these might change over time and between countries or regions. It also entails "investigation" of various factors (such as smoking, diet or exposure to asbestos) which might increase or decrease the risk for cancer. Cancer is a collective term which embraces different malignant tumors which may be defined primarily by their site within the body (e.g. breast cancer) or solely by histological type (e.g. Kaposi's sarcoma). Strategies for cancer control rely on knowledge of incidence and mortality rates for individual tumors as well as information on their specific risk factors. Only through epidemiological studies can definitive data be provided on the existence, extent and nature of cancer risks in humans and on the effectiveness of preventive and intervention strategies.

CLASSIFICATION OF CANCERS

In categorizing neoplasms the three most important items of information are the location of the tumor in the body (site, topography), the histological (morphological) or cytological appearance and the behavior of the tumor (benign, malignant; *in situ*, invasive).[1] Cancer registries and national statistics agencies which code death certificates generally use the International Classification of Diseases (ICD) which is revised regularly. Data in this book are based on the 9th revision.[2]

MOST COMMON CANCERS

Estimates of worldwide incidence and mortality for the year 1985 have been made at the International Agency for Research on Cancer.[3,4] Excluding non-melanocytic skin cancer, there were 7.6 million new cases (52% in developing countries) and 5.0 million cancer deaths (56% in developing countries). Lung cancer was the most common (22% of male cancers in developed countries), stomach

---

Box 1.1. Sources of cancer data.

Incidence: Population-based cancer registries

Mortality: Population-based cancer registries
National Bureau of Statistics

Comprehensive texts

Cancer Incidence in Five Continents — incidence data from more than 120 cancer registries worldwide; published every five years by the International Agency for Research on Cancer.[5]

World Health Statistics Annual — mortality data from many countries; published annually by the World Health Organization.[6,7]

---

cancer ranked second in frequency and breast cancer, by far the most important cancer in women, was third. Other major cancers were those of colon/rectum and prostate in developed countries and cervix uteri, mouth and pharynx, liver, and esophagus in developing countries. Contrasts were apparent in the relative importance of various cancers in different regions of the world. If mortality rates estimated for 1985 continue to prevail, there will be 20% more deaths in developed, and 18% in developing countries by the year 2000 simply as a consequence of aging and population growth.[3,4] Sources of routinely collected cancer statistics are presented in Box 1.1.

VARIABLES AFFECTING FREQUENCY OF CANCERS

Age

The incidence of most cancers increases greatly with age; for example, in the USA colon cancer is more than 200 times as common in white males aged 80–84 years than in those aged 30–34 years, and the rate of prostate cancer in black males aged 80–84 years is 450 times that in those aged 40–44 years.[5] In developed countries about 60% of new diagnoses of cancer occur in those aged 60 years and over. Not only does cancer incidence vary with age, but the way in which it does so also varies. For example, the incidence of stomach cancer rises in each successive age group in New South Wales but in The Gambia it changes little after the age of 45 years.[5]

Sex

Most cancers are more frequent in men than in women, a difference which can be explained by known exposures only for the minority. A few cancers (e.g. thyroid) predominate in women.[5]

Race

Ethnic background influences the risk of some malignancies. For example, nasopharyngeal cancers occur with a markedly higher frequency among those of Chinese origin and, in some regions of the USA, prostate cancer is almost twice as common among black as white men.[5]

Box 1.2.   Measures of disease frequency.

Number of new cases in defined period — indicates public health burden.

Population at risk: generally approximated by mid-year population obtained from census.

Incidence rate: frequency of new cases occurring in a defined population of disease-free individuals in a specified period of time; for cancer, conventionally expressed per 100,000 person-years.

Crude incidence rate: total number of new cases divided by total population at risk.

Age-specific incidence rate: number of new cases in particular age group divided by population at risk in that age group (usually determined separately for males and females).

Age-standardized incidence rate: enables comparison of rates in populations with different age structures.

Cumulative rate: for ages 0–74 years approximates the lifetime risk of developing cancer.

Place of residence

Certain cancers (e.g. lung, breast) have a higher recorded incidence among urban than rural residents[5] but to some degree this may reflect less complete registration.

MEASURES OF CANCER

Commonly used measures of incidence[8–11] are described in Boxes 1.2 and 1.3; comparable measures of mortality are calculated in the same way.

Cancer epidemiology often involves the comparison of rates for a particular cancer between two different populations or for the same population at different times. Comparison of *crude rates* can be misleading because of variations in the age structure of the populations. If one population is younger than another, then even if age-specific rates were the same in both populations, more cases would appear in the older population. Thus, it is important to allow for the changing or differing age structure and this is done through age-standardization using either the 'direct' or the 'indirect' method.

A *directly age-standardized rate* is a theoretical rate which would have occurred if the observed age-specific rates applied in a reference or standard population[8] (see Box 1.3 for calculations). The

Box 1.3. WORKED EXAMPLE of the most common statistical calculations.

This example uses data for new cases of lung cancer (ICD-9 code 162) diagnosed in females in NSW, Australia in 1992.[9]

Table. Cancer of the lung in females

Age group	Number of cases (1)	NSW female population 1992 (2)	Age-specific rate per 100 000 $(3) = (1) \div (2) \times 10^5$	Standard population World (4)	Expected no. in standard population $(5) = (3) \times (4)/10^5$
0–4	0	212,156	0	12,000	0
5–9	0	208,823	0	10.000	0
10–14	0	203,468	0	9,000	0
15–19	0	214,241	0	9,000	0
20–24	0	232,704	0	8,000	0
25–29	0	232,577	0	8,000	0
30–34	5	246,282	2.0	6,000	0.12
35–39	3	227,215	1.3	6,000	0.08
40–44	15	215,545	7.0	6,000	0.42
45–49	35	184,243	19.0	6,000	1.14
50–54	42	146,812	28.6	5,000	1.43
55–59	45	128,802	34.9	4,000	1.4
60–64	94	130,766	71.9	4,000	2.88
65–69	115	127,104	90.5	3,000	2.72
70–74	119	106,122	112.1	2,000	2.24
75–79	121	82,721	146.3	1,000	1.46
80–84	59	54,142	109.0	500	0.55
85 & over	40	40,503	98.8	500	0.49
All ages	693	2,994,226	Crude rate = 23.1	100,000	14.93

Total number of cancers for all ages: 693   *(Total of column 2)*

Percent of all cancers in women:

$$\frac{Number\ of\ lung\ cancers\ in\ women}{Total\ number\ of\ all\ cancers\ in\ women} = \frac{693}{10,474} \times 100 = 6.62\%$$

Age-specific incidence rates:

$$\frac{Number\ of\ cases\ in\ age\ group}{Population\ in\ age\ group} \quad \frac{121}{82,721} = 146.3 \quad for\ ages\ 75–79$$

$$(Column\ 3\ in\ Table\ above)$$

Crude rate per 100,000:

$$\frac{Total\ number\ of\ female\ lung\ cancers}{Total\ female\ population} = \frac{693}{2,994,226} \times 100,000 = 23.1\ per\ 100,000$$

Age-standardized rate (by 'direct' method):

$$\frac{Total\ expected\ number}{Total\ standard\ population} \times 100,000 = \frac{14.93}{100,000} \times 100,000 = 14.93\ per\ 100,000$$

Cumulative rate and cumulative risk[11]:
The cumulative rate for ages 0–74 years approximates the lifetime risk of developing cancer.

Cumulative rate (0–74 years) = 5 × (sum of age-specific rates for ages 0–74) × 100 / 100 000
$= 5 \times (0 + 0 + 0 + 0 + 0 + 0 + 2.0 + 1.3 + 7.0 + ... + 90.5 + 112.1) / 1000 = 5 \times 367.3 / 1000 = 1.84\%$

This method may be used to calculate cumulative rates for any period (e.g. 0–14, 35–64 yr).
$$Cumulative\ risk = 100\ (1 - e^{-cumulative\ rate/100})\%$$

For female lung cancer the cumulative risk (0–74 years) is:
$$100\ (1 - e^{-1.84/100}) = 1.82\%$$

For female lung cancer: $\dfrac{1}{cumulative\ risk} = \dfrac{1}{1.82\ /\ 100} = 1\ in\ 55$

That is, 1 in 55 women will develop lung cancer during their first 75 years providing they continue to experience the age-specific rates applying in 1992.

"World" standard population[1] is in widespread use by cancer registries and greatly facilitates the comparison of cancer rates. Use of different standard populations will produce different 'standardized rates'.

An alternative method of *indirect age-standardization* is equivalent to comparing observed and expected numbers of cases. The expected number of cases is calculated by applying a standard set of age-specific rates to the population of interest. The observed to expected ratio is generally expressed as a percentage by multiplying by 100 and is known as the *standardized incidence ratio (SIR)* or the *standardized mortality ratio (SMR)*.[8,11]

Prevalence is a measure of the amount of cancer present in the community at a particular time.[12] It will depend on the definition of cancer — under active surveillance; under active treatment, thus excluding those apparently cured; ever have had a diagnosis of cancer and currently alive. This last definition is most commonly used when cancer registries publish data on prevalence.

Survival can be expressed as the percentage of those cases alive at a 'starting date' who were still alive after a specified interval. The choice of interval is arbitrary and will depend upon the prognosis of the cancer concerned. A detailed explanation of the actuarial or life-table method can be found in Parkin and Hakulinen (1991).[13] Survival based on data from population-based cancer registries will represent the average prognosis in the population and provide, theoretically at least, an objective index of the effectiveness of cancer care for the community as a whole. However, evaluation of the effectiveness of different forms of treatment can be determined only by a properly conducted clinical trial.

Relative survival is the ratio of the observed survival rate to that expected for a group of people in the general population who are similar to the patient group with respect to race, sex, age and calendar period of observation.[13] Thus, this measure takes into account (or adjusts for) other causes of death.

Kaplan-Meier survival[13] is widely used particularly in the clinical setting. It is similar to the actuarial method but, instead of calculating only the cumulative survival rate at the end of each year of follow-up, it allows determination of the proportion of patients still surviving at shorter intervals.

TYPES OF EPIDEMIOLOGICAL INVESTIGATIONS

Descriptive epidemiology

The essential feature is that cancer rates are compared within or between populations — for example, trends over time[14,15] and differences between birth cohorts, geographical areas, or cultural or racial groupings.[12]

International variation in cancer rates has led to the recognition that much of human cancer is related to environmental factors and is therefore theoretically preventable.[16–18] The term 'environment' covers all exogenous factors that affect human health, whether physical, chemical, biological or cultural. Correlation or ecological studies have been undertaken to see if the international variation was associated with demographic, industrial or other global indices, such as *per capita* use of tobacco.[12] Examples include plotting national mortality rates from colon cancer against *per capita* consumption of fat, death from bladder cancer in different states of the USA against the density of industry, and incidence of melanoma against the latitude. The strength of the correlation between the two measures is an indication of their association at the population level. These studies are limited in that they use surrogate measures of exposure to environmental risk factors and do not necessarily take into account the latent period of cancer. However, geographical variation has suggested clues to risk factors that can be investigated further by analytical epidemiology.

Migrant studies compare rates of a particular cancer in migrants with that of native-born residents in their host country and their country of origin.[12] The patterns of cancer risk in migrants are highly site-specific and may depend on the age at which migration occurred. For example, mortality from stomach cancer is high in Japanese in Japan, lower in Japanese-born Americans, and much lower in US whites while the reverse pattern is seen for breast cancer. Further, the risk of melanoma in migrants to Australia from the British Isles is greatest if migration occurred before 15 years of age, being close to that in native-born Australians; however, if migration occurs after 15 years of age, the risk of melanoma is about one third of that in the Australian-born.[19,20]

Analytical epidemiology

Essentially, analytical epidemiology collects information about disease and exposure in individuals in such a way as to provide clues to causal relationships.[21,22] In the observational case-control and cohort studies, the investigator examines the relationship between disease and exposure but does not intervene. In a clinical trial, the investigator intervenes and observes the effect on the disease process.

A case-control study is an investigation into the extent to which persons selected because they have a specific disease (cases) and comparable persons who do not have the disease (controls) have been exposed to risk factors that are thought to be causal.[21] The cases and controls are ascertained first and their exposures during some defined period of time in the past are obtained retrospectively, usually by means of a questionnaire with the addition, in recent research, of biological marker(s) of exposure. Cases are commonly ascertained through a population-based cancer registry and controls through a population register such as an electoral roll.

A cohort (or follow-up) study starts with a defined population about whom certain exposure information is collected; the group is then followed forward in time to ascertain which persons go on to develop the disease and which do not.[22] One example is the cohort of British male doctors, assembled in 1951 by Doll and Hill, in whom smoking status was assessed at baseline and subsequently on five occasions; mortality from lung cancer originally was the main outcome of interest but this project has also provided information about the risks of additional cancers and other diseases.[23] Further examples include cohorts of workers, where employment records and/or measures of the work environment are used to assess exposure to occupational hazards; subsequent mortality from cancer is determined.

In a clinical trial subjects are allocated randomly to one of at least two alternative treatments (which may include a placebo) and followed to determine the occurrence of specific outcomes.

MEASURES OF ASSOCIATION

In analytical epidemiology measurements are made (or attempted) of exposures which are known or suspected to be linked with cancer. Measurement of

---

Box 1.4. Measure of disease-exposure relationship.

In a *cohort* study:

Relative risk (RR) of cancer associated with an exposure = cancer rate in exposed group divided by cancer rate in unexposed group.

In a *case-control* study:
Odds ratio (OR), an estimate of the relative risk, = ad/bc
   where:

	Cases	Controls
Exposed	a	b
Non-exposed	c	d

---

exposures is complex for several reasons.[24] The suspected agent may be only a contributing, rather than the sole, etiological factor; there is usually a long latent period between exposure and development of cancer; and there may be no measurable indicator of past exposure. The effect of the suspected etiological factor will also depend on its intensity, duration and timing, and the ability to demonstrate an effect will be influenced by the presence of bias or of confounding factors which may distort the exposure–disease relationship. Examples of different "levels" of measurement are: tobacco (never, ex-smoker, current smoker); acetylation phenotype (fast, slow); level of adducts in blood; mutations in DNA.

The *relative risk* (RR) of cancer associated with an exposure can be calculated directly in a cohort study.[22] However, in a case-control investigation direct calculations of the absolute rates and the relative risk of cancer cannot be made.[21] In this case, the relative risk is estimated by the *odds ratio* (OR). Calculations for the relative risk and odds ratio are given in Box 1.4.

By combining information on the distribution of exposures with the estimates of relative risk, it is possible to determine the degree to which cases of disease occurring in the population are explained by the exposure. Two such measures are the *attributable risk for exposed persons* (proportion of cases of disease occurring among exposed persons which is in excess of that in the non-exposed) and the *population attributable risk* (proportion of cases occurring in the total population which can be explained by the risk factor).[21]

CAUSE-AND-EFFECT

In evaluating a cause-and-effect hypothesis in epidemiology it is necessary firstly to determine whether an association found between an exposure and a disease is valid. Alternative explanations include *chance, bias* and *confounding*. If there had been systematic error (bias) in the way in which the subjects of a study were selected or the information about the exposure and/or the disease was obtained, then the association would be invalid. If a third factor was linked both to the exposure and the disease, then it could confound the relationship, producing a spurious result. Statistical tests are used to quantify chance associations.

Once a valid exposure–disease relationship has been established certain criteria have to be met in judging causality — these are the strength of the association, dose–response relationship, temporal sequence, consistency with other investigations and biological plausibility.

PRIMARY PREVENTION OF CANCER

Primary prevention implies elimination of risk factors so that cancer does not occur. Avoidance of exposure to UV solar radiation (for melanoma of skin) and of cigarette smoking (for lung cancer) are examples of preventive strategies. Neither require complete knowledge of carcinogenic mechanisms to be effective. While it is possible to prevent some occupationally-associated cancers by reduction of hazardous exposures in the workplace, primary prevention usually requires active involvement of the individual. We have had evidence for several decades that tobacco in its various forms causes a significant proportion of cancer deaths (e.g. lung, larynx, pancreas, bladder, mouth, pharynx) and that alcohol abuse increases the risk of cancers of the upper respiratory and alimentary tracts, yet people continue to drink alcohol and smoke cigarettes.

Cancers of the liver and uterine cervix are major problems in developing countries. Both could be substantially reduced — liver cancer by immunization against hepatitis B virus infection and cervical cancer by early detection of preneoplastic lesions through Pap smears.

SECONDARY PREVENTION OF CANCER — SCREENING. See Chapter 2.

Site-specific Information in Later Chapters

At the end of most of the following chapters which deal with individual cancers is a box summarizing epidemiological data. The information has been obtained from a variety of sources including the most recent volume of *Cancer Incidence in Five Continents* which covers the period 1983–87.[5] The age-specific graphs depict incidence data for New South Wales in the period 1990–92[9] and are typical of those for most developed countries with one exception — New South Wales rates of melanoma are far higher than those seen in Europe or North America. Five-year relative survival refers in most instances to the white population in the USA[25] and occasionally to South Australia.[26] Much of the information on risk factors came from Higginson et al., 1992.[18]

References

1. Jensen, O.M., Parkin, D.M., Maclennan, R., Muir, C.S. and Skeet, R.G. (eds) (1991). *Cancer Registration: Principles and Methods*. Sci Publ No 95, Lyon: International Agency for Research on Cancer.
2. World Health Organization. (1976). *Manual of the International Statistical Classification of Diseases, Injuries, and Causes of Death. Ninth Revision*. Geneva: World Health Organization.
3. Parkin, D.M., Pisani, P. and Ferlay, J. (1993). Estimates of worldwide incidence of eighteen major cancers in 1985. *International Journal of Cancer*, **54**, 594–606.
4. Pisani, P., Parkin, D.M. and Ferlay, J. (1993). Estimates of worldwide mortality of eighteen major cancers in 1985. Implications for prevention and projections of future burden. *International Journal of Cancer*, **55**, 891–903.
5. Parkin, D.M., Muir, C.S., Whelan, S.L., Gao, Y-T., Ferlay, J. and Powell, J. (eds) (1992). *Cancer Incidence in Five Continents*. Vol VI. Sci Publ No 120. Lyon: International Agency for Research on Cancer.
6. World Health Organization. (1995). *World Health Statistics Annual 1994*. Geneva: World Health Organization.
7. Aoki, K., Hayakawa, N., Kurihara, M. and Suzuki, S. (eds) (1992). *Death Rates for Malignant Neoplasms for Selected Sites by Sex and Five-Year Age Group in 33 Countries 1953–57 to 1983–87*. Nagoya: UICC.
8. Esteve, J., Benhamou, E. and Raymond, L. *Statistical Methods in Cancer Research. Vol IV. Descriptive Epidemiology*. Sci Publ No 128. Lyon: International Agency for Research on Cancer.
9. Coates, M.S., Day, P., McCredie, M., Taylor, R. (1995). *Cancer in New South Wales. Incidence and Mortality. 1992*. Sydney: NSW Cancer Council.

10. Day, N.E. (1987). Cumulative rates and cumulative risk. In *Cancer Incidence in Five Continents, Vol V*, edited by C. Muir, J. Waterhouse, T. Mack, J. Powell, and S. Whelan. Sci Publ No. 88. Lyon: International Agency for Research on Cancer.

11. Armitage, P. and Berry, G. (1994). *Statistical Methods in Medical Research*, 3rd edn. London: Blackwell.

12. Schottenfeld, D. and Fraumeni, J.F. Jr. (1996). *Cancer Epidemiology and Prevention*. Oxford: Oxford University Press.

13. Parkin, D.M. and Hakulinen, T. (1991). Analysis of survival. In *Cancer Registration: Principles and Methods*, edited by O.M. Jensen, D.M. Parkin, R. Maclennan, C.S. Muir and R.G. Skeet. Sci Publ No 95, pp. 159–176. Lyon: International Agency for Research on Cancer.

14. Doll, R., Fraumeni, J.F. and Muir, C.S. (eds) (1994). *Trends in Cancer Incidence and Mortality*. Cancer Surveys Vol 19/20.

15. Coleman, M., Esteve, J., Damiecki, P., Arslan, A. and Renard, H. (1993). *Trends in Cancer Incidence and Mortality*. Sci Publ No 122. Lyon: International Agency for Research on Cancer.

16. Doll, R. and Peto, R. (1981). *The Causes of Cancer*. Oxford: Oxford University Press.

17. Tomatis, L. (ed-in-chief) (1990). *Cancer: Causes, Occurrence and Control*. Sci Publ No 100. Lyon: International Agency for Research on Cancer.

18. Higginson, J., Muir, C.S. and Munoz, N. (1992). *Human Cancer: Epidemiology and Environmental Causes*. Cambridge: Cambridge University Press.

19. Holman, C.D.J. and Armstrong, B.K. (1984a). Pigmentary traits, ethnic origin, benign nevi, and family history are risk factors for cutaneous malignant melanoma. *Journal of National Cancer Institute*, **72**, 257–266.

20. Holman, C.D.J. and Armstrong, B.K. (1984b). Cutaneous malignant melanoma and indicators of total accumulated exposure to the sun: an analysis separating histogenetic types. *Journal of National Cancer Institute*, **73**, 75–82.

21. Breslow, N.E. and Day, N.E. (1980). *Statistical Methods in Cancer Research. Vol I. The analysis of case-control studies*. Sci Publ No 32. Lyon: International Agency for Research on Cancer.

22. Breslow, N.E. and Day, N.E. (1987). *Statistical Methods in Cancer Research. Vol II. The design and analysis of cohort studies*. Sci Publ No 82. Lyon: International Agency for Research on Cancer.

23. Doll, R., Peto, R., Wheatley, K., Gray, R. and Sutherland, I. (1995). Mortality in relation to smoking: 40 years' observations on male British doctors. *British Medical Journal*, **309**, 901–911.

24. Armstrong, B.K., White, E. and Saracci, R. (1992). *Principles of Exposure Measurement in Epidemiology*. Oxford: Oxford University Press.

25. Miller, B.A., Ries, L.A.G., Hankey, B.F., Kosary, C.L. and Edwards, B.K. (eds) (1992). *Cancer Statistics Review: 1973–1989*, NIH Pub No 92–2789. Maryland: National Cancer Institute.

26. Bonett, A., Dickman, P., Roder, D., Gibberd, R. and Hakulinen, T. (1992). *Survival of Cancer Patients in South Australia 1977–1990*. Adelaide: South Australian Health Commission.

2. Screening for Cancer

NICHOLAS ARMITAGE

Department of Surgery, University Hospital, Queen's Medical Centre, Nottingham, UK

DEFINITION

Screening may be defined as "the presumptive identification of unrecognized disease or defects by the applications of tests, examinations or other procedures which can be applied rapidly". This definition covers screening for all health problems from color blindness to heart disease but can certainly be used for cancer and contains a number of key points of screening. In the first section of this chapter, the definition, principles, objectives and application of screening will be examined before going to subsequent sections which will explore screening for specific cancer sites.

PRINCIPLES OF SCREENING

Characteristics of the disease screened

Prevalence of the disease

To be worthwhile, screening needs to offer a substantial impact within a population. This will mean either that the disease is common, such as breast cancer, or that a subset of the population can be defined in whom the prevalence is high, i.e., esophageal cancer in columnar lined esophagus (Barratts).

Outcome for symptomatic disease

The disease should have serious implications in terms of morbidity and mortality when detected symptomatically. For instance, in patients with advanced stomach cancer, there is a poor outlook with few surviving beyond five years whereas, even when presenting late, most patients with non-melanoma skin malignancy may have a good outlook.

Outcome for early disease

Following from the previous section, there should be evidence that patients treated for early disease have a good prognosis. It is well accepted that patients with colorectal cancer confined to the bowel wall (Stage A) have a good prognosis, in excess of 80% surviving for five years or more.

Characteristics of an ideal screening test

Simplicity

Since such a test will be used by individuals who in the main do not have the disease, it must be simple, free from unwanted side effects, easy to interpret and inexpensive. In most screening programs, the costs are twofold. There is usually an initial test which is individually cheap but incurs a high cost due to the large numbers of tests done. The second cost is that of investigating those people shown to have a positive test in order to arrive at a final diagnosis.

Performance

It is therefore essential to use a test which has an optimal *sensitivity*, i.e. to detect as high a proportion

		DISEASE	
		PRESENT	ABSENT
TEST RESULT	POSITIVE	(1) TRUE POSITIVE	(2) FALSE POSITIVE
	NEGATIVE	(3) FALSE NEGATIVE	(4) TRUE NEGATIVE

$$\text{SENSITIVITY} = \frac{\text{TRUE POSITIVE (1)}}{\text{TRUE POSITIVE (1)} + \text{FALSE NEGATIVE (3)}}$$

$$\text{SPECIFICITY} = \frac{\text{TRUE NEGATIVE (4)}}{\text{TRUE NEGATIVE (4)} + \text{FALSE POSITIVE (2)}}$$

Figure 2.1.

of individuals in the screened group who have the disease as possible but also with a reasonable *specificity* to avoid large numbers of individuals who do not have the disease being put through the anxiety, discomfort and cost of the secondary investigation. In all screening programs there is a "trade-off" between sensitivity and specificity and this needs to be considered in evaluating a screening test (Figure 2.1).

Acceptability

In addition to these criteria, a screening test must be acceptable to the population screened. This is referred to as *Compliance*, which is the proportion of individuals offered a screening test who actually complete it. Many factors influence compliance. The age, sex and social class of the individuals are important determinants depending on which type of cancer is being screened for. In general women tend to have a higher compliance as do younger individuals and those of higher social class. This may be related to health awareness and will be mentioned later. In addition, general perceptions of the disease are important in determining the compliance. These will include the general level of knowledge of the disease, attitudes towards its curability and the potential benefits of early treatment. These perceptions may be influenced by health education both on a general level via the media and on a more individual level by health care workers, e.g. practice nurses, particularly in the context of "well person" checks. It has been shown for bowel cancer screening by fecal occult blood testing that the source of the invitation is important with a higher compliance when the individual is invited by their family doctor compared with a public health department. These considerations may have important implications for the structure and running of cancer screening programs.

In the United Kingdom, breast cancer screening is organized separately and initially as a specified service with its own personnel, protocols and quality assurance while cervical cancer screening is generally carried out locally with the family doctor's surgery and referral etc organized by the family doctor. The optimal mechanism for screening may be different for different cancers. The screening test itself may determine the mechanisms for maximizing compliance.

Identification of a suitable group for screening

Population screening

In a tumor which has a high prevalence, e.g. breast cancer in the UK, USA, Australia or stomach cancer in Japan, programs have been introduced to cover the population. Even then there is a degree of selection, e.g. only women are screened for breast cancer and generally women over 50 years are offered screening since both the HIP and Two Counties studies showed no benefit to women screened between the ages of 40 and 49 years.

Risk group screening

This type of screening is aimed at individuals who are at an increased risk of developing a particular cancer.

Family screening: This may be due to a genetic predisposition. It is well recognized that affected individuals with Familial Adenomatous Polyposis, inherited in autosomal dominant manner, have a 100% chance of eventually developing colorectal cancer. Similarly, certain familial forms of breast cancer have been identified. Genetically predisposed tumors tend to develop at an earlier age than the "sporadic" variety. Members of these families merit screening at a relatively early age and in a more intensive fashion than for population screening.

Increased risk screening: Certain groups of individuals have an increased risk of developing tumors but which is not as high as that conferred by the genetic predisposition outlined above. These include patients with total ulcerative colitis who have an increased risk of colorectal cancer, heavy smokers who have an increased risk of lung cancer, patients who have had one breast cancer treated have a higher than population risk of developing cancer in the contralateral breast. These individuals at increased risk may constitute a suitable group for screening.

Evaluation of cancer screening

Evaluation of the screening test

Before undertaking any form of screening, it is essential to have a test which is capable of detecting asymptomatic disease. Clearly the test must perform well in terms of sensitivity and this may be tested in patients with symptomatic disease or in those undergoing the investigation for other reasons. For instance, fecal occult blood (FOB) testing using a particular FOB test may be done by individuals with known cancer prior to operation. In addition FOB tests may be done prior to bowel preparation by individuals who are undergoing colonoscopy for whatever reason.

These methods will give some idea of the sensitivity of the test but extrapolation to sensitivity in asymptomatic disease must be done with some caution. In general it is necessary to conduct a pilot study in order to determine the performance of the test in the screened population with regard to the rate of positivity and the number of true positives within those initially identified by the screening test. The sensitivity, however, will generally have to await prolonged follow up. This is in order to determine the number of individuals who are subsequently identified with the disease who initially had negative tests (*False Negatives*). The difficulty here is knowing whether these tumors were present and not detected by the test or whether they developed *de novo* after the completion of the test. This will be influenced by the natural history of the particular cancer being screened and by the interval between screening tests.

In evaluating the test, the specificity will also be of crucial importance. A test with low specificity will have considerable implications by producing a large number of false positives which will result in many individuals who do not have the disease undergoing uncomfortable (e.g. repeat mammography) or potentially harmful (colonoscopy) investigations. In addition there is a considerable cost implication to the screening program determined by the performance of the test since the investigation of a positive test is usually expensive. A useful measure in evaluation is the *positive predictive value*. This is the proportion of individuals with a positive test who are found to have the disease when investigated further.

Evaluation of a screening program

End points: The only true end point for a screening program is a reduction in mortality from that disease within the population screened. This will usually take many years to become apparent and various measures are available sooner to gauge whether a program is likely to succeed. The first is an improvement in the stage at which the disease is detected by the screening test. An increase in the proportion of early stage cancer and a reduction in advanced disease found by screening is a prerequisite for an improvement in mortality. In addition, many screening programs produce an appreciable yield of preinvasive disease, e.g. breast carcinoma *in situ*, severe dysplasia in intestinal lesions, which intuitively should reduce the subsequent incidence of invasive cancer. A further point to be remembered is that in order to evaluate the usefulness of a program, the whole population must be studied rather than just those individuals whose tumors were detected. This will include those whose tumors were missed by screening (*False Negatives*) and those people who did not do the test (*Non Acceptors*).

Biases

In evaluating the effectiveness of screening, it must be recognized that there are various biases in favor of the screened groups. The first of these is generally referred to as *Selection Bias*. The group of individuals who complete screening tests will in general be those who are more health conscious, e.g. more likely to attend the dentist regularly, wear car safety belts, etc., and will therefore have selected themselves as a group more likely to have a good outlook. Some screening studies have been based on volunteer rather than population groups

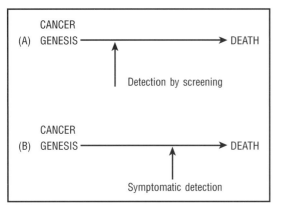

Figure 2.2. Lead time.

and will tend to reflect this "more healthy" group. The second bias is referred to as *Lead Time Bias*. This concept is that if a cancer has a natural history which brings about the death of the patient, then detecting it earlier will have an apparent lengthening in survival from diagnosis with no effect on the natural history (Figure 2.2).

Figure 2.2 depicts diagramatically the effect of lead time giving an apparent survival advantage to patient A over patient B with no real effect on natural history. The third bias towards screening is that of *Length Bias*. By their natural history, slower growing, less aggressive tumors will be present asymptomatically in the individual for longer and therefore are more likely to be detected by screening than aggressive tumors which will tend to produce symptoms earlier. This effect may produce an imbalance of good prognosis tumors within a screen detected group. Such an imbalance will tend to skew the prognosis for patients with screen detected cancers.

The biases detailed above will have the effect of giving patients with screen detected cancers an improved prognosis. However, as stated earlier, in order to evaluate a screening program, it is essential to study the effect of screening on the whole of the group or population offered screening rather than a specified subset.

Methods of determining effect

As mentioned earlier, the true end point in determining the effectiveness of a screening program is a reduction in mortality in the group offered screening. In some situations, such as cervical cancer screening, it is not possible to conduct a randomized

study since this type of screening has already been introduced widely. It is necessary therefore to compare mortality in screened and non-screened groups in different ways. Such non-randomized studies may compare mortality from the particular cancer in the population before and after the introduction of screening. Alternatively one could study two populations, one in which screening was widely adopted and one in which it was not. Such comparisons are difficult to interpret as studying the same population over time will have to take into account changes in the demographics of that population as well as changes in health care and other social aspects over the time period, Similarly, comparing two populations, even if they are adjoining counties, provinces or countries, may be open to error as the population studied will have differences other than the application of cancer screening.

An alternative approach is the *Case Control Study*. This is a complex method of evaluation which takes a group of patients who have died of the particular cancer and a control group who have not. The screening history of the two groups are then compared. The complexity of this technique is in making appropriate allowances for the other variables within the two groups to show the effect of screening. The two approaches above do give some ability to evaluate screening, particularly if there are a number of studies all of which are giving consistent results. However, some bias is not eliminated.

The most powerful method of determining the effect of screening is the *Randomized Controlled Trial*. In such a trial, screening is offered to one group within a population while a second age/sex matched group act as a control group and are observed. The group offered screening are selected from the whole population in a random manner. The end point is mortality from the particular cancer. In order to show significant differences, such trials require large numbers of subjects to be randomized and studied over a prolonged period of time. Such trials have been conducted for breast and colorectal cancer and will be detailed later in this chapter.

Economic and logistic evaluation

The previous sections have examined whether screening can reduce mortality and how this may be evaluated. This may be shown in trials but before moving from a trial to a national or population screening program, two questions need to be asked and answered. Firstly, can it be done and secondly is it cost effective? Screening programs have major implications for resources. This is not just for the initial test which, while it may be individually cheap, such as a FOB test, will be expensive when large numbers are sent out. In addition, a new infrastructure may need to be put in place for identifying individuals to be invited for screening, informing screenees and family doctors about results and ensuring that appropriate investigations are undertaken. This implies that screening will be centrally organized such as breast cancer screening in the UK. it is more likely that such a program with inbuilt quality control measures will bring about the mortality reduction necessary to maximize the effect of screening. As well as the mechanisms for initial screening being established, it is essential that adequate facilities are available to investigate fully any individual found to have a positive screening test as expeditiously as possible. Any person informed of a positive screening test will inevitably be anxious that they have cancer. Such anxiety in screenees, many of whom will not have cancer, is one of the unwanted effects of screening. The time to reaching a final diagnosis either to the certainty of cancer with a subsequent treatment plan or to the reassurance that the individual does not have cancer should therefore be minimized. To complete investigations over a short time, it may be necessary to increase diagnostic facilities. This may involve providing more equipment, e.g. mammography apparatus, but frequently will involve recruiting and training extra personnel, e.g. cytologists or specifically trained radiologists for breast cancer screening or colonoscopists for colorectal cancer screening. The infrastructure must be in place before a widespread cancer screening program is introduced.

The second question relates to the cost effectiveness of a screening program. Clearly if screening does not reduce mortality, it should not be introduced. A modest reduction in mortality from one of the common cancers, e.g. breast or colorectal, will bring about a greater number of "lives saved" than a similar reduction in less common tumors e.g. esophagus in the UK. Since the goal is reduction in cancer mortality, the costs of achieving this reduction by cancer screening must be compared between different forms of screening and between cancer screening and improvements in the treatment of symptomatic disease. It is therefore important in any screening trial or pilot study to perform an economic evaluation of that type of screening so that subsequent projections on cost may be made. The eventual introduction of a screening program needs a decision at a national level and therefore will be influenced by health care, cost effectiveness and political factors.

SITE-SPECIFIC CANCER SCREENING

Screening for specific cancers can be broadly subdivided into three categories:

- female cancers (cervix uteri, ovary and breast)
- gastrointestinal cancer (esophagus, stomach, large bowel)
- others (lung, prostate, melanoma and other less common tumors)

Screening for these malignancies will be considered separately. In most countries, the two best developed screening programs are for cervical and breast cancer and these will be considered first.

SCREENING FOR CERVICAL CANCER

Although only the eighth most common malignancy in women, screening for cervical cancer continues as the earliest established mass screening program since its introduction in the 1960s in many countries (UK 1964). The five-year survival for women with localized disease is almost 80% while that for advanced disease is less than 10%. Cervical cancer has a premalignant phase of dysplasia and the cervix is relatively accessible. These factors suggest that screening should be feasible.

Screening for cervical cancer involves cytological examination of smears taken from the cervix. These are then classified depending on the cytological appearances into Inadequate, Normal, Dyskaryosis (borderline, mild, moderate or severe) or carcinoma. The presence of cytological abnormality will prompt further investigation. It is recognized that in the precancerous phase both progression and regression are possible. Two studies from Canada have shown that;

(1) for women with mild or minimal dysplasia, subsequent smears have shown normal cytology;

(2) an estimated 61–77% cases of carcinoma *in situ* regressed particularly in younger women.

It is necessary to appreciate this natural history of the preinvasive phase of cervical cancer to plan investigation of women with abnormal smears. In addition, the presence of human papilloma virus in a cervical smear adds another variable to be considered in deciding upon management. Generally the investigation of an abnormal smear will involve colposcopy with biopsy where appropriate. Women with moderate or severe dyskaryosis or suspected neoplasia referred for treatment should be colposcoped immediately. There is some debate as to whether women with mild or borderline changes should be colposcoped or have repeat smears with referral if a second smear is abnormal. The latter strategy has been shown to be relatively inefficient by a study from Aberdeen in which three-quarters of such women required colposcopy and many women defaulted in the surveillance group.

The best evidence of effectiveness of screening in cervical cancer comes from the Scandinavian countries. Although the data is not from randomized trials, the reduction in mortality ranges from 18% in Norway to 60% and 62% respectively in Finland and Iceland. In the UK, until recently, there has been little if any improvement in mortality. The screening program is organized through General Practitioners and the factors cited for this underperformance have been the relatively low compliance and a poor call/recall system. Over recent years changes have been made:

(1) in the organization, e.g. with improvements in practice registers, call/recall systems, the follow-up of non-responding women and monitoring of the effectiveness of the system.

(2) increasing the proportion of women screened by setting targets for General Practitioners with payments for 50% and 80% coverage of the women targeted. Between 1990 and 1993 the proportion of GPs achieving 80% rose from 53% to 83%. In addition, women of lower social class, i.e. those at greater risk, are now participating in cervical screening.

Cervical cancer screening in the UK offers a contrast to breast cancer screening in its organization and with the improvements now undertaken it is expected that a reduction in mortality will be seen in the future.

SCREENING FOR OVARIAN CANCER

Ovarian cancer presents a problem in that the majority of women, about 60%, present with Stage III and Stage IV disease with a poor outlook, while in only a small minority of women is the tumor confined to the ovary when adequate treatment can achieve a good five-year survival rate. Some 4360 women died of ovarian cancer in the UK in 1992 which accounted for 6% of all cancer deaths in women and more than the combined total of the other gynecological malignancies.

Since the ovary is an intra-abdominal organ, detection of malignant change is difficult and two main approaches have been adopted to achieve early detection. These have been by serum markers and ultrasound scanning. Of the serum tumor markers examined that which detected by the monoclonal antibody, CA125, holds the most promise. Overall in patients with ovarian cancer, 81% will have elevated serum CA125 levels compared with only 4% of unaffected women. However, in women with Stage I disease, only 44% have elevated levels compared with greater than 85% in more advanced stages. This low sensitivity may not be sufficiently able to detect early disease to change mortality. In addition, a specificity in the range of 97% would result in some 50 false positive results for each cancer detected by screening. Since the detection of a screening abnormality may result in a laparotomy, it is crucial to keep the specificity as high as possible, in excess of 99%. A combination of tests — CA125 followed by abdominal ultrasound — achieves a specificity of 99.9% with a positive predictive value of 27% in the general population of postmenopausal women. Multiple markers may increase sensitivity without a large rise in specificity; however, further study is required. Ultrasound scanning may be done transabdominally or transvaginally, the latter being more comfortable since it does not require the bladder to be full. When combined with colour Doppler flow imaging, a low false positive rate can be achieved. As yet, however, there is no data that screening for ovarian cancer results in reduced mortality. A multicenter European randomized trial of transvaginal ultrasound screening has recently started and the results are awaited.

SCREENING FOR BREAST CANCER

Breast cancer is estimated to affect 1:12 women over their lifetime, making it a major health problem. In 1992, there were 15,000 deaths in the UK, comprising 5% of all deaths in women. Therefore it fulfills the criteria of being an important and common disease. It is also clear that patients with small, node negative tumors have a better outlook than those with more advanced disease. Various methods of early detection have been investigated but only mammography has been conclusively shown to reduce mortality for breast cancer. The two main pillars of evidence are the Health Insurance Plan (HIP) study from New York and the Swedish Two Counties study. In the former, two-view mammography was randomly offered to 62,000 women aged 40–64 years together with a clinical examination on an annual basis over four years. Two-thirds of the women accepted the tests and there was a significant reduction in the number of deaths from breast cancer of about 30%. This benefit was confined to women aged 50–64 with no benefit derived to those women aged 40–49 years. In the Two Counties trial, 77,000 women aged 40–74 years were randomized to single-view mammography while 56,000 were controls. Compliance was age related with 93% of younger women attending compared with 79% of women aged 70–74 years. Compliance also reduced with subsequent screening rounds. The rate of detection of cancers smaller than 2 cm and without nodal or distal metastases was significantly higher in the screened group. There was a reduction in mortality from breast cancer at 6, 8 and 10 years of follow-up with a relative risk of death of 0.7. This was again apparent in the women aged 50–69 years with no such benefit being shown in the women aged 40–49 years. The trials from the UK and Sweden indicated an overall reduction in mortality of 28% in women aged 50 and over. In women aged 41–49 a recent meta analysis has shown a statistically significant benefit if the Canadian study is excluded. Further studies continue in this age group.

Mammographic screening for women aged 50–64 was introduced in the UK as a national program in 1988. Unlike screening for cervical cancer, the screening program was centralized, being organized by screening centers which were specifically set up and which had clearly identified teams of radiologists, radiographers, pathologists and surgeons. The systems for identification, recall and follow-up of screenees were carefully developed. A set of quality standards were set and for the prevalence rounds, these were all achieved except the proportion of invasive cancers detected less than 1 cm, i.e. standard 1.5/1000 screened, achieved 1.4/1000. The compliance to the screening round was 71% of those invited which varied between 58 and 81% depending on the region. The recall rate was 6.2% with 6.2/1000 women having cancer detected. A recent report, seven years after the introduction of the program, has demonstrated that the incidence of breast cancer rose steeply in the screening age group but has levelled off at 25% higher than that for 1987. Breast cancer mortality which had been rising since the 1950s had already begun to fall in the mid-1980s in younger women and in women aged 50–69 years started to fall three years after the introduction of screening, i.e. 1990. This reduction in mortality is thought unlikely to be due to the effect of screening which seems to take about seven years to appear. It is more likely that the reduction is due to changes in treatment, particularly in the use of hormone and chemotherapy. Certainly one of the effects of the screening program has been to identify more clearly, specialist teams with specific interest and skills in managing breast disease. It has been demonstrated that clinicians with a specific interest in and with a reasonable caseload of breast cancers tend to achieve improved survival rates for their patients.

A recent report, also from the UK screening program, has shown that two-view mammography is better than single view in that it detects more cancers and reduces recall rates while having a similar cost effectiveness. The question of compliance to mammographic screening is crucial in maximizing its effectiveness and is an important area for study with particular attention to co-operation between the primary health care team and the screening center. Despite mammographic screening, the majority of women who present with breast cancer do so symptomatically. There has been considerable effort in early detection by Breast Self Examination (BSE). However, there is no evidence of a reduction in mortality as a result of taught self-examination which certainly results in more referrals for specialist evaluation of young women in particular and in more benign biopsies. Against this, however, it seems reasonable for women to be "breast aware" and to report changes such as a new lump or skin dimpling early.

SCREENING FOR COLORECTAL CANCER

Large bowel cancer is a common cancer affecting about 2% of the population. It is the second commonest cause of death from malignant disease in the UK with 19,600 deaths in 1992. The genesis of colorectal cancer is better understood than most tumors. There is strong evidence that most cancers develop from benign precursors (adenomas). There is a long time period from the first changes which seem to be a disturbance of the proliferation of the colonic epithelium through adenoma to invasive cancer. This time period may be between five and ten years and is associated with recognized genetic changes. Symptoms generally occur late in the natural history of the disease. A large proportion of patients still present with metastases to lymph nodes (Stage C) or distant sites (Stage D) when the outlook tends to be poor. However, if treated before it has progressed through the bowel wall (Stage A), colorectal cancer has an excellent prognosis. There seems to be a good opportunity to decrease mortality by screening since colorectal cancer is a common lethal disease with a long asymptomatic phase and good results for treatment of early disease.

The main questions in setting up a screening program for colorectal cancer are who to screen and how to screen them. Apart from particular small subgroups at high risk, most deaths occur in patients over the age of 55 years. Most population screening programs therefore have chosen to screen individuals aged 50 years and older. Some high risk groups would appear to merit earlier and more intensive screening than the population. Familial Adenomatous Polyposis (FAP) is a condition which is autosomal dominantly inherited and characterized by hundreds or thousands of polyps throughout the large bowel. The genetic defect has been located in Chromosome 5. The FAP gene is a large gene and the exact site of the mutation will determine the pattern of disease which may be associated with extracolonic manifestation, e.g. duodenal polyps, desmoids, tumors etc. A further autosomal dominant condition is Hereditary Non Polyposis Colon Cancer (HNPCC). With a 1 in 2 chance of developing cancer at a young age, members of FAP and HNPCC kindreds require intensive early screening by colonoscopy. Genetic tests have been developed for FAP which will identify affected individuals in informative families and conversely identify non-affected individuals who do not require such intensive screening. In HNPCC, some progress has been made in identifying the genetic abnormalities which holds promise for the future. Outside these syndromes, individuals with a first degree family history of colorectal cancer have an increased personal risk, the magnitude of which is related to the number and age of relatives involved. As such, they constitute a group at increased risk who may be screened, as are patients with inflammatory bowel disease and those who have had previous colorectal neoplasia. The screening for these will tend to be less intensive than for FAP and HNPCC.

The second issue to be discussed is the method of screening, Essentially this will be by some form of endoscopy or by a preliminary test to detect tumor/associated substances in the stool followed by endoscopy of those found to be positive. Taking this latter approach first, the most usually detected tumor product is fecal occult blood (FOB) which may be detected by a chemical test such as the Guaiac reaction. The most common FOB test uses a Guaiac impregnated paper (Haemoccult) which is simply developed by the addition of hydrogen peroxide to give a blue color. This relatively insensitive test detects about two-thirds of tumors if individuals with known cancer are tested. Sensitivity may be increased (i.e. reducing false negatives) by rehydrating the slides, testing for longer or by using a more sensitive test. However, with increased sensitivity the specificity will decrease (i.e. increasing the rate for false positives). In population screening 1 or 2% will have positive tests when unhydrated which rises to 6–12% when the slides have water added before developing. As discussed in the first section, sensitivity and specificity are crucial to the effectiveness of screening. Theoretically, immunological tests for fecal occult blood should increase sensitivity and specificity but are limited like Haemoccult by tumors which do not bleed. Other tumor products may be detected in stool such as tumor associated antigens, e.g. Carcino Embryonic Antigen (CEA), and tumor DNA protein products, e.g. the product of the ras oncogene. It is likely that detection of tumor DNA itself in the stool may be more promising and research is ongoing into this.

Digital rectal examination is part of the screening protocol in Germany but the mucosa examined is only a small proportion of the whole. Rigid sigmoidoscopy examines the rectum and Gilbertson showed that sigmoidoscopic examinations with removal of adenomas reduced the subsequent number of cancers. Two recent studies, a case control study from the USA and a retrospective analysis of patients with rectal polyps treated at St Mark's Hospital, have indicated the efficacy of rigid sigmoidoscopy in reducing mortality. However, only the rectum is examined and more recently, screening by flexible fibreoptic sigmoidoscopy has been advocated. A 60 cm instrument will examine the left colon in most patients and detect the majority of neoplasms. The examination is expensive compared with FOB tests and will detect small (less than 1cm) polyps in a large number of individuals. The acceptability of the test in a population has not been determined. Pilot studies for a proposed randomized controlled trial of flexible sigmoidoscopy are under-way in the UK. A trial of screening for prostate, lung and colorectal cancer in men is ongoing in the USA with flexible sigmoidoscopy as the screening modality.

Randomized trials of FOB testing have been conducted in the USA and Europe over the past two decades. All have used Haemoccult as the screening tool. A major trial began in Minnesota in 1975 and has recently been reported. 46,550 volunteers were randomized into one of three groups — annual screening by Haemoccult, alternate year screening by Haemoccult and a control group. A high compliance was achieved with an overall positivity of 7.4%. This study is now mature and shows a reduction in mortality for the group offered annual screening but not those offered biennial screening over the control group. Four large trials are ongoing in Europe, of which two have very similar protocols (Nottingham, UK and Odense, Denmark). The Nottingham study enrolled 150,000 subjects randomized into test and control groups. The compliance was lower than in the Minnesota study at 54% with a Haemoccult positivity of 2%. An excess of Stage A cancers (20 %) was detected in the test group as a whole compared with the control group (11%) and this has been translated into a mortality reduction of 15% at median follow-up of eight years. The Danish study randomized 31,000 subjects, achieved a higher compliance than Nottingham (67%) but the mortality reduction was similar.

In summary, screening for colorectal cancer by FOB testing has been shown to reduce mortality. Haemoccult is not the ideal test and other FOB tests and tests for fecal tumor products are being investigated. Screening by flexible sigmoidoscopy offers an alternative screening modality and is the subject of current investigation which will include assessment of efficacy and cost effectiveness.

SCREENING FOR STOMACH CANCER

Stomach cancer is the second most common gastrointestinal malignancy in most developed countries. The exception is Japan which has the highest incidence in the world (75–100/100,000 men and 38–51/100,000 women). The etiology of stomach cancer is not yet fully determined but diet appears to be the most important factor. Diets containing a high content of salt, especially in preserved food, have been implicated. The increase in refrigeration and reduction in consumption of preserved food may in part explain the general decline in the incidence in stomach cancer.

The key to reduction in mortality in stomach cancer appears to lie in increasing the proportion of early gastric cancer (EGC). This form of the disease is limited to the mucosa or submucosa of the stomach. A follow-up study from Japan documented a group of patients with EGC whose resection was delayed for more than six months. At an average interval of 29 months (6–88 months), 28 (51%) had progressed to advanced cancer and the median five-year survival for untreated EGC was 64%. This compares with patients undergoing resection for EGC in Japan who have a five-year survival greater than 90%. In Europe and the USA, the proportion of EGC is only 5–10% of those patients presenting symptomatically.

The methods of screening are: radiology by barium meal with a limited number of views taken, endoscopy, cytology of endoscopic brushings or gastric washings or tumor markers in gastric juice. In Japan the incidence is high enough to justify population screening. Individuals over the age of 40 years are offered a barium meal usually performed by technicians in mobile units with detailed endoscopic examination limited to those shown to have an abnormality. Of 4.6 million screened in 1983, 14% were recalled and 4598 (0.1%) found to have stomach cancer of which nearly half was EGC.

No randomized studies were carried out before the introduction of screening and it is not now possible to carry them out, Therefore other methods are necessary to assess effectiveness. A reduction in mortality of 25% has been estimated in the intensively screened areas.

In areas such as the UK with a medium risk of stomach cancer, population screening is not justified. Higher risk groups may be identified (and offered surveillance) such as individuals who have had previous gastric surgery. However, it is recognized that most (70–90%) of patients with EGC have had dyspepsia and early referral and investigation of such symptoms may lead to an increased diagnosis of EGC. Open Access Endoscopy Services for GPs may help in this but as yet no firm evidence is available for a mortality reduction.

SCREENING FOR ESOPHAGEAL CANCER

In most countries esophageal cancer is only of moderate incidence with some 5000 deaths in the UK in 1986. In certain parts of the world (Northern Iran and China) it is one of the commonest cancers affecting 100–200/100,000 men aged 35–64 years. Clearly a different approach to screening is necessary between high and low risk areas.

The screening modalities available are barium swallow which is not particularly suitable, esophagoscopy and blind esophageal cytology. Blind esophageal cytology has been employed in population screening in China when a balloon covered with fine mesh was swallowed, the balloon inflated and withdrawn. The sample is examined cytologically and in Chinese studies the accuracy was 95%. Esophagoscopy gives the opportunity for direct visualization of the mucosa as well as take both biopsies and brushings for cytology. The combination can consistently achieve a high degree of accuracy and in addition identify individuals with dysplasia who may require surveillance.

In high risk areas mass screening is reasonable since the disease is common and in screening studies 74% of cancers diagnosed were early (compared with only 17% early cancer in patients with upper GI symptoms). In patients with early cancer a five-year survival rate of 90% can be achieved.

In low risk areas, mass screening cannot be justified but is reasonable in individuals at high risk, e.g. those with Columnar Lined Esophagus

(BARRATTS). Endoscopic screening is usually advocated at yearly intervals with the presence of dysplasia on biopsy reducing the interval between screening examinations.

SCREENING FOR TESTICULAR CANCER

Testicular cancer is the commonest tumor in men aged 20–34 years in the UK. Over recent decades the outcome of treatment has improved greatly and patients with localized disease have a good outlook. Even with advanced metastatic disease modern combination chemotherapy can bring about high cure rates. This being so, any effect of screening on mortality can only be small and not justified at present Any impact will be on detecting disease at an earlier stage when less toxic treatment may be used. Public health education and testicular self-examination may reduce delay in diagnosis but may also bring about large numbers of "false positives" which raise anxiety and require evaluation. The unusual condition of cryptorchidism is associated with a three to fourfold increase in risk if unilateral and tenfold if bilateral If coffected below the age of 10 years, the risk is reduced in unilateral cryptorchidism but not if bilateral. Surveillance is appropriate in this condition.

SCREENING FOR PROSTATIC CANCER

The incidence of prostatic cancer is the second highest of non skin cancers in men in the UK and is rising. Some of the increase is due to improved diagnosis and increased age but in addition, there is a real increase in incidence. In autopsy studies, prostatic cancer has been shown to be very common in men over the age of 50 years but most of this disease is occult. This highlights one of the potential problems for screening, i.e. a capacity for overdiagnosing clinically insignificant disease. There are several other problems which include the low sensitivity and specificity of the tests and that the appropriate treatment for early disease is still uncertain in view of the side effects of radical surgery.

The tests for screening men for prostatic cancer are: digital rectal examination, transrectal ultrasonography and the serum marker Prostatic Specific Antigen (PSA). Digital examination has a relatively low sensitivity for detecting early disease. Transrectal ultrasound is more sensitive than digital examination, particularly for localized disease. PSA levels may be raised in 25% of benign prostatic hypertrophy and normal values will be found in a quarter of men with localized cancer. Improvements are being sought in sensitivity and specificity and currently the "best buy" approach appears to be a combination of digital examination and PSA with a transrectal ultrasound for evaluating a positive test. A reasonable proportion of screened subjects will have to undergo an unnecessary prostatic biopsy due to screening detected abnormalities which is both unpleasant and potentially hazardous.

Screening for prostatic cancer has yet to be shown to reduce mortality and as indicated there are some major problems in screening. Screening is being evaluated, by randomized trials in the USA and Europe.

SCREENING FOR SKIN CANCER

The commonest skin cancers, Basal Cell and Squamous Cell carcinomas, have a good outlook from current treatment However, malignant melanoma, which is less common, has a less favorable outlook. The factors which have an impact on survival in melanoma are the thickness of the tumor (Breslow thickness), the type of melanoma (Superficial spreading, Nodular, Lentigo Maligna Acral) and the presence or absence of metastases. Melanoma is associated with exposure to sunlight particularly at an early age, in individuals with a fair skin which burns easily and those with many moles. There is an increase in the number of people dying of melanoma in recent years. Various measures may be taken to reduce the risk of exposure especially to ultraviolet rays of which the most damaging are ultraviolet B and C. These include avoidance of strongest sunlight (between 11 a.m. and 3 p.m.), hats and light clothing and the use of sunscreen creams. Since the risk is greatest when exposure happens at a young age, these measures are particularly important in children. Such measures should reduce the number of people developing melanoma particularly in those at greatest risk.

Population screening for malignant melanoma is not feasible even in Australia (ten times greater incidence than the UK) but considerable effort has been directed at earlier diagnosis. Screening by full view examination is unproven with regard to benefit and if taken up would be extremely costly in time of health professionals. Delay occurs in the patient reporting suspicious change in a naevus (changes in size, shape or color, bleeding, inflammation or sensory change) and in their family practitioner referring for expert advice. Various campaigns to reduce delay in a diagnosis have used a combination of professional and public health education. In the UK these have been associated with the inception of Pigmented Lesion Clinics. Preliminary results from Australia and the West of Scotland suggest a benefit. Increasing public awareness will have an impact on General Practitioners' workload but seems to be acceptable.

SCREENING FOR LUNG CANCER

Lung cancer is the most common malignancy in most developed countries and in the USA accounts for some 100,000 new cases annually with 93,000 deaths in 1988. In addition the mortality from this cancer continues to rise. There is clear evidence linking smoking and lung cancer, This being so, most of the effort from a public health point of view is aimed at reducing the number of individuals smoking with bans of tobacco advertising, messages on cigarette packs and public awareness campaigns. Lung cancer is however a major cause of death and efforts have been made to achieve diagnosis at an earlier stage by screening.

The main modalities for screening for lung cancer are chest X-ray and sputum cytology. A number of trials were conducted in the 1950s, and 1960s in the USA and UK which were, in the main, nonrandomized and uncontrolled. In some an increased survival was shown for screen detected cases compared with expected outcome but there was no overall improvement in mortality due to screening. Recent reports from Europe — a randomized trial from Czechoslovakia and a case control study from East Germany — showed no difference in the death rate. Further studies from the Mayo Clinic, John Hopkins University Hospital and Memorial-Sloan Kettering Cancer Institute in the USA have used chest X-ray either four-monthly or annually as well as sputum cytology. In the Mayo Clinic study of heavy smokers, the cancers tended to be at an earlier stage but again no mortality reduction was demonstrated.

Recently further interest has been expressed in lung cancer screening since the earlier studies may have had insufficient power to detect small reductions in mortality, e.g. 10–15% which in a common disease would represent a substantial number of patients. For this reason, a further trial of annual chest X-ray in men aged 60–74 is one arm of the Prostate, Lung and Colorectal Cancer (PLC) trial initiated by the National Cancer Institute in the USA designed to recruit 100,000 subjects and to run over 16 years.

3. Basic Aspects of Cancer Pathology

C. SOON LEE

Head of Anatomical Pathology, University of Newcastle (NSW, Australia); Staff Specialist and Head of Teaching and Research, Hunter Area Pathology Service

INTRODUCTION

Neoplasia is the new growth of tissue which has some form of resemblance to its tissue of origin. Specific tumors produce certain systemic complications more than others but the approach to the clinico-pathological problem of a cancer remains the same. The immediate and late effects of the tumor, both locally and systemically, have significant prognostic implications. These effects are related to the different types of proteins and hormones that can be elaborated by certain tumors.

Some knowledge of the basic aspects of cancer development will assist in the understanding of cancer behavior and in the diagnosis and management of this condition. This chapter attempts to provide a brief discussion on the pathological aspects of malignancies that are relevant to surgical practice and aims to familiarize the student on the current concepts on the pathogenesis and the laboratory tests used in the investigation of neoplasia.

MORPHOLOGICAL APPEARANCES OF NEOPLASIA

Grossly malignant tumors have poorly defined growth margins due to their infiltrative behavior and they tend to destroy surrounding native tissues. Their external surfaces are frequently irregular and indurated. They tend to be large and grow rapidly. On the other hand, benign tumors are often encapsulated by variably thick fibrous tissue and have a smooth external surface. These tumors have pushing growth margins and compress the adjacent native parenchyma. They grow slowly and tend to be small, although some can be large.

The histologic hallmarks of a neoplasm are characterized by its growth pattern and cytologic features. Malignant tumors have a disordered growth pattern and in their least differentiated form, bear no resemblance to their origin from the involved primary organ. Malignant cells have enlarged, hyperchromatic nuclei with an increased nuclear:cytoplasmic (N:C) ratio. The nuclei are crowded and stratified, the nuclear chromatin may be clumped, nucleoli are enlarged and mitotic activity is increased, often with abnormal forms. Tumor necrosis and hemorrhage are commonly found. In advanced stages of disease progression, tumor cells may aggressively infiltrate and destroy surrounding normal tissues and invade nerves, lymphatic or vascular channels. Lymph node or distant organ metastases may be present.

In contrast, benign tumors appear highly differentiated and resemble the normal tissue from which they originate. Benign tumor cells have abundant cytoplasm with a low N:C ratio, regular normochromatic nuclei and lack nuclear stratification. Nucleoli are usually inconspicuous. Mitoses may

21

Table 3.1.   Examples of various carcinogenic agents and associated human tumors.

Carcinogen	Tumors
Chemical	
Cigarette smoke	Oropharynx, esophagus and bladder
Aromatic amines	Bladder
Aflatoxin	Liver cell carcinoma
Vinyl chloride	Liver angiosarcoma
Arsenic	Liver angiosarcoma, cutaneous squamous cell carcinoma
Nitrosamine	Gastric
Betel leaf	Oral
Anticancer chemotherapeutic agents	Leukemia
Asbestos	Mesothelioma, bronchogenic carcinoma
Radiation	
Ultraviolet radiation	Skin — squamous and basal cell carcinomas, melanoma
X-ray	Skin cancers, leukemia, sarcomas
Radioisotopes	
Radioactive iodine	Thyroid
Thorotrast (no longer used)	Liver angiosarcoma, hepatoma, cholangiocarcinoma
Radium	Osteosarcoma
Viruses	
DNA viruses:	
Human papilloma viruses (HPV)	Cervical and vulvar squamous cell carcinoma
Hepatitis B & C	Hepatocellular carcinoma
Epstein-Barr virus (EBV)	Burkitt's lymphoma, nasopharyngeal carcinoma
RNA viruses:	
Human lymphocyte virus type I	Adult T-cell leukemia/lymphoma
(HTLV-1)	
Human immunodeficiency virus	Hodgkin's lymphoma (rare), B-cell non-Hodgkin's lymphoma, Kaposi's sarcoma
Hormones	
Estrogen	Endometrial adenocarcinoma, liver angiosarcoma (rare)
Oral contraceptive steroids	Liver cell adenoma, liver cell carcinoma (rare)
Diethylstilbesterol (DES)	Vaginal adenocarcinoma

be present but are few. Tumor necrosis is rare but variable degenerative changes are common. Benign tumors do not infiltrate into but may compress the surrounding normal tissues. Metastasis does not occur with benign tumors.

ETIOLOGY OF NEOPLASIA

A number of agents (*carcinogens*) are known to be associated or directly involved in causing specific cancers. Carcinogens can be classified as: chemical, radiation, viral hormonal and genetic.

Chemical carcinogens act on the DNA directly causing mutations or act as promoters for other carcinogens. The best known and most commonly encountered carcinogen is cigarette smoke. The active carcinogens in cigarette smoke are polycyclic hydrocarbons. Cigarette smoking increases the risk of various human cancers. Other documented carcinogens and the associated tumors are listed in Table 3.1.

Excessive exposure to ultraviolet (UV) *radiation* from the sun can cause DNA damage due to the formation of pyrimidine dimers and if these are not repaired, transcriptional errors with malignant cellular transformation can occur. UV radiation also inhibits cell-mediated immunity due to activation of suppressor T-cells which can result in the development of cutaneous cancers. On the other hand, ionizing radiation from X-rays and radioiosotopes cause carcinogenesis from genetic mutations either by direct effect of the radiation or indirectly through the interaction with oxygen or water to produce toxic free radical species.

Some *viruses* can cause cancer development. When DNA viral genes that are transcribed early in the viral replicative cycle persisting as episomes or become integrated into the host cell genome are expressed, neoplastic cell transformation can occur. Some gene products induce tumor growth either by enhancing normal growth factor proteins or inhibiting the actions of tumor suppressor gene proteins. *Slow transforming* oncogenic RNA viruses cause malignant transformation of cells by synthesizing a cDNA by reverse transcription that becomes integrated into the host genome close to a host proto-oncogene, whose expression can cause cancer. On the other hand, *acute transforming* RNA oncogenic viruses infect a host cell and proto-oncogenes from the host cell become incorporated into the viral genome, a process known as *transduction*, forming viral oncogenes or *v-oncs*. Mutations can occur during this process and the products of these v-oncs can have malignant transforming effects on the host cell. Carcinogenesis can also be induced during transduction when proto-oncogenes become located close to retroviral promoters resulting in abnormal expression of oncogenes.

Some tumors are caused by the effect of exogenously administered *hormones*. Unopposed estrogen effect can cause endometrial hyperplasia and adenocarcinoma. The progression of some tumors can also be influenced by hormonal balance. Certain breast carcinomas are hormone responsive and their progression can be arrested by hormonal therapy such as tamoxifen. The estrogen or progesterone receptor status of these tumors has important prognostic and management implications.

PATHOGENESIS OF NEOPLASIA

The development of neoplastic tissue involves a multistage process. *Initiation* of the neoplastic process occurs when a cell is exposed to a carcinogen and the time required for the cell to develop into the malignant phenotype is known as the *latent period*. The sequence of cellular and molecular events following the initiation process is known as *promotion* during which several agents act on the cell to promote it to develop into the malignant stage.

Chromosomal changes in neoplasia

Malignant cells have karyotypic changes with one or several chromosomal abnormalities and abnormal DNA content such as aneuploidy and polyploidy. There is increasing data on certain chromosomal abnormalities that are found in specific tumors. The chromosomal abnormality is often in the form of a translocation between break-away segments of 2 chromosomes, deletion of part(s) of an arm of a chromosome or even the acquisition of an additional chromosomal segment. Some of the well-known examples of chromosomal rearrangements characterized for human malignancies include t(9;22) (Philadelphia chromosome) in chronic myeloid leukemia, t(11;14) in chronic lymphocytic leukemia, t(14;18) in follicular non-Hodgkin's lymphoma, t(8;14) in Burkitt's lymphoma and acute lymphocytic leukemia, t(11;22)(q24;q12) in Ewing's sarcoma, del(3p) in renal cell carcinoma, del(3) (p14p23) in small cell lung carcinomas and del (13q14) in retinoblastoma. The significance of cytogenetic analysis of tumor tissue is that some of the known abnormalities are sufficiently specific to allow definitive diagnosis.

MOLECULAR GENETICS OF CANCER DEVELOPMENT

Several genetic mechanisms can be involved in the development of neoplasia. Alteration of a gene (*oncogene*) can intrinsically cause uncontrolled cell growth or by producing *growth factors*. Inactivation of a gene or its function that is normally involved in preventing or suppressing cell growth (*tumor suppressor genes*) can result in uncontrolled cell proliferation and subsequent neoplastic growth. Cells can be preprogrammed to 'commit suicide' by some genes (*apoptosis genes*) to prevent undesirable overgrowth. Finally, *DNA repair genes* that are responsible for repairing other genes can be mutated resulting in loss of prevention of the latter genes from becoming oncogenic. These genetic changes may be due to chromosomal translocation, gene mutations, gene deletions or gene amplification. Some of the better characterized oncogenes, tumor suppressor genes and growth factors involved in the development of various human tumors are outlined in Table 3.2.

Table 3.2.   List of various genes associated with human tumors.

Genetic abnormalities	Tumor
Oncogenes and growth factors	
ras	Colorectal, pancreatic, lung, bladder, melanoma, stomach, ovary etc.
c-erbB-1	Gastric, lung, brain
c-erbB-2	Breast, ovary
c-fos	Pancreaticobiliary, colorectal
myb	Colorectal, gastric
N-myc	Neuroblastoma
L-myc	Lung
myc	Gastric, pancreatic, colorectal, lung, breast, cervical, testis, prostatic, Burkitt's lymphoma
EGFR	Various epithelial tumors e.g. pancreaticobiliary, laryngeal, colorectal, gastric, lung, breast etc.
TGF-alpha	Breast, hepatocellular carcinoma, oral, lung, renal cell, neuroendocrine, gastrointestinal
sis	Brain
Tumor suppressor genes	
Rb1	Retinoblastoma
NF1	Neurofibromatosis type 1
p53	Wide range of tumors e.g. breast, colorectal, pancreatic, lung, melanoma, gliomas etc.
APC	Colorectal (familial adenomatous polyposis coli)
WT1	Wilm's tumor
p16 (MTS1)	Gliomas, melanomas, leukemia, osteosarcoma, various carcinomas such as bladder, breast, lung, ovarian, renal, esophageal
BRCA 1 & 2	Breast
nm23	Breast, colorectal, pancreatic, lung, melanoma, laryngeal
Metastasis suppressor genes	
nm23	Breast, colorectal, pancreatic, lung, melanoma, laryngeal
Apoptosis inducing genes	
p53	
myc	
Apoptosis suppressing genes	
bcl-2	Follicular non-Hodgkin's lymphoma
Activated ras	
DNA repair genes	
DNA polymerase B	Colorectal

Oncogenes

Cellular oncogenes are involved in the neoplastic process through a positive growth regulatory pathway on the cell involving activation of the gene through a combination of mechanisms such as: (1) *gene amplification*, resulting in overproduction of a protein which enhances cell growth; (2) loss of gene *transcriptional activity* from gene rearrangement during a chromosomal translocation; and (3) specific *structural changes* in the gene by point mutations or chromosomal translocation resulting in the production of abnormal proteins.

Excessive growth promoting proteins (*growth factors*) or their corresponding *receptor* proteins on the cell membrane encourage the cell in the resting phase to proceed through the cell cycle. This involves a complex series of events in which the growth factor binds onto its receptor which also has an intracellular tyrosine kinase component that is important in *signal transduction* for the mitogenesis.

In some tumors the number of growth factor receptors may not be increased but may be abnormal and do not require a growth factor protein to stimulate the cell into proliferating. Various abnormal proteins produced by oncogenes can also interact with or bind to the tyrosine kinase or guanosine triphosphatase (GTP) binding proteins leading to increased activities of these enzymes with subsequent increase in signal transduction and cell proliferation. Oncogenic products can also act on the cell nucleus by binding to the DNA and alter its properties which can result in DNA replication and cell proliferation.

Tumor suppressor genes

Tumor suppressor genes inhibit cell proliferation and uncontrolled cell growth occurs when these genes are inactivated or their functions inhibited. Inactivation of tumor suppressor genes can occur with either gene mutation, allelic loss of the gene (loss of heterozygosity) or regional DNA hypermethylation that terminates gene transcription or predisposes it to allelic loss.

Metastasis suppressor genes

Tumor progression and metastasis also involves a complex, multi-step series of genetic events. One of the recently discovered genes with anti-metastatic activity is the nm23 gene. The nm23 protein is found in both the cytoplasm and nucleus of the cell and is important in the regulation of cell growth and differentiation. The protein has nucleoside diphosphate (NDP) kinase activity and is able to supply nucleoside triphosphates (except ATP) to cells, regulate microtubule polymerization in the mitotic spindle and cytoskeleton, and provide GTP to the G-proteins involved in signal transduction. Reduced expression of nm23 is seen in several tumors with high metastatic potential although more recent data also suggests that overexpression of nm23 can occur in some tumors. Other possible genes involved in tumor metastasis may be located in chromosomes 11p and 17p.

Apoptosis genes

The genetic alterations that initiate apoptosis are currently not fully characterized. Some of the genes important in the normal regulation of cell growth, such as p53 and myc, are also involved in the control of apoptosis that prevents uncontrolled cell proliferation. The activated bcl-2 and ras genes are known to cause neoplasia by preventing cells from undergoing apoptosis resulting in cellular immortalization.

COMPLICATIONS OF NEOPLASIA

Local invasion and spread

The *immediate* consequences of neoplasia are due to the local mechanical effects of the growth and functional loss of the affected organ. The *local* mass effect of the tumor may be direct compression or destruction of normal tissue. Tumor invasion of the primary organ may result in perforation of the organ. Hemorrhage is often found in tumor tissue and may be a result of invasion and destruction of a nearby blood vessel or abnormal angiogenesis that accompanies tumor growth. Obstruction of a hollow organ occurs when it is extensively involved by tumor and may affect other organs, e.g. bronchial obstruction by tumor may result in pneumonia or lung collapse. In some aggressive malignancies, vascular infiltration by tumor cells can result in vascular obstruction leading to ischaemic changes or infarction of an affected organ. With progression of tumor growth, eventual functional deficit of an involved organ occurs. Host response to a tumor is often found in the form of inflammation with accompanying edema and effusions involving body cavities such as pleural or pericardial effusions and ascites.

The destruction and local effects of tumor metastases are the same as in the primary tumor except that these occur at distant and multiple sites. When vital organs are involved, *death* will ensue.

Paraneoplastic syndromes

Some tumors, without evidence of metastatic disease, may cause clinical signs or syndromes at sites distant from the primary lesion due to the elaboration of hormones or hormone-like proteins. These are the paraneoplastic syndromes.

Several endocrinopathies are seen in some tumors. Pulmonary small cell carcinoma can produce ACTH and ACTH-like substances resulting in Cushing's syndrome, or antidiuretic hormone (ADH) or ADH-like substances causing syndrome of inappropriate

ADH secretion. Hypercalcemia can be caused by secretion of parathyroid hormone-like protein in bronchogenic squamous cell carcinoma or the osteoclast activating factor-like substances in the case of multiple myeloma. Hypoglycemia is present in some sarcomas and liver cell carcinoma due to the production of insulin or insulin-like substances. Polycythemia is noted in renal cell carcinoma and some other tumors due to production of erythropoietin.

Neurological disorders such as dementia, cerebellar degeneration and peripheral neuropathy can be encountered in various cancers. Musculoskeletal disorders such as myasthenia gravis may be associated with bronchogenic carcinoma (Eaton-Lambert syndrome), but the exact mechanism for this association is not fully elucidated. Similarly, the pathogenesis for hypertrophic osteoarthropathy seen in lung cancer is unknown.

Some visceral cancers can give rise to skin lesions such as acanthosis nigricans and dermatomyositis. Coagulation disorders such as disseminated intravascular coagulation and thrombophlebitis migrans (Trousseau's phenomenon) can be seen in several malignancies, possibly as a result of hypercoagulability.

Tumor metastasis

As primary tumor growth progresses, a metastatic subclone may develop and attaches to the stromal connective tissue matrix via binding of tumor cell surface receptors to laminin and fibronectin. Tumor cells secrete proteolytic enzymes such as type IV collagenases and plasmin, to degrade the stromal connective tissue and matrix. Eventually, tumor cells reach, invade and penetrate the basement membrane of blood vessels or lymphatics. Tumor cells which enter vascular or lymphatic channels are transported to a distant site as emboli. Some of these cells are destroyed by host lymphoid cells within the channels but those that survive will penetrate the basement membrane of the vessels and into the stroma, in a similar mechanism involving receptor binding to laminin and fibronectin and degradation with proteolytic enzymes, leading to the establishment of a metastatic tumor deposit in the distant site.

Metastatic spread via lymphatic channels is more common in carcinomas and melanoma whereas hematogenous spread is favored by sarcomas.

However, some carcinomas, such as renal cell carcinoma, can show early spread via both vascular and lymphatic routes. Depending on the site and tumor type, the common target organs for metastasis are the liver, lungs, adrenal glands, lymph nodes, bone marrow and brain. Tumor metastasis can also occur by spreading along body cavities such as the pleural, pericardial and peritoneal cavities or the subarachnoid space. Not all tumor metastatic foci will result in death as some tumor metastasis can remain dormant and clinically undetectable for prolonged periods. This may be related to the host immune response to the tumor.

Cachexia

A common manifestation of cancer-related complication is cachexia. One of the underlying mechanisms for its development is the production of tumor necrosis factor (TNF)-alpha by activated macrophages in response to tumor antigens. TNF-alpha stimulates body fat catabolism.

IMMUNOPATHOLOGY OF NEOPLASIA

Two types of antigens present on tumor cells are important in the host immune response: tumor-specific antigen (TSA) and tumor-associated antigen (TAA). TSAs are present only in tumor cells but their exact nature, particularly in humans, is not known. TSA may develop as a result of either: (1) mutation of cellular proteins, not normally recognized as foreign, which bind to MHC class I antigens to form complexes that can be recognized as foreign; (2) mutation of cellular proteins that do not normally bind to MHC class I antigens resulting in binding of these proteins to the MHC antigens to manifest as TSA; or (3) activation of a normally silent gene during cell transformation to synthesize new proteins that can act as TSA. The various oncogene and anti-oncogene products are some of the examples of TSAs. On the other hand, TAAs can be found in both tumor and some normal cells and they do not evoke an immune reaction. Many of these antigens are used for diagnostic aids and for follow-up. Some examples of TAAs include carcinoembryonic antigen (CEA), alpha-fetoprotein (AFP), blood group antigens, prostate specific antigen (PSA), mucins and CD10.

Host immune response to neoplasia

The host immune response to tumor, consisting of both cell mediated and humoral immunities, is variable and is dependent on the tumor type, grade and antigenicity. However, some oncogenic agents, tumors and tumor products can have immunosuppressive effects. Several cell types are involved in the host defense against invasive tumor cells.

Cell mediated immunity to tumor is characterized by tumor cell destruction by *cytotoxic T-cells* sensitized against tumor antigen and *natural killer (NK)* cells. NK cells destroy tumor cells either directly or by activation of the antibody-dependent cellular cytotoxicity (ADCC) mechanism with destruction of antibody-coated tumor cells. LAK cells, which are derived from precursors of NK cells but enriched for CD3-expressing cells, can destroy NK-resistant tumor cells. Similarly, humoral immunity against tumor cells may be mediated via ADCC or activation of the complement system.

Macrophages, activated by gamma-interferon (IFN), a cytokine produced by T-cells, destroy tumor cells by secreting tumor necrosis factor (TNF) alpha, which is cytolytic and cytostatic, or by direct killing and production of reactive oxygen-derived free radicals. However, macrophages can also stimulate angiogenesis and produce growth factors which can promote tumor cell growth. Consequently, the balance between these inhibitory activities and promoting functions of macrophages may be critical in the regulation of tumor cell growth and progression.

Mast cells tend to accumulate at tumor periphery and they produce histamine which has mitogenic effects. Mast cells also produce various cytokines such as TNF-alpha, interleukin (IL)-3, IL-4, GM-CSF, leukotrienes, proteinases and heparin which are important in angiogenesis, tumor growth and progression.

Several *cytokines,* such as the various interleukins, interferons, tumor necrosis factors, colony-stimulating factors and transforming growth factors, are produced by lymphocytes, macrophages, monocytes, splenic cells, thymocytes, fibroblasts, epithelial cells and even tumor cells. The cytokines are signaling proteins which have overlapping actions with a complex network of interactions and are involved in the regulation of tumor cell turnover or destruction by the host. Elucidation of the cytokine network will be needed so that the effects of cytokines can be successfully exploited for the treatment of neoplasia.

LABORATORY APPROACH TO THE DIAGNOSIS OF NEOPLASIA

Serum and urinary biochemical markers

There is as yet no single entirely specific marker for any tumor type although a number of tumor markers may be useful in the clinical management of a patient with malignancy. Some of these serologic markers include the various ectopic hormones produced by bronchogenic carcinomas such as ACTH, ADH, PTH, calcitonin. Prostaglandins can be produced by some colonic and breast carcinomas. Some of the clinically useful markers include prostate specific antigen (PSA) and human chorionic gonadotrophin (HCG) produced by prostatic carcinoma and choriocarcinoma respectively. HCG is also raised in nonseminomatous germ cell tumors. Hormones (eutopic hormones) that are produced by the tissue of origin of the tumor can also serve as tumor markers. These include serum calcitonin in medullary carcinoma of the thyroid, urinary catecholamines in phaeochromocytoma and homovanilic acid in neuroblastoma. The oncofetal proteins such as carcinoembryonic antigen (CEA) and alpha-fetoprotein produced by various gastrointestinal tumors are only useful for predicting prognosis and monitoring therapy. CA 19-9 and DUPAN-2 are apparently raised in pancreatic carcinomas while a high serum level of CA-125 is more in favor of a diagnosis of ovarian carcinomas. However, the detection of urinary paraproteins is very suggestive of plasma cell myeloma.

Cytogenetic analysis

As mentioned earlier, the presence of certain chromosomal abnormalities may be diagnostic for some tumors.

Cytologic diagnosis

In *fine needle aspiration (FNA) biopsy and cytology,* tumor cells from solid organs or bodily fluids from organ lumens and cavities are aspirated using a needle and syringe, to achieve a cytologic diagnosis. The technique is popular due to the ease in obtaining cellular material, lack of complications and fairly high accuracy of diagnosis. It is inexpensive and a result can often be obtained quickly. Tumor cells can also exfoliate spontaneously or can be scraped and smeared onto a slide for cytologic examination. This is *exfoliative cytology*; any bodily fluids that contain tumor cells such as sputum, urine, effusions from the peritoneal, pleural and pericardial cavities, or cysts, can be collected and examined for tumor cells. A well-known example is the cervical (Papanicolaou) smear for screening cervical carcinoma.

Histologic diagnosis

Surgically excised tumor tissue sent to pathology departments for histologic diagnosis is fixed in formalin, processed through a series of formalin and alcohol solutions and embedded in paraffin. Tissue sections are then cut and stained with hematoxylin and eosin (H&E) for histologic examination. A number of clinically useful prognostic parameters are included in the histopathologic report such as tumor size, differentiation, grade, mitotic count, lymphocytic infiltrates, presence or absence of vascular and lymphatic invasion, lymph node metastases and disease stage.

Frozen section

A rapid intraoperative diagnosis can be made with frozen sections of fresh tissue stained immediately with H&E so that further surgical procedures may be performed (e.g. mastectomy for a confirmed case of breast carcinoma) or aborted (e.g. metastastic colorectal carcinoma in the liver). Often a high degree of accuracy can be achieved. Sometimes information on the adequacy of surgical clearance of a tumor may be requested by the surgeon using the frozen section technique. The major problem is that the histology is not as good as in a paraffin section and occasionally a diagnosis may not be achievable.

Immunohistochemistry

Immunohistochemistry is a technique in which an antibody reaction is raised against a specific tumor antigen on a histologic section, and is immensely useful for the diagnosis and classification of tumors.

Electronmicroscopy

The role of electronmicroscopy for the diagnosis of human neoplasia is now mostly replaced by immunohistochemistry.

Molecular biological studies

Southern blotting is used for gene rearrangement studies for the diagnosis of B and T cell non-Hodgkin's lymphomas. The polymerase chain reaction (PCR) technique can be used for the detection of certain gene products which can be diagnostic for some tumors such as Ewing's sarcoma and various leukemias. The application of molecular biological techniques in the diagnosis of neoplasia is progressing rapidly and newer more sensitive and specific techniques that are being developed may be useful for the diagnosis and study of human neoplasia.

Further Reading
1. Cawkwell, L., Quirke, P. (1994). Molecular genetics of cancer. In *Recent advances in histopathology no. 16*, edited by P.P. Anthony and R.N.M. MacSween, pp. 1–20. Edinburgh: Churchill Livingstone.
2. Chandrasoma, P. and Taylor, C.R. (1992). *Pathology Notes*, pp. 170–206. Connecticut: Appleton and Lange.
3. Cotran, R.S., Kumar, V. and Robbins, S.L. (1994). *Robbins Pathologic Basis of Disease*, 5th Edition, pp. 241–303. Philadelphia: W.B. Saunders.
4. Gatter, K.C. (1992). Morphology of neoplasia. In *Oxford Textbook of Pathology*, Vol. 1, edited by J.O'D. McGee, P.G. Isaacson and N.A. Wright, pp. 577–586. Oxford: Oxford University Press.
5. Harnden, D.G. (1992). Carcinogenesis. In *Oxford Textbook of Pathology*, Vol. 1, edited by J.O'D. McGee, P.G. Isaacson and N.A. Wright, pp. 633–673. Oxford: Oxford University Press.
6. Harnden, D.G. and McGee, J.O'D. (1992). Neoplasia. In *Oxford Textbook of Pathology*, Vol. 1, edited by J.O'D. McGee, P.G. Isaacson and N.A. Wright, pp. 571–577. Oxford: Oxford University Press.
7. Lewis, C.E. (1992). Cytokines in neoplasia. In *Oxford Textbook of Pathology*, Vol. 1, edited by J.O'D. McGee, P.G. Isaacson and N.A. Wright, pp. 709–715. Oxford: Oxford University Press.
8. Mitchison, N.A. (1992). Immunology of cancer. In *Oxford Textbook of Pathology*, Vol. 1, edited by J.O'D. McGee, P.G. Isaacson and N.A. Wright, pp. 706–709. Oxford: Oxford University Press.
9. Ratcliffe, J.G. (1992). Endocrine effects of tumors. In *Oxford Textbook of Pathology*, Vol. 1, edited by J.O'D. McGee, P.G. Isaacson and N.A. Wright, pp. 694–703. Oxford: Oxford University Press.

10. Tarin, D. (1992). Tumor metastasis. In *Oxford Textbook of Pathology*, Vol. 1, edited by J.O'D. McGee, P.G. Isaacson and N.A. Wright, pp. 607–633. Oxford: Oxford University Press.

11. Woolley, D.E. (1993). Tumor cell growth and metastatic spread: an introductory overview. In *Histamine in Normal and Cancer Cell Proliferation*, edited by M. Garcia-Caballero and L.J. Brandes, S. Hosoda, pp. 1–29. Oxford: Pergamon Press.

4. Principles of Surgical Oncology

DAVID L. MORRIS

UNSW Department of Surgery, The St. George Hospital, Kogarah, Sydney, Australia

Surgery has many roles in oncology — perhaps these could be categorized:

- Diagnostic/staging
- Curative
- Palliation

The concept of surgical excision is fundamental — that is, that complete removal of the tumor, sometimes with adjacent structures or the lymphatic drainage, may be helpful to the patient either by curing them entirely, by significantly elongating their life or by preventing or ameliorating symptoms. The role of surgery in cure is considerable — the *only* curative treatment for cancer of the stomach, pancreas, liver and colon is surgery. The role of surgery in palliation is also often considerable either in bypassing obstruction, for example in gastric outlet obstruction, or by debulking cancer either as a prelude to chemotherapy in ovarian cancer or to reduce symptoms from hormone secreting tumors. All treatments have some risks and surgery must be achieved with a minimum of mortality and morbidity for the risk/benefit equation to work in the patient's favor.

PREPARATION

Consent

The patient must understand the procedure, its potential benefits and its risks. The risk of death, even if small, must be understood, and the possible need for unexpected procedures. If a stoma is contemplated it should be discussed and its site marked. Common short-and long-term complications should be explained to the patient. Prognosis should be understood by the patient. Risks of anesthesia must be covered; it may be appropriate to ask the anesthetist to explain this aspect of risk directly.

Counseling

The surgeon should, if the patient is agreeable, discuss the procedure with the patient's family or close friends. Specific counseling may involve special groups, for example if a stoma is planned, a visit to the stoma therapist.

Fit

An important part of preparation is the assessment of the ability of the patient to undergo surgery. As well as a full history and examination, most patients over 40 years of age will need a chest X-ray, ECG and simple hematological and biochemical testing. Formal assessment by an anesthetist will be required for patients thought to be at risk, and is certainly not a bad routine policy. It also gives the anesthetist the opportunity to inform risks of anesthesia and discuss the type of post-operative analgesia which is to be used (patient-controlled analgesia/epidural/infusion or on-demand narcotic).

Thromboembolism

This potentially fatal complication of surgery is a particular risk in cancer patients and while there are many different risk groups, all cancer patients undergoing intra-abdominal surgery deserve prophylaxis. We routinely use Heparin 5000 units s/c twice daily (three times in obese patients) starting with the pre-medication, as well as graded compression stockings on the legs and intra-operative calf compression.

Pre-medication

Typically used to sedate the patient and also sometimes to inhibit secretion.

Starve

Pre-operative fasting of at least six hours must be observed (other than in an emergency setting) to reduce risks of aspiration pneumonia. In the presence of gastric outlet problems or bowel obstruction, a pre-operative nasogastric tube is required to empty the stomach.

Blood transfusion

Patients who may need a blood transfusion should have their blood group established and serum held (group and hold) to enable cross-match of blood to occur rapidly. If blood transfusion is very likely to be needed then a suitable number of units of blood will be *cross-matched* and held available for the procedure.

Shave

Removing hair from where the incision (by shaving or clipping) will be placed is usual. For operations on the head, axilla and groin, such as lymph node dissection, it would be essential. There is some evidence that clipping causes less skin injury and preparation should only be done immediately prior to surgery, otherwise the tiny shaving injuries may become colonized and the risk of sepsis increased.

Pre-operative staging

Every effort must be made to avoid unnecessary surgery. An "open and close" laparotomy may still be a very unpleasant, even fatal, experience for the patient and a significant waste of money to the health system. The converse, however, is perhaps even more disastrous, if we overstage disease with our investigations and deny potentially curative treatment to our patient. One example of this is lymphadenopathy on pre-operative abdominal CT scans — in stomach cancer. The prognostic value of lymph nodes below 2 cm in diameter in this situation is low. Inaccurate investigations must be recognized; CT portography (angio CT) can overdiagnose the number of liver metastases because of misinterpretation of flow artefact, so we may decide a patient is inoperable because there is one too many liver metastases for a possibly curative liver resection. A solitary abnormality on bone scan does not reliably indicate metastasis. Great care and more than a little experience is required.

OPERATION

Individual operations are considered in this book in the specific chapters.

POST-OPERATIVE CARE

Post-operative care has many aspects which are specific for the type of procedure. However, there are some generalizations of post-operative care which could be dealt with here:

Monitoring

Temperature, pulse, blood pressure are recorded at defined and regular intervals. In some patients, far more invasive monitoring is needed, with continuous monitoring of blood pressure, central venous pressure and ECG.

Pain

For the patient post-operative pain is perhaps the most unpleasant part of having an operation. Commonly used methods of relief include:

(a) *Intermittent intramuscular opiate* — (e.g. pethidine 1 mg/kg four hourly as required) together with an anti-emetic (e.g. stemetil 12.5 mg).

(b) *Opiate infusion* — A continuous IV infusion. This is often a good choice if the patient is unsuitable for PCA but there is some risk of respiratory depression. If concerned, check pupils, turn off opiate, give NARCAN (0.1–0.2 mg every 2–3 minutes until reversal of depression is achieved).

(c) *Patient Controlled Analgesia (PCA)* — In this type of system, the patient has a button which administers a small, predetermined bolus of analgesic. The pump machine is programmed so as not to allow the patient to take more than a perceived safe total dose/time.

(d) *Regional analgesia* — for example using epidural morphine infusion, provides excellent pain relief without the central effects of morphine. Complications include infection, respiratory paralysis and inadvertent spinal administration of opiate.

Fluid balance

A good chapter could be written on this alone. The first requirement is for accurate fluid balance (output/intake) charts. If the patient cannot take oral fluids, then IV fluid and electrolyte therapy will be required. Volume required will depend on losses (e.g. urinary output, nasogastric aspirate, drain losses, fistula loss, loss into bowel in ileus). The type of fluid required will vary — blood transfusion may be needed to replace intra- or post-operative loss. Plasma protein may be severely depleted due to loss and reduced production. Intravenous fluids can perhaps be divided into blood, volume expanders (e.g. plasma protein fraction, Haemacel, Dextran) and electrolyte solutions. The amount and type of electrolyte replacement required will clearly depend on losses but normal daily requirements are as follows:

Na 1–2 mmol/kg
K 0.5–1 mmol/kg

Nutrition

Most patients will be unable to eat for at least a few days after abdominal surgery. This does not constitute a need for expensive and potentially dangerous parenteral nutrition: this should only be considered when there is significant pre-existing nutritional deficit or after approximately two weeks without food. Severely malnourished patients do have a higher incidence of post-operative complications and, in particular, failure of healing. If the patient has a functioning gastrointestinal tract, enteral feeding is preferable because of the cost and risks of parenteral nutrition. Most surgeons wait until gastrointestinal function has returned, as evidenced by bowel sounds or the passage of flatus before recommencing significant oral intake, otherwise the paralytic ileus can cause considerable distension.

Renal function

Urinary output is usually measured hourly in patients after major procedures, which allows early recognition of reduced function. This must then rapidly be assessed and appropriate action taken, perhaps increasing parenteral fluids or giving diuretic.

Communication

Post-operative communication with the patient and family is important. They will want to know what has been done, were there any unexpected findings, has the prognosis altered?

Outcome of surgery

There are some general principles of surgical oncology. Clearly, if a cancer is being removed with hope of cure, then the excision margins must be free of tumor. Cancer cells can implant into wounds or anastamoses; care is needed not to spill them or to use cytocidal washouts to destroy them (e.g. cetrimide rectal washout).

Adjuvant therapy

Both radiotherapy and chemotherapy are used with surgery in particular tumors to improve outcome. They may be given prior to surgery, e.g. neo-adjuvant chemotherapy in oesophageal cancer and pre-operative radiotherapy prior to excision of fixed rectal cancer. Post-operative adjuvant chemotherapy improves survival in colonic cancer, radiotherapy allows breast lumpectomy to achieve similar results as mastectomy. A prohibitively high rate of local recurrence occurs in this situation if radiotherapy is omitted.

Access surgery

Surgery is sometimes just the means of providing access for chemotherapy. In long-term systemic chemotherapy, a port can avoid many cannulae for the patient. The use of regional chemotherapy is of established value in the liver and requires a small catheter to be placed into the hepatic artery through a side branch of the gastroduodenal artery.

Prophylactic palliation

While this sounds incongruous, some lesions have a predictable course which can best be influenced by preventing progress. Lytic long bone lesions can cause pathological fracture and this can be prevented by internal fixation. Bowel cancers which are causing obstructive symptoms or have a radiological appearance which suggests that obstruction is very likely, should be resected before obstruction occurs, as this would often commit the patient to a higher risk procedure and perhaps a stoma.

Why follow-up?

Follow-up can be of value to both patient and surgeon. Put simply, it's good for surgeons to know what their results are, both to be reminded of their failures and encouraged by their triumphs. Follow-up can identify and allow management of post-operative complications. Patients often value reassurance and support. Early diagnosis of recurrence of cancer can be useful; but may not be because recurrence is less often curable than the primary tumor. Follow-up may mean more than a history and examination. In fact, in colorectal cancer, the serum tumor marker, CEA, is probably the most useful means of detection of recurrence and with a considerable lead time over symptomatic disease. Another good example of the value of follow-up is lower GI endoscopy following colorectal cancer resection. The finding of metachronous (second primary) cancers will be achieved at an early stage.

Success

The measures of success of a surgical procedure are, first, the morbidity and mortality. Overall survival is a useful measure and is often expressed as % at five years. A Kaplan Meier survival plot is a common method of representing survival where

Table 4.1. The general complications of surgery might be categorized into the following organ list.

CNS
Anoxic brain death
Epileptic fit
Brain abscess
Post-op confusion (common in the elderly)

Cardiac
Arrhythmia
Infarction (an important cause of death after major procedures due to pre-existing heart disease)

Respiratory
Airway obstruction
Atelectasis (lung collapse) first 24 hours or so due to sputum retention
Chest infection/pneumonia
Pulmonary embolism (prevention: heparin 5000 units s/c TDS; TED stockings; intra-operative calf compression)

GI
Ileus
Peritonitis — often due to anastamotic leak
GI bleeding due to gastric erosions
Fistula due to the tumor or a leak
Intra-abdominal abscess — often due to a haematoma becoming infected
Anastomotic leak

Renal
Retention of urine
Acute renal failure — frequently pre-renal (avoid by careful monitoring, not only using output)

Locomotor
DVT
Pressure ulcers
Back pains

Soft tissue
Wound sepsis (avoid with technique, preparation, prophylactic antibiotics); (treat by drainage? antibiotics)

100% of patients are alive on day 1 and there is a progressive fall thereafter. Tumor marker response or time until relapse can be a meaningful interim measure of the outcome of surgery. Tumor-free survival may also be quoted.

COMPLICATIONS OF SURGERY

There are general conplications of all operations (Table 4.1) and specific complications of a procedure which cannot be covered here. The most important specific complication of all oncological surgery, however, is *recurrence*, which can either be local or be in the form of distant metastases. While biological factors and tumor stage influence the risks of both, surgical technique has an important role in minimizing local recurrence by achieving adequate margins — one of the best examples of this is low anterior resection where both complication rates and recurrence rates have been found to be very surgeon-dependent and to relate closely to the number of procedures being performed annually. Mortality rates of more challenging procedures (esophagectomy, pancreatic resection, liver resection) have now all fallen to under 5% in centers with large experiences of such procedures; mortality rates of 4 or 5 times as great have been reported. Sarcoma surgery is probably another good example of widely varying results. While specialization may make surgical life a little less varied ... it does seem to matter!

5. Radiotherapy

J.H. KEARSLEY and H.R. WITHERS

The St. George Hospital, Kogarah, Australia

INTRODUCTION

Radiotherapy (radiation oncology) refers to the clinical specialty of medicine in which ionizing radiation, either alone or combined with other modalities, is used to treat cancer. The radiation oncologist is a highly specialized clinician whose training spans the entire spectrum of malignant disease and who requires an in-depth knowledge of the biologic and physical basis of radiation therapy as well as a fundamental knowledge of the natural history of human malignancy. On rare occasions radiotherapy is used to treat benign conditions, e.g. pituitary adenomas, pterygium, or to prevent hypertrophic bone formation following hip replacement. Radiotherapy is the most important non-surgical therapy and is used to treat approximately one-half of all common cancers; it may be used with either curative or palliative intent.

The aim of radiotherapy is to deliver a precisely measured dose of radiation to a defined tumor volume with as little damage as possible to surrounding healthy tissues, resulting in eradication of the tumor, a high quality of life and prolongation of survival at reasonable cost.

THE IMPORTANCE OF LOCAL CANCER CONTROL

There is no doubt that for many cancers, the principal cause of treatment failure (and consequently, patient death) is distant metastatic disease. Indeed,

the advent of modern aggressive cytotoxic chemotherapy regimens for selected metastatic cancers such as testicular cancer, lymphoma and choriocarcinoma has resulted in many cures which would not have been possible 20 years ago. However, because of an emphasis on the treatment of systemic disease, the important role of loco-regional cancer control has been relatively underemphasized. Table 5.1 illustrates the fact that loco-regional recurrence of cancer is just as common (68% of the patients dying with disease) as are distant metastases. A large proportion of patients (50%) have both loco-regional recurrence and distant metastases.

Suit and Westgate (1986) estimated that elimination of loco-regional failures in patients without distant metastases at the time of diagnosis would result in a significant increase in survivors per year. These authors presented data to indicate that in a variety of cancers, a correlation exists between the incidence of loco-regional failures and the development of distant metastases. Not only is there an urgent need to develop new approaches to the treatment of systemic metastases, but further research initiatives in radiation oncology are needed to define therapeutic strategies which will increase the chances of local cancer control.

RADIOBIOLOGY

X-irradiation produces breaks in the DNA. Single-strand breaks are of little consequence because the cell has sufficient mechanisms for repairing them,

Table 5.1.   Estimated incidence, mortality and sites of recurrence for the most common types of cancer in USA (1990).

Organ	New cases/yr	Deaths/yr	Distribution of failures (deaths)			
			L-R Only	Comb. L-R + DM	DM Only	Total deaths L-R Tumor
Lung	157,000	142,000	49,700	49,700	42,600	99,400
Colon and rectum	155,000	60,900	6090	14,225	39,585	21,315
Breast	150,900	44,300	6645	26,580	11,075	33,225
Prostate	106,000	30,000	4500	19,500	6000	24,000
Uterus*	46,500	10,000	2000	5000	3000	7000
Oral, pharynx, larynx	42,800	12,100	6050	3630	2420	9680
Bladder	49,000	9700	2910	2425	4365	5335
Lymphomas	54,800	28,700	5740	5740	17,220	11,480
Pancreas, biliary	42,700	36,900	7380	22,140	7380	29,520
Esophagus, stomach	33,800	23,200	6960	11,600	4640	18,560
Leukemia	27,800	18,100	7240	7240	3620	14,480
Ovary	20,500	12,400	11,160	620	620	11,780
Brain, CNS	15,600	11,100	10,711	278	111	10,989
Total	902,400	439,400	127,086	169,678	142,636	296,764 (68%)

*Cervix, invasive and endometrium
L-R: local-regional tumor
DM: distant metastases
(Data from American Cancer Society, Cancer Facts and Figures, 1990)

presumably evolved to protect us against accumulating injury from environmental radiation and other toxins. However, if the dose of X-rays is high enough, two single-strand breaks will be close enough to one another to cause a double-strand break. Without intact templates for their mutual repair, double-strand breaks may be misrepaired and disrupt the integrity of the chromosome. Chromosomal aberrations do not normally affect the survival or function of cells between the time they are irradiated and the time they attempt to replicate themselves; cell death usually ensues at the first or early subsequent mitotic divisions. Thus, normal tissues and tumors show a radiation response at a rate which is proportional to their rate of proliferative turnover.

Tumors, like normal tissues, also respond to X-irradiation at different rates. Tumors with a high proliferative activity and a high rate of cell loss diminish in size quickly, whereas more indolent tumors may take months to become smaller in size. The rate at which a tumor regresses is not a reliable index of its radiocurability. Some tumors that regress quickly may also recur quickly, whereas other tumors may remain detectable for weeks or even months after the end of radiotherapy and yet ultimately disappear and never recur. Therefore, as long as a tumor is regressing after radiotherapy, biopsy is contraindicated. A positive result from a biopsy specimen may lead to unnecessary "salvage" surgery, and repeated biopsies interfere with the healing of normal tissues.

Why treatment takes so long

Radiotherapy is commonly given as a series of equal-sized doses, usually five times a week for several weeks, a process called fractionation. Each daily dose "fraction" kills the same proportion of cells. For instance, a commonly used daily dose is 200 centiGray (cGy; previously expressed as 200 rad) and, as a reasonable approximation, that dose reduces tumor cell survival to about 50%. A similar dose the next day will further reduce survival by 50% — i.e. to 25% of the original population. This equal proportionate effect results in a logarithmic (geometric) decline in total surviving cell number with increase in number of dose fractions.

A series of fractionated doses amplifies the therapeutic differential between normal tissue and tumor for several reasons, easily remembered as the 4 R's: **R**epair of cellular injury, **R**epopulation by surviving viable cells, **R**edistribution within the division cycle, and **R**eoxygenation of the tumor.

Repair

Repair of DNA damage is completed over a few hours, but the extent of repair is not equal in all tissues. In general, slowly responding normal tissues (e.g. connective tissue, kidney, spinal cord) are capable of greater repair than are malignant tissues. Thus, by spacing dose fractions by at least 6 hours (normally 24 hours) the recovery in slowly responding normal tissues is relatively greater than that in tumors. Because cell killing is logarithmic rather than linear, the difference in each day's effect is amplified exponentially — e.g. if the greater repair taking place in critical "target" cells of a slowly responding normal tissue leads to 60% of them surviving each dose fraction compared with only 50% of the cancer cells, then, after 30 dose fractions, the relative survival will be $(60/50)^{30} = 237$, a major therapeutic differential.

Repopulation

Repopulation by surviving cells in proliferative normal tissues takes place as a homoestatic response to injury and provides an important reason for extending treatment over several weeks. This regenerative response allows acutely responding tissues (e.g. mucosa) to tolerate an increased dose given to the tumor.

Treatment-induced acceleration of growth has also been identified and quantified in some cancers. This response to injury was unexpected since most tumors were thought to grow autonomously, although hormone-sensitive tumors were an exception. The mechanisms underlying the accelerated regrowth of tumor cells are unknown, just as they are for normal tissues. It seems reasonable to assume that growth factors are involved, and that their effect may be supplemented by improved vascularization of residual tumor as it shrinks. Also, like normal tissues, the delay between irradiation and a regenerative response, and its rate once it has begun, may vary widely from tumor to tumor. The rate of repopulation in the average tumor is less than that in acutely responding normal tissues, and the difference determines the therapeutic advantage for extending treatment. However, rapid regeneration is not a factor in the therapeutic differential between late-responding normal tissues and the tumor; it is therefore desirable to deliver the radiation dose in as short an overall time as is compatible with acceptable acute toxicity. Within the frame-work of keeping dose fractions small and limiting the total duration of therapy, the exact pattern of dose fractionation for a given patient can vary.

Redistribution within the mitotic cycle

Cells show large changes in their radiosensitivity as they progress through the division cycle. In general, cells are most radiosensitive in M and G_2 phases and most resistant in late S phase. Only a small radiation dose to the tumor is necessary to kill preferentially most cells in the more radiosensitive phases of the division cycle. This selective killing leaves the surviving cell population partly "synchronized" in more radioresistant phases immediately after each daily dose fraction. By stopping the dose and waiting, say 24 hours, one allows cells in radioresistant phases of the division cycle to progress into more radiosensitive phases. Eventually they will return to being an asynchronous population because of the wide range of division cycle times in most tumors. A population of asynchronous cells is more radiosensitive, on average, than the population surviving a dose of 200 cGy from which the more radiosensitive cells have just been eliminated. This self-sensitizing effect of cell-cycle redistribution applies to both tumors and normal tissues that show acute effects from multi-fraction radiotherapy; it is not, however, a feature of the normal tissues that show only late effects, whose cells are essentially static within the division cycle (in a phase that permits repair). The division cycle redistribution that takes place between successive doses in a course of radiotherapy enhances the differential effect between the critical late-responding normal tissues and the cancer.

Reoxygenation

When solid tumors grow, they often outstrip their blood supply and acquire areas of hypoxia and necrosis. Hypoxic cells are two-to-three times as radioresistant as normoxic cells (for radiochemical and not metabolic reasons). Hence, even a small proportion of hypoxic cells could limit radiocurability of the tumor. When multiple small doses of X-rays are given over a period of days or weeks, the normoxic cells, being more radiosensitive, are killed selectively by each dose fraction. During the interval between dose fractions, killed normoxic cells are eliminated and the previously hypoxic cells gain better access to oxygen. This process of

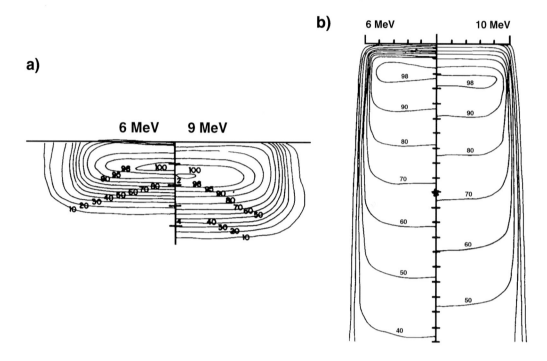

Figure 5.1. Typical isodose curves for (a) 6 meV and 9 meV electrons, (b) 6 meV and 9 meV photons. Note the rapid dose falloff with electrons and the higher penetrating power of 10 meV photons.

reoxygenation limits the negative effect of hypoxic cells on radiocurability.

The notion of fractionating the total radiation dose into many smaller doses — thereby repeatedly eliminating the radiosensitive subpopulation of cells and allowing surviving radioresistant cells to become sensitive during the interval — thus depends on both cell-cycle redistribution and reoxygenation.

RADIATION DOSIMETRY

The amount of radiation dose absorbed by material, e.g. human tissues was designated as the rad (radiation absorbed dose) by the International Commission on Radiological Units (ICRU) in 1956. One rad was defined as the absorption of 10^{-2} joules of radiation energy per kilogram of material. Under the current SI units, the unit of absorbed dose is the gray (Gy) which is defined as the absorption of 1 joule of radiation energy per kilogram of material i.e. it is 100 times larger than the previous unit, the rad. In some radiotherapy departments it has been found convenient to use the centigray (cGy) which is, exactly the same as the rad. Therefore,

one gray is equivalent to 100 rad which is equivalent to 100 centigray.

Isodose curves provide a visual representation of the absorbed dose at various positions across the radiation field within tissue. These curves are obtained by determining all the points within a radiation field in a water phantom where the percent depth dose is the same. Isodose distributions are extremely useful for visualizing the dose distribution for multiple beams in clinical practice. Typical examples of isodose plots are shown in Figure 5.1. The goal of treatment planning is to produce an appropriate isodose plan for the site to be irradiated in each patient. Typically, this process results in a plan being generated by the summing of several different beams directed at the target volume. This process is usually performed by a computer but can also be carried out manually. The shape of an isodose distribution is modified by the contour of the patient, and if the patient's contour changes within the radiation field during treatment, unacceptable and inaccurate isodose distributions may result.

Modern megavoltage machines (linear accelerators) usually operate in the region 4–10 MV and have significant advantages over kilovoltage machines used prior to the 1960s. Firstly, megavoltage radiations are far more penetrating in tissue and allow more effective treatment of deep-seated malignancies in the chest or pelvis. Secondly, megavoltage radiations have a significant "skin sparing" effect; the maximum dose from a single field usually occurs one to several cm below the skin surface. The skin surface usually receives approximately 30% of the given dose. Radiation from older kilovoltage machines generated maximum dosage on the skin surface which resulted in frequent examples of unacceptable skin reactions. Thirdly, megavoltage radiations result in significantly less "side scatter" of radiation and the beam edge tends to be considerably better defined and "sharper". This attribute enables very accurate placement of smaller fields to be used with megavoltage radiations and less radiation exposure to adjacent normal tissues.

DOSE AND TUMOR CONTROL

Some patients abandon their courses of radiotherapy before completion. This outcome is serious because to cure a cancer requires killing every cell that is capable of indefinite proliferation. An inadequate total dose will result in few or no cures. For instance, if 80% of the full dose is given, it will not achieve an 80% cure rate. If a tumor contained 10^{10} malignant clonogenic cells capable of indefinite proliferation, then a dose that was only 80% of that thought to be curative would reduce survival by a factor of only about 10^8; 100 (10^2) malignant cells capable of causing a recurrence would remain.

The relation between dose and the probability of curing the tumor is shown in Figure 5.2. There is a threshold dose below which no tumors are controlled but above which control increases steeply. The same curve applies to normal tissue injury but, through dose fractionation and other biological and physical maneuvers, it is displaced to the right. The greater the distance between the curves for tumor control and complications, the greater the therapeutic ratio. The aim of research is to increase the separation further.

The art of clinical radiotherapy practice is to determine the most appropriate risk–benefit ratio. Major complications such as myelitis must be avoided, but it is not in the best interests of patients to choose doses so low that there is no risk of complications.

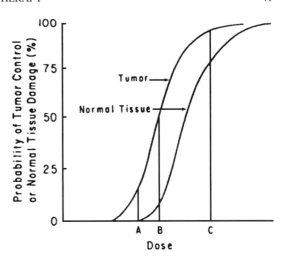

Figure 5.2. Typical dose-response curves seen with radiotherapy. Dose A results in a tiny probability of tumour control, but no side-effects. Given the sigmoidal shape of the curves, a small increment in dose (B) produces significantly higher cell kill with only a small risk of side-effects. Dose C represents the level at which most curative radiotherapy courses operate.

NORMAL TISSUE TOLERANCE

Curative radiotherapy usually implies an attempt to deliver the maximum dosage which the irradiated normal tissue can tolerate before the onset of significant acute and/or late complications. The dose which may safely be administered to a particular type or volume of tissue is known as the tolerance dose. Normal tissues which commonly limit the amount of radiotherapy able to be delivered include the gastrointestinal tract, bone marrow, lens and to a lesser extent, skin.

A detailed knowledge of tolerance doses for different normal tissues is essential for the safe practice of radiotherapy. Tolerance doses need to be known by radiation oncologists for each different tissue, quality of radiotherapy beam, the volume of tissue irradiated, the number and size of radiation fractions and the overall treatment time (Table 5.2). The severity of early or late radiation-induced lesions varies greatly from disfiguring change in the skin to transection of the spinal cord. Side effects may relate simply to severe atrophy and telangiectasia of the skin, or more seriously to frank necrosis or ulceration.

High doses of radiotherapy that carry some small risk of serious morbidity are regularly used in the treatment of many common cancers of limited

Table 5.2.   Tolerance doses for various "critical" organs when radiation is delivered with standard fractionation.

Organ	Injury	$TD_{5/5}$*	$TD_{50/5}$†	Whole or partial organ (field size or length)
Bone marrow	Aplasia, pancytopenia	250	450	Whole
		3000	4000	Segmental
Liver	Acute and chronic hepatitis	2500	4000	Whole
		1500	2000	Whole (strip)
Stomach	Perforation, ulcer, hemorrhage	4500	5500	100 cm
Intestine	Ulcer, perforation, hemorrhage	4500	5500	400 cm
		5000	6500	100 cm
Brain	Infarction, necrosis	5000	6000	Whole
Spinal cord	Infarction, necrosis	4500	5500	10 cm
Heart	Pericarditis, pancarditis	4500	5500	60%
		7000	8000	25%
Lung	Acute and chronic pneumonitis	3000	3500	100 cm
		1500	2500	Whole
Kidney	Acute and chronic nephrosclerosis	1500	2000	Whole (strip)
		2000	2500	Whole
Fetus	Death	200	400	Whole

radio-sensitivity. The level of risk of radiation morbidity in normal tissues which experienced clinicians may be prepared to accept is determined by a number of considerations. The most important of these is the clinical significance of the particular high dose effect. If the site of radiation necrosis is a vital center, such as the mid-brain, the lesion will be fatal and is clearly unacceptable. Similarly, irreversible injury to the spinal cord that would produce paraplegia may not be a justifiable hazard of radical radiotherapy unless the risk is very small indeed, and no other form of management can be offered. Most radiation oncologists would be prepared to accept levels of 3–5% necrosis in many sites, and in the treatment of advanced laryngeal cancer a necrosis rate of 10% is often taken as the limit of acceptable morbidity when laryngectomy is feasible.

DAILY ROUTINE

Patients having radiotherapy are usually required to attend the Radiotherapy Department for up to one hour per day on a Monday–Friday basis for periods which may vary from one to several weeks. Patients who are being treated with curative intent will usually attend for 4–7 weeks. Patients requiring palliative irradiation may only require treatment for 1–3 weeks, or occasionally, only a few treatment sessions. In some cases, however, an "incurable"

patient may be prescribed high doses of radiotherapy over a 4–5 week period if a large volume of cancer requires palliation.

During the radiotherapy planning process, patients are taken to the simulator room where their tumor can be accurately localized, and various measurements, e.g. physical contour of the patient, can be made. Computerized planning is used to produce a final draft plan within 24 to 48 hours. The isodose requires approval by the attending radiation oncologist before the patient can commence treatment. In many modern departments, resources and manpower limitations require a waiting period of 2–6 weeks between completion of a treatment plan and commencement of radiotherapy.

During treatment, patients are usually reviewed on at least a weekly basis by their radiation oncologist so that side effects can be anticipated and treated appropriately.

TREATMENT PLANNING

Before a patient commences a course of radiotherapy, the following steps must be considered:

1. What is the volume and location of the tissue to be treated? The use of planning CT scans has made the planning process very accurate.
2. What dose should be delivered to the target volume over what period of time? In general,

large target volumes require a prolongation of overall treatment time in order to prevent the development of significant side effects.

3. What normal tissues will be irradiated, and what dose is acceptable on these irradiated sites? In many instances, critical sites such as spinal cord, lens, testis will require special shielding to prevent serious side effects.

4. How will the external beams or brachytherapy be orientated to produce the maximal dose to the cancer but minimal dose to surrounding normal tissues?

EFFICACY OF RADIOTHERAPY

Highly sensitive (response occurs at modest radiation dose)

1. Seminoma (and dysgerminoma in the female).
2. Hodgkin's disease.
3. Non-Hodgkin's lymphoma.
4. Myeloma.
5. Small cell carcinoma.
6. Many pediatric malignancies, e.g. Wilms' tumor, neuroblastoma.

Moderately sensitive (response occurs at high radiation dose)

1. Squamous cell carcinoma.
2. Basal cell carcinoma.
3. Large cell carcinoma.
4. Adenocarcinoma.
5. Transitional cell carcinoma.
6. Non-seminomatous germ cell tumors.
7. Low grade astrocytoma.

Poorly sensitive (response may not occur within limits of normal tissue tolerance)

1. Melanoma.
2. Osteosarcoma.
3. Gastrointestinal adenocarcinomas, e.g. pancreas, stomach.
4. Soft tissue sarcoma.
5. Glioblastoma multiforme.
6. Renal cell (clear cell) carcinoma.

There is a wide variation in radiosensitivity amongst adenocarcinomas. Response to radiotherapy also depends on the amount of residual disease present following surgical resection. Microscopic amounts of moderately or poorly sensitive disease may be curable with radiotherapy administered post-operatively.

CAUSES OF CANCER RECURRENCE AFTER RADIOTHERAPY

1. Geographical miss, e.g. part of the cancer was not included in the irradiated volume. There may have been inadequate appraisal of the full extent of cancer in surrounding tissues, or failure to irradiate adjacent draining lymph nodes involved with tumor. In other cases, unreliable patient positioning and immobilization techniques may contribute to a geographical miss.

2. Underdosage. It is possible that the dose prescribed by the radiation oncologist was insufficient to sterilize all the cancer cells. Alternatively, a poor isodose treatment plan can reveal "cold spots" or areas of significant underdosage within the treated volume, even though the prescribed dose may otherwise have been satisfactory.

3. Poorly radiosensitive cancer, e.g. melanoma, some adenocarcinomas.

4. Other cancer-related factors:
   • Areas of hypoxia.
   • Accelerated clonage and repopulation.
   • Poorly vascularized cancers.

5. A new primary cancer.

RADIATION INDUCED SIDE EFFECTS

The cytotoxic effects of radiotherapy on normal host tissues result in the development of side effects. As is the case with cancers, normal tissues demonstrate a radiation response at a rate proportional to their rate of proliferative turnover. For instance, the mucosa of the respiratory and digestive tract, which is actively proliferative, develops a detectable reaction within 2 to 3 weeks of first exposure to a course of radiation therapy. Damage to bone marrow may be signaled by a fall in platelet and white cell counts within a few days if large volumes of the bone marrow are exposed. Skin reactions are reported only rarely with modern high energy, highly penetrating X-ray beams, but when the skin dose is raised intentionally or unavoidably, desquamation and/or hair loss begin to appear about three weeks after the start of treatment. The rate of appearance of injury depends not only on the proliferative activity of "stem", or germinal cells, but also on the lifetime of the differentiating progeny of these cells. Thus, although the platelet and white cell count may decrease quickly after irradiation, anemia is uncommon because of the slow turnover of mature erythrocytes and the ability of the surviving erythropoietic precursor cells to compensate for injury before the effects of radiation injury become obvious.

Slowly proliferating tissues such as connective tissue, kidney, cartilage, bone, lung and oligodendrocytes respond slowly to X-irradiation with signs of injury occurring only months or years after exposure.

The treatment of specific side effects includes:

Skin

The most common side effect is itchiness and irritation of the skin within the irradiated field due to the effect of radiation on sweat and sebaceous glands. Moisturisers containing sorbolene, vitamin E or aloe vera usually provide good relief. If the radiation dose is sufficiently high, acute inflammation will occur and may require regular application of hydrocortisone cream until the acute reaction resolves. If frank moist desquamation occurs, then saline/ bicarbonate bathing, good ventilation and nursing applications are extremely useful.

Oral cavity

Dry mouth, loss of taste, thickened saliva, taste perversions and a painful mucositis often respond to regular bicarbonate mouth washes, soluble aspirin or panadol, local anesthetic gels or liquid morphine if the pain is severe. Artificial saliva may alleviate xerostomia. Patients are also advised to take prophylactic nystatin drops orally to prevent the development of candidiasis. Liquid food supplements and the opinion of a dietitian are important to maintain weight and nutritional support. A soft toothbrush should be used to clean the teeth, and an electric shaver, not a razor, used to shave facial hair.

Esophagitis

Esophageal inflammation is a common side effect seen in the treatment of patients with lung,

esophageal or mediastinal tumors. Treatment usually requires soft foods with a high caloric/protein content, local anesthetic gel, soluble aspirin and occasional liquid morphine.

Cystitis

This is a common symptom in the treatment of bladder, prostate and other pelvic malignancies. Treatment requires a high oral fluid intake, urinary alkalinization and occasionally anti-inflammatory antibiotics, e.g. sulfonamides. Occasionally, propantheline is useful to reduce bladder tone, spasm and urinary frequency.

Proctitis

A common symptom in patients receiving radical radiotherapy for prostate cancer. Patients are advised to maintain a good liquid intake and to avoid constipation and to insert corticosteroid and/or local anesthetic suppositories for clinically troublesome proctitis.

Other side effects, e.g. nausea, diarrhea, etc. are treated along standard symptomatic lines with appropriate medication. Alopecia is universal within the irradiated area of skin and usually commences 2–3 weeks following the commencement of a radiotherapy course. Hair may re-grow 6–8 weeks after completion of radiotherapy.

Quite apart from local specific side effects, most patients will also notice lethargy and tiredness during a radiotherapy course. This symptom may take many weeks to resolve, and there is no specific antidote.

CURATIVE RADIOTHERAPY

Radiotherapy may be used as a curative treatment modality in either of two situations: macroscopic cancer and sub-clinical (microscopic) cancer.

Macroscopic cancer

Patients with clinically obvious cancer may be cured by radiotherapy alone. Several factors can influence the chance of cure.

The size of the cancer

In general, most common cancers, e.g. squamous cell carcinomas, adenocarcinomas, have a high chance of cure if the size of the primary lesion is small (usually < 3 cm in diameter). The larger the size of the primary cancer, the higher the dose of radiotherapy required to kill all tumor clonogens, and the higher the chance of severe early and late normal tissue complications. It is important to realize that cancers generally become smaller in size at a rate which is proportional to their cellular kinetics. Therefore, while squamous cell cancer may become considerably smaller by the completion of a course of high dose radiotherapy, adenocarcinomas may not have changed significantly in size until several weeks have passed. The rate at which the primary tumor shrinks in response to radiotherapy is therefore not a good indicator of the chances of ultimate cure.

Tumor radiosensitivity

Malignancies such as lymphoma and germ cell tumors are generally very sensitive to the effects of ionizing radiation, and large volumes of tumor may be sterilized during a course of treatment. For instance, a patient with a large lymphomatous abdominal mass may experience a complete response to relatively modest doses of radiation.

The volume requiring treatment

As a general rule, when small volumes of tumor are irradiated, higher radiation doses may be used, and therefore the chances of cure become higher. However, as the volume requiring radiotherapy becomes larger e.g. whole pelvis, the amount of radiation which can be administered is limited by the extent of normal tissue tolerance, e.g. intestine within the proposed field.

Sub-clinical (microscopic) cancer

Curative radiotherapy may also be undertaken to sterilize microscopic cancer following surgery. Common examples include the use of pelvic radiotherapy following surgery for locally advanced rectal cancer, or the application of radiotherapy to the residual breast tissue following a lumpectomy. Similarly, patients with head and neck squamous cell cancers may require prophylactic radiotherapy to neck nodes in an attempt to sterilize microscopic nodal disease following definitive surgical resection of the primary cancer.

PALLIATIVE RADIOTHERAPY

Although 40% of patients receiving radiotherapy are treated with curative intent, the majority (i.e. 60%) are referred with advanced cancer, and often require palliation of their symptoms.

Indications for palliative radiotherapy include:

(a)   Bony pain — this is the most common indication for radiotherapy. Results from treatment are usually very satisfactory although some pain may not be relieved if the cancer is radio-resistant and/or structural changes, e.g. crush fracture with weight-bearing bones, have occurred. Very occasionally, bony pain may be exacerbated for 12 to 48 hours following commencement of radiotherapy, and in this case, a short course of corticosteroids may be indicated.

(b)   Obstruction to hollow viscera, e.g. esophageal cancer, bronchogenic carcinoma. Associated symptoms of increasing shortness of breath, cough and hemoptysis usually respond well to radiotherapy.

(c)   Spinal cord compression. This is a radiotherapeutic emergency and urgent consultation between radiation oncologist and neurosurgeon is highly desirable in order to prevent permanent paraplegia and sphincter dysfunction. Concomitant corticosteroid usage should be considered. Patients with established paraplegia and sphincter dysfunction are unlikely to respond to radiotherapy.

(d)   Superior vena cava obstruction. Although usually due to right upper lobe bronchogenic carcinoma, SVC obstruction may be the result of other malignant conditions, e.g. lymphoma. Treatment of concomitant tracheal/bronchial obstruction is usually considered an emergency situation.

(e)   Prevention of or treatment of fungating tumors in order to improve nursing care.

(f)   Cerebral metastases. Secondary deposits to the brain often result in symptoms related to raised intracranial pressure. While treatment with corticosteroids often produces short-term symptomatic improvement, long-term use is undesirable because of side effects including proximal myopathy, oral candidiasis, significant weight gain and bruising. Radiotherapy is useful in reducing the size of brain metastases and controlling raised intracranial pressure. However, in patients with rapidly-progressive malignancy, radiotherapy may not be considered appropriate.

Radiotherapy is not usually recommended for the treatment of metastatic disease involving lungs or liver, given the potential for serious side effects when these organs are irradiated.

BRACHYTHERAPY

Brachytherapy refers to the use of sealed gamma-ray emitting radioactive sources in the treatment of small volumes of malignant tissue. By placing radioactive sources inside, or immediately adjacent to, the tissue to be treated, radiation dosage to other nearby tissues is minimized. Brachytherapy is usually limited to accessible sites where relatively small tissue volumes require treatment.

Three types of brachytherapy are used clinically. For *interstitial* treatments, the sealed sources are inserted directly into the tissue to be treated, e.g. tongue, brain. In *mold* treatments, the radioactive sources are mounted on a plastic carrier which is then applied to the patient's skin. *Intracavitary* treatments refer to the placement of sources in a natural body cavity, e.g. uterine canal, anal canal.

In elderly or infirm patients, brachytherapy is advantageous in that the treatment time is relatively short (a few days only) and toxicity to nearby normal tissues is minimized. Patients will normally require hospitalization during brachytherapy treatments.

USE OF UNSEALED RADIOACTIVE SOURCE

In some conditions, radioactive isotopes can be either ingested or injected into the body to treat disease. Examples include I-131 for thyroid cancer, Sr-89 for prostate/breast cancer metastases and P-32 for polycythemia rubra vera. As is the case for brachytherapy procedures, special radiation protection precautions must be taken to ensure the safe delivery of unsealed isotopes to patients.

THE FUTURE

The need to improve local control while minimizing treatment-related toxicities continues to represent a major challenge in the management of local human cancer. The limited success in controlling localized disease with currently available modalities and the association of local failure with incurable metastatic disease have stimulated a search for improved methods to accomplish permanent control of the primary tumor at the initial therapeutic attempt. The following initiatives have been, or are being, actively investigated at the present time to address the issue of improved local cancer control:

- Strategies to reduce hypoxia within cancers
- Radiotherapy combined with cytotoxic drugs
- Altered radiotherapy fractionation
- Heavy particles
- Hyperthermia
- Intra-operative radiotherapy
- Predictive assays of radiosensitivity
- Technical advances
- Radiosensitizing drugs
- Targeted radiotherapy

Reference
Suit, H.D. and Westgate, S.J. (1986). Impart of improved local tumor control on survival. *Int. J. Radiat. Oncol. Biol. Phys.*, **12**, 453–458.

6. Medical Oncology

MICHAEL BOYER

Department of Medical Oncology, Royal Prince Alfred Hospital, Missenden Road, Camperdown, Australia

INTRODUCTION

The specialty of medical oncology has evolved over the past three decades in parallel with the development of effective pharmaceuticals for the treatment of cancer. As a discipline, medical oncology is concerned primarily with the management of cancer by the use of drugs (both cytotoxics and hormonal agents). However, the role of the medical oncologist typically goes far beyond this. Not uncommonly, the medical oncologist becomes the health professional who co-ordinates the care of the cancer patient. Given their training in internal medicine, medical oncologists are in an ideal position to manage not only the patient's cancer, but also the various other illnesses, problems and complications that may be associated with it. This chapter will provide an overview of the practice of medical oncology, as well as the principles of the chemotherapeutic treatment of cancer.

HISTORY

Although medical oncology is a relatively "young" specialty, the basis for the pharmacological treatment of cancer with either hormones or cytotoxic agents extends back into the first half of this century.[1,2] Considerable experimentation was carried out with alkylating agents during both World Wars.

The cytotoxic and myelosupressive properties of the mustard gases were first recognized in 1919, but clinical use was not made of this observation until 1942. At that time, treatment with alkylating agents was attempted in patients with Hodgkin's and non-Hodgkin's lymphomas; however, because of secrecy surrounding chemical warfare programs, the results were not reported until 1946.[3] A good deal of excitement was produced by the dramatic regressions that were observed, followed by disappointment, as tumors inevitably recurred.

Soon after, in 1948, the use of folic acid analogs was pioneered by Farber and associates, with encouraging results in the treatment of childhood acute lymphoblastic leukemia.[4] The development of cytotoxic chemotherapy then began in earnest, and the succeeding two decades saw the development of many of the agents that are in common use today. In addition, this period witnessed a growing awareness of the importance of the use of combinations of chemotherapeutic agents (as opposed to single drugs used alone). In the early 1960s, chemotherapy came of age, with the recognition that certain advanced malignancies, such as Hodgkin's disease and choriocarcinoma in women, could be cured by chemotherapy.

In contrast to the relatively recent development of cytotoxic chemotherapy hormonal manipulation has been used in the management of malignancy since the end of the nineteenth century. In 1896,

Beatson reported the regression of metastatic breast cancer in some pre-menopausal women following oophorectomy. Similarly, in prostate cancer, androgen ablation has been in use for over 50 years, since the pioneering work of Huggins.

THE PRACTICE OF MEDICAL ONCOLOGY

Uses of chemotherapy

The practice of medical oncology is based on the use of medications to cure or control cancer. The drugs used to achieve this include not only cytotoxics, but also hormonal agents and modulators of immune function.

Chemotherapy is generally used in four different ways. These include: induction treatment for advanced disease; primary treatment for patients with localized cancer; adjuvant treatment following other local methods of treatment; and regional treatment in specific sites.

Induction chemotherapy refers to the use of chemotherapy in patients with advanced cancer, where the aim of such therapy is to induce remission. This may be part of a curative strategy, or a component of palliative therapy (such as in women with symptomatic, metastatic breast cancer). Typically, treatment comprises the use of combinations of drugs, which have been developed and shown to be effective in the particular disease in question.

Adjuvant therapy refers to the use of hormonal therapy or chemotherapy following local treatment of malignancy by surgery or radiotherapy. The aim of adjuvant therapy is to increase the likelihood of cure by controlling systemic, micrometastatic disease, and thus preventing relapse. Examples include the use of systemic therapies in women with resected breast cancer, and the use of chemotherapy in patients with resected colon cancer. In some situations, combinations of chemotherapy and radiotherapy may be used as adjuvant therapy (for example, in rectal cancer).

Adjuvant therapies are usually distinguished by the need to treat relatively large numbers of patients in order to benefit a few. This is because those patients who were already cured by local therapy alone do not benefit from adjuvant treatment; unfortunately, it is not usually possible to identify such patients prospectively and spare them the need for adjuvant treatment. The magnitude of absolute benefit of adjuvant therapies is determined not only by the efficacy of the therapies themselves, but also by the underlying risk of disease recurrence. For a therapy of given efficacy, the higher the risk of relapse, the greater the absolute benefit of adjuvant treatment.

Chemotherapy may be used as primary treatment for localized malignancy in certain situations. This is often referred to as neo-adjuvant treatment. This approach, where initial chemotherapy is followed by planned definitive local treatment with surgery or radiotherapy, has been explored in several disease types but has only been demonstrated to be of benefit in a small number of these. Examples include the use of primary chemotherapy followed by radiotherapy in locally advanced laryngeal cancer, and the use of chemotherapy prior to radiotherapy in some patients with stage IIIB non-small cell lung cancer.

Regional administration of drugs can be achieved in several ways and for a range of purposes. Chemotherapeutic agents can be instilled directly into body cavities, such as the peritoneal cavity or the bladder, or injected into the cerebrospinal fluid. Alternatively, chemotherapy can be given directly into an artery which supplies a tumor (for example, intra-arterial chemotherapy for osteosarcoma) or organ (for example, hepatic arterial infusion for the treatment of hepatic metastatic disease). The rationale for regional chemotherapy is to achieve higher local drug concentrations, minimization of systemic exposure, and in some circumstances, the role of a first-pass effect. The place of regional chemotherapy is still being evaluated, and there are few situations where these approaches are clearly superior to systemic chemotherapy.

Assessing the effectiveness of chemotherapy

The effects of chemotherapy (along with other anticancer therapies) may be measured in several different ways, which vary in their relevance to clinical outcome. In the development of new cytotoxics, response rate is the most commonly used indicator of drug activity. This is a measure of the ability of a drug to cause objective tumor shrinkage, in accordance with pre-defined criteria.[5] Typically, complete response is defined as the total disappearance of all tumor, while partial response requires a >50% decrease in the cross-sectional areas of known tumor deposits. Any tumor that increases in size by

>25% is considered as having progressed, and all other situations are classified as stable disease.

While providing a useful guide to the activity of a drug, response is not a direct measure of patient benefit. It is, however, true that most therapies which are beneficial (as measured by some other criteria) usually also produce high response rates. More direct measures of patient benefit include survival (or disease-free survival) and palliative measures, such as quality of life or symptom scores, both of which may be incorporated into clinical trials.[6,7] Although survival is an appropriate endpoint in settings where cure or prolongation of life is the goal of treatment, when the intent of therapy is to control symptoms, palliative endpoints may provide a better indication of the usefulness of therapy.

CHEMOTHERAPEUTIC AGENTS

Since the initial use of the mustards as cytotoxic agents in the 1940s, many thousands of compounds have been screened for anti-neoplastic activity. A small number of these have been developed, and are in common clinical use. The origins of these drugs are diverse. Relatively few of the cytotoxics in use today have been designed rationally. Most have been identified by chance, or as a result of mass drug screening programs. Included amongst them are drugs derived from plants, drugs derived from fungi, analogs of the heavy metal platinum, and several rationally designed antimetabolites. For convenience, anticancer drugs are usually classified into groups based on their origin, or mechanism of action. Table 6.1 contains a list of commonly used cytotoxic drugs. A brief description of the mechanism of action of some of the more important anticancer drugs is to be found below. Full details are available in standard reference texts.[8]

Anticancer drugs may cause cell death by a variety of mechanisms; in some cases, a single agent may have several mechanisms of action. Alkylating agents, which were amongst the first drugs to be used in the treatment of cancer, cause damage to DNA by forming adducts (the result of the binding of the drug to DNA), which disrupt its structure and function. The platinum-based drugs, cisplatin and carboplatin, also have DNA as their target, and are able to cause adducts, as well as crosslinks between the two strands of DNA. Other agents which have DNA as their major target include bleomycin, and the anthracyclines, doxorubicin and daunorubicin.

Other drugs may inhibit cellular replication by interfering with microtubules (which are needed to form the mitotic spindle). The vinca alkaloids inhibit the formation of microtubules, while paclitaxel has the opposite mechanism of action, causing stabilization of these structures. A further important intracellular target for cytotoxics is the enzyme topoisomerase II. This enzyme is involved in the unwinding of DNA during replication, and interference with it halts this process. Etoposide and teniposide have topoisomerase II as their target. In addition, the anthracyclines may also interfere with the operation of this enzyme.

The antimetabolites typically act to interfere with DNA or RNA synthesis. Methotrexate, by binding to the enzyme dihydrofolate reductase, depletes intracellular reduced folate pools, and thereby impairs *de novo* synthesis of purines and pyrimidines. 5-Fluorouracil (FU), another commonly used antimetabolite, binds to, and inhibits, the enzyme thymidylate synthetase. This results in the depletion of thymidine based precursors, necessary for DNA synthesis. FU may also interfere with RNA synthesis, though the relative contribution of these different mechanisms to cytotoxicity is unknown.

PRINCIPLES OF COMBINATION CHEMOTHERAPY

Early in the development of cytotoxic chemotherapy, it became clear that in order to produce durable remissions, combinations of chemotherapeutic agents rather than single drugs needed to be used. Although a few diseases (e.g. gestational trophoblastic disease) provide an exception to this general principle, most curative chemotherapeutic strategies, such as those used in the treatment of the lymphomas, leukemia and testicular cancer, are based on drug combinations. Furthermore, in the adjuvant setting, combinations are probably more effective than single agents in the treatment of diseases such as breast cancer and osteogenic sarcoma.[9] Compared to single agents, the use of drug combinations allows greater cell kill, provides a broader range of cytotoxic activity against heterogeneous clonal populations within tumors, and prevents or slows the development of resistant lines.

In order to develop effective drug combinations, certain principles have been followed. Combina-

Table 6.1. Commonly used chemotherapeutic agents.

	Common Uses*	Major Side Effects
Alkylating agents		
Busulfan	Chronic myeloid leukemia	Most alkylators produce infertility
Chlorambucil	Chronic lymphoid leukemia, ovarian cancer	Myelosuppression Myelosuppression
Cyclophosphamide	Breast cancer, non-Hodgkins lymphoma, ovarian cancer, paediatric sarcomas	Myelosuppression, alopecia, nausea, hemorrhagic cystitis (dose dependent)
Ifosfamide	Pediatric sarcomas	Hemorrhagic cystitis
Melphalan	Multiple myeloma	Myelosuppression
Nitrogen Mustard	Hodgkins disease	Myelosuppression, nausea
Nitrosoureas (BCNU, CCNU)		
Anthracyclines		
Daunorubicin	Acute leukemia	As for doxorubicin
Doxorubicin	Breast cancer, pediatric sarcomas, lymphoma, gastric cancer, sarcomas	Myelosuppression, alopecia, nausea and vomiting, mucositis, cardiomyopathy
Epirubicin	As for doxorubicin	As for doxorubicin
Idarubicin	Acute myeloid leukemia	
Antimetabolites		
Cytosine Arabinoside	Acute myeloid leukemia	Cerebellar dysfunction, myelosuppression
5-Fluorouracil	Colon cancer, breast cancer, gastric cancer, head and neck cancers	Diarrhoeas, mucositis, chest pain
Methotrexate	Breast cancer, sarcoma	Mucositis
Antitumor antibiotics		
Bleomycin	Testicular cancer, lymphoma	Pneumonitis, pulmonary fibrosis, flu-like syndrome
Dactinomycin	Pediatric sarcoma	Mucositis, nausea
Mitomycin C	Anal cancer, colon cancer, breast cancer	Myelosuppression
Drugs derived from plants		
Vincristine	Lymphoma, small cell lung cancer, acute lymphoblastic leukemia	Peripheral neuropathy
Vinblastine	Testicular cancer, lymphoma	Myelosuppression, abdominal cramps
Vinorelbine (synthetic)	Non small cell lung cancer	Myelosuppression
Vindesine (synthetic)	Non small cell lung cancer	Myelosuppression
Etoposide	Small cell lung cancer, non-small cell lung cancer, lymphoma, testicular cancer	Alopecia, hypotension, myelosuppression
Teniposide	As for etoposide	As for etoposide
Paclitaxel	Breast cancer, ovarian cancer, non-small cell lung cancer	Alopecia, myelosuppression, peripheral neuropathy, cardiac arrythmias, hypersensitivity reactions
Docetaxel	As for paclitaxel	Alopecia, myelosuppression, fluid retention
Platinum analogs		
Carboplatin	Ovarian cancer, non-small cell lung cancer, small cell lung cancer	Myelosuppression
Cisplatin	Testicular cancer, gastric cancer, ovarian cancer, non-small cell lung cancer, small cell lung cancer, head and neck cancers	Anemia, nausea and vomiting, peripheral neuropathy, tinnitus, hearing loss
Miscellaneous agents		
Asparaginase		
Dacarbazine	Hodgkin's lymphoma, melanoma	Nausea and vomiting
Procarbazine	Hodgkin's lymphoma	

*The list of common uses is not a complete list, but provides examples of some of the diseases in which these drugs are used.

tions are constructed from drugs which possess single agent activity against the disease in question. Furthermore agents are chosen which have qualitatively different normal tissue toxicities, but additive (or greater than additive) therapeutic effects. This is relevant because the combination of drugs has the potential to increase normal tissue toxicity. If both the toxicity and the anticancer activity of a combination are greater than for the respective single agents, the overall therapeutic effect may be inferior.

The selection of agents which have non-overlapping toxicities is also important in allowing the use of effective doses of each of the drugs that comprise the combination. Most of the commonly used chemotherapeutic drugs exhibit a dose–response relationship, and reductions in dose are often associated with lower response rates.[10] As a result, if a combination requires that the doses of individual agents be reduced, the net effect may be a lower response rate than that achievable with single agents given in full dose. This situation is most likely to occur when the toxicities of the drugs within the combination are similar. For example, if a combination contains two drugs, both of which have myelosuppression as their dose limiting toxicity, it is unlikely that both agents could be given simultaneously at full dose. By contrast, successful combination regimens, such as the cisplatin, etoposide and bleomycin program for testicular cancer, contain drugs with differing toxicities, allowing all of the agents to be delivered in full dose and on schedule.[11]

Tumor heterogeneity provides one of the most compelling theoretical reasons for the use of combination, rather than single agent, chemotherapy. Although tumors are clonal in origin, the genetic instability that is associated with the malignant process results in variation in the phenotypic characteristics of daughter cells. Thus cells with a greater proliferative, invasive or metastatic potential may evolve with time. Part of this evolution may also involve changes in the target sites for the action of chemotherapeutic agents, so that within a single tumor, there may be subpopulations with varying levels of sensitivity to different cytotoxics (see the subsection *Resistance to chemotherapy*, below). The early use of combination, rather than single agent, chemotherapy may slow or prevent the emergence of clinically overt resistant tumor populations.

Biochemical modulation has been of increasing importance in recent years, and represents a special example of combination therapy. This approach involves the combination of a cytotoxic drug with a modulator, which is usually not a cytotoxic in its own right. The modulator acts to change or enhance the biochemical processes necessary for the action of the drug. A clinically important example of biochemical modulation is the addition of folinic acid (leucovorin) to the chemotherapeutic agent, 5-fluorouracil (FU). The biochemical rationale for the modulation is based on the mechanism of action of FU. Intracellularly, FU is converted into FdUMP, which binds to the substrate site of thymidylate synthetase, inhibiting its activity, and ultimately interfering with DNA synthesis. The stability and duration of this inhibition is related to 5–10 methylene-tetrahydrofolate, a metabolic product of folinic acid. The administration of folinic acid results in enhanced inhibition of thymidylate synthetase. This has translated into higher tumor response rates in the clinical setting, for example in the treatment of metastatic colon cancer.[12]

TUMOR BIOLOGY AND CHEMOTHERAPY

The use of anticancer therapies should be based on a sound understanding of the biology of malignancy. A detailed discussion of the biology of tumors is beyond the scope of this chapter, and can be found in Chapter 3. However, some aspects of tumor biology that relate particularly to the use and effects of chemotherapy will be discussed here.

The cell cycle, tumor kinetics and chemotherapy

In populations of cells, both normal and neoplastic, there are three distinct subpopulations. The first comprises those cells that are actively passing through the cell cycle (see below). These cells are proliferating continuously, passing from one mitosis to the next, and represent the growth fraction of the tumor or tissue. A second subpopulation comprises cells that have terminally differentiated, having lost the capacity for further division. These cells have irreversibly left the cell cycle. The final subpopulation is composed of cells that are quiescent, and have temporarily left the cell cycle. These

Table 6.2. Mechanisms of drug resistance.

Mechanism	Examples
Decreased cellular uptake	Methotrexate, Nitrogen Mustard
Decreased intracellular drug activation	5-Fluorouracil, 6-Mercaptopurine, Cytosine Arabinoside
Increased drug efflux	Doxorubicin, Etoposide, Vinca Alkaloids, Cisplatin
Altered targets (qualitative or quantitative)	Methotrexate, 5-Fluorouracil, Etoposide, Amsacrine
Increased DNA repair	Cisplatin, Alkylating Agents

cells, often referred to as G0 cells, can re-enter the cell cycle following an appropriate stimulus. Stem cells, contained within normal bone marrow, fall into this category and, with stimulation, are capable of reproducing themselves and re-populating the bone marrow following chemotherapy. Unfortunately, stem cells within tumors may also fall into this subpopulation, producing difficulties in the chemotherapeutic treatment of cancers.

The growth and division of cells, both normal and neoplastic, follows an orderly progression of events which comprise the cell cycle. The cell cycle is divided into four phases, known as G1 (gap 1), S (synthesis of DNA), G2 (gap 2, the premitotic interval) and M (mitosis). In some tumors and normal tissues there is a prolonged G1 or resting phase, which is commonly referred to as G0, where cells are effectively out of the cycle.

The effect of most anti-neoplastic agents is determined by the phase of the cell cycle. Thus, antimetabolites such as methotrexate and 5-fluorouracil act predominantly in S phase, while agents affecting microtubules, such as the vinca alkaloids and the taxanes, act in M phase. Some drugs, such as the alkylating agents, are active throughout the cell cycle, including in G0; however, in order for cells to actually die, they must return to the cell cycle.

Since the effects of most chemotherapeutic agents are dependent on processes associated with cell growth and division, the response of tumors (in terms of tumor shrinkage) to chemotherapy is generally enhanced by a large growth fraction. By contrast, cure of a tumor by chemotherapy is dependent on the elimination of all clonal stem cells, which may or may not be contained within the growth fraction. This difference between the requirements to produce response and cure is one explanation for the common clinical observation of tumors which are highly responsive to chemotherapy, but rarely cured by it (for example, small cell carcinoma of the lung).

Resistance to chemotherapy

The development of resistance by tumors represents one of the limiting factors in the successful use of cytotoxic chemotherapy. Despite initial responses to chemotherapy, many tumors eventually become resistant to this form of treatment. The clinical manifestation of this is that of tumor growth despite continued treatment. Several mechanisms may lead to the clinical syndrome of drug resistance and are summarized in Table 6.2. These mechanisms include both *de novo* (or intrinsic) resistance, and, more commonly, resistance following exposure to anti-cancer agents (acquired drug resistance).

The development of resistant clones within populations of tumor cells is believed to be a function of the genetic instability of the tumor, and the number of cells present. Goldie and Coldman proposed a mathematical model to account for the development of resistance within tumors.[13] Their model suggests that resistance may occur in even relatively small tumors, although the absolute number of resistant cells in this situation would be relatively small. A corollary of this is that if multiple drugs are available with which to treat a tumor, as many as possible of these agents should be administered as early as possible. This approach has led to the development of alternating schedules of non cross-resistant drugs, where drugs with different putative resistance mechanisms are given in alternating cycles. Despite the appealing theoretical basis for this approach to treatment, there is little convincing clinical data to support it.

Several different mechanisms may produce drug resistance (Table 6.2). These include changes in the uptake, metabolism, and excretion of the drug, alterations in the cellular targets for the drug, and enhanced repair mechanisms. Decreased drug uptake may occur as a consequence of changes to drug transporters. This is a common cause for resistance to both methotrexate and nitrogen mustard.[14,15]

Table 6.3. Strategies for overcoming drug resistance.

Combination chemotherapy (rather than single agents)
High dose chemotherapy
Rational design of drugs using different transporters, or not requiring active transport
Inhibition of efflux pumps
Biochemical modulation

Alterations in drug metabolism can result in decreased levels of active drug. Similarly, enhanced drug excretion may cause low intracellular drug levels, and hence resistance. The discovery of the p-glycoprotein, an energy-dependent efflux pump coded for by the *mdr*1 gene, has focused attention on this as a mechanism of resistance.[16] The novel feature of p-glycoprotein is its ability to mediate cross-resistance to several, structurally unrelated drugs. Thus cells selected for resistance to adriamycin as a result of overexpression of p-glycoprotein are also resistant to the vinca alkaloids. Several agents (for example, verapamil and cyclosporin) have been identified that can inhibit the action of this transport protein and overcome resistance *in vitro*; however, clinical trials have thus far failed to reveal meaningful benefit in humans.[17]

Changes in the intracellular targets upon which cytotoxics act is a further cause for drug resistance. Resistance to agents which act on specific enzyme targets may occur due to qualitative or quantitative changes in these enzymes. Alterations in dihydrofolate reductase, thymidylate synthetase and topoisomerase II have all been reported to produce resistance in the drugs that target these enzymes (methotrexate, 5-fluorouracil and etoposide, respectively). Even when drugs are able to exert their effects, resistance may still occur due to enhanced ability of cells to repair drug-induced damage. This has been demonstrated for both alkylating agents and cisplatin.

Since drug resistance is believed to play a part in the failure of chemotherapy to control or eradicate human cancer, approaches are being developed to circumvent resistance. These are summarized in Table 6.3, and include the use of combination chemotherapy and high dose chemotherapy. In addition, the use of specific inhibitors of p-glycoprotein is being investigated.

TOXICITY OF CHEMOTHERAPY

One of the limitations to the use of chemotherapy in the treatment of cancer is the occurrence of normal tissue toxicity. The patterns and severity of toxicity resulting from chemotherapy are determined by several factors including the drugs used, the dose, and the general condition of the patient. In addition, the presence of specific pre-existing conditions may predispose to particular complications. In order to limit the impact of chemotherapy toxicity, strategies have been developed to minimize specific side effects. Common toxicities and the interventions used to prevent or treat them are listed in Table 6.4.

Table 6.4. Toxicities of chemotherapy and strategies to minimize them.

Toxicity	Drugs commonly implicated	Minimization strategies
Alopecia	Doxorubicin, Daunorubicin, Etoposide, Cyclophosphamide, Paclitaxel	Ice cap (to reduce scalp blood flow); rarely used
Arrhythmia	Doxorubicin, Daunorubicin, Paclitaxel	
Cardiac failure	Doxorubicin, Daunorubicin, Mitoxantrone	Limit cumulative dose of these agents
Interstitial pneumonitis/fibrosis	Bleomycin, Alkylating agents, Nitrosoureas	
Myelosuppression	Dose related, but caused by most drugs, except vincristine, cisplatin, methotrexate, bleomycin	Colony stimulating factors
Nausea and vomiting	See Table 6.5	Serotonin antagoists, other anti-emetics
Neuropathy (peripheral or autonomic)	Cisplatin, Paclitaxel, Vincristine, Vinblastine	
Renal failure	Cisplatin, Methotrexate (high dose)	Forced diuresis (cisplatin), Urinary alkalinization (methotrexate)

Myelosuppression

Myelosupression is one of the most common, and potentially most dangerous side effects of chemotherapy. Although cytotoxic agents vary in the extent to which they suppress the bone marrow, most produce some suppression. Typically, this is most marked 7–14 days following treatment, and recovers relatively rapidly, although some agents, such as the nitrosoureas and mitomycin C, produce myelosuppression that is delayed in onset and more prolonged in duration. A small number of drugs produce little or no myelosupression; examples include cisplatin, vincristine, and methotrexate (when used in conjunction with folinic acid rescue).

All hematological elements may be affected by chemotherapy, though the most common problem is leucopenia. In particular, neutrophil production is impaired resulting in neutropenia, which is associated with a risk of bacterial sepsis. The risk of infection is related to both the severity and the duration of neutropenia. Absolute neutrophil counts of less than 0.5×10^9 per litre are associated with a significant risk of infection, which most commonly presents as fever (febrile neutropenia).[18] Although causative organisms are only identified in 40% of cases of febrile neutropenia, the high mortality rate when infection is untreated in this setting means that all patients should be treated with empirical broad spectrum antibiotics. The specific combinations used vary depending on the local bacterial isolates, but typically include a broad spectrum penicillin (such as ticarcillin or piperacillin) together with an aminoglycoside, or a third-generation cephalosporin alone.[19]

The frequency and importance of neutropenia as a side effect of cancer chemotherapy has prompted the development of agents which may abrogate this side effect. The identification and pharmacological development of the colony stimulating factors has resulted in the availability of compounds that can either prevent or limit the severity of chemotherapy-induced neutropenia. Granulocyte colony stimulating factor (G-CSF) is effective in reducing the degree of neutropenia, and the occurrence of febrile episodes.[20] At present, however, its cost limits the situations in which it is used.

Thrombocytopenia may occur as a result of treatment with cytotoxics, but is a less common complication than neutropenia. The major risk associated with the development of thrombocytopenia is that of spontaneous hemorrhage. This becomes a particular risk when the platelet count falls below 20×10^9 per litre, and platelet transfusions are usually administered when this level is reached. In the future, thrombopoietin, a cytokine with specific effects on platelet production, may limit the occurrence and severity of this complication.

Anemia is also a complication of chemotherapy, although in patients with advanced malignancy, its etiology may be multifactorial. While any of the cytotoxics may cause or contribute to anemia, cisplatin in particular may produce severe anemia. Chemotherapy-induced anemia is commonly treated with transfusion, which in addition to producing symptomatic benefit may also enhance the response to other cancer treatments such as radiotherapy.

Nausea and vomiting

Nausea and vomiting are amongst the most distressing side effects of cytotoxic chemotherapy. The mechanism(s) by which chemotherapy causes emesis is not completely understood, but probably involves both effects in the central nervous system and direct effects on the gastrointestinal tract. Within the central nervous system, cytotoxics probably exert their influence on the chemoreceptor trigger zone, which is located within the medulla. Two separate emetic syndromes are recognized to result from chemotherapy. Acute emesis usually commences 1–2 hours after starting chemotherapy and lasts for up to 24 hours. Delayed emesis, occurring 48–72 hours following chemotherapy, is particularly a problem following treatment with high dose cisplatin, and may occur despite successful treatment of acute emesis.

Chemotherapeutic agents vary greatly in their propensity to cause nausea and vomiting. Cisplatin, dacarbazine and nitrogen mustard are the most emetogenic of agents while vincristine, fluorouracil and methotrexate rarely cause significant nausea or vomiting (Table 6.5). In addition, patient factors may contribute to the likelihood of nausea and vomiting. Typically, it is easier to control nausea and vomiting in men than in women, in patients with a history of chronic heavy alcohol use, and in older rather than younger patients.

The recognition of the importance of serotonin in the genesis of chemotherapy-induced emesis has led to the development of a new generation of highly effective anti-emetics, the serotonin antagonists.

Table 6.5. Emetic potential of chemotherapeutic agents.

High emetogenic potential
  Cisplatin
  Dacarbazine
  Dactinomycin
  Nitrogen Mustard
Intermediate emetogenic potential
  Doxorubicin (adriamycin)
  Carboplatin
  Cyclophosphamide
  Carmustine
  Etoposide
Low emetogenic potential
  Bleomycin
  Methotrexate
  5-Fluorouracil
  Vincristine
Vinblastine

Drugs such as ondansetron and tropisetron are able to control completely acute post-chemotherapy emesis in 60–70% of patients.[21,22] The addition of dexamethasone adds to emetic control, and is now part of routine treatment. Delayed nausea and vomiting remains a problem which is difficult to control, even with these newer agents.

Other toxicities

Cytotoxic agents may produce a variety of other toxic effects, in many organ systems. These are summarized in Table 6.4. Amongst the more important of these is the cumulative cardiotoxicity of the anthracyclines (doxorubicin, daunorubicin and epirubicin) which can result in cardiomyopathy and cardiac failure. This is particularly a problem in patients with pre-existing cardiac failure, in whom these drugs are contraindicated. Other toxicities which may limit treatment are hearing loss and tinnitus caused by cisplatin, and ischemic chest pain, which may rarely result from several drugs, including fluorouracil, vincristine, vinblastine, and cisplatin.

HORMONAL THERAPY OF CANCER

In addition to the use of cytotoxic chemotherapy, hormonal treatments may be useful in the treatment of malignant disease. Not surprisingly, the diseases in which hormonal therapies have been of the greatest use are those arising in organs which are normally under hormonal control, such as carcinoma of the breast, prostate and endometrium. Several different approaches to hormonal therapy have been used, including the ablation of physiological hormone production, the use of hormone receptor blockers, and the administration of pharmacological quantities of hormones.

Ablation of hormonal production has been used in the treatment of both breast cancer, with the elimination of estrogens, and prostate cancer with the elimination of androgens. Hormonal ablation can be achieved by removing the source of the steroid hormone (for example, by oophorectomy or orchidectomy). An alternate approach has been to interfere with the hormonal control mechanisms which are necessary for steroid synthesis. The LHRH agonists, such as goserelin and leuprorelin, decrease the pituitary secretion of gonadotropins, which in turn abolishes gonadal androgen or estrogen production.

Hormone antagonists have found widespread use in the management of hormonally sensitive malignancy. Examples of these agents include the anti-estrogen, tamoxifen, and the anti-androgens, cyproterone acetate and flutamide. In general, this class of agents is well tolerated, and have relatively few side effects.

The third approach to hormonal therapy is the use of additive hormonal treatment. The use of progestational agents in the treatment of breast and endometrial cancer is the most frequently used example of this. Although other forms of additive therapy have been used in the past (for example, high dose estrogens in breast cancer) these are rarely employed now.

The recognition and characterization of receptors for steroid hormones has aided in the hormonal management of some cancers. In breast cancer, receptors for estrogen and progesterone can be measured, both biochemically and by using immunocytochemical techniques. Information obtained from these measurements allows prediction of the likelihood of response to treatment to be made, with tumors that are rich in receptors being more likely to respond to treatment.

References
1. Marshall, E.K.J. (1964). Historical perspectives in chemotherapy. In *Advances in chemotherapy*, edited by A. Goldin, I.F. Hawkin, pp. 1–8. New York: Academic Press.

2. DeVita, V.T. (1978). The evolution of therapeutic research in cancer. *N. Engl. J. Med.*, **298**, 907–910.

3. Goodman L.S., Wintrobe, MM., Dameshek, W., Goodman, M.J., Gilman, A. and McLennan, M. (1946). Nitrogen mustard therapy: use of methylbis (B-chlorethyl)amino hydrochloride for Hodgkin's disease, lymphosarcoma, leukemia and certain allied and miscellaneous disorders. *JAMA*, **132**, 126–132.

4. Farber, S., Diamond, L.K., Mercer, R.D., Sylvester, R.F. and Wolff, V.A. (1948). Temporary remissions in acute leukemia in children produced by folic antagonist 4-amethopteroylglutamic acid (aminopterin). *N. Engl. J. Med.*, **238**, 787–793.

5. WHO (1979). *WHO handbook for reporting results of cancer treatment*. WHO offset publication no. 48. Geneva: WHO.

6. Coates, A.S., Gebski, V.J., Bishop, J.F., *et al.* (1987). Improving the quality of life during chemotherapy for advanced breast cancer. A comparison of intermittent and continuous treatment strategies. *N. Engl. J. Med.*, **317**, 1490–1495.

7. Moore, M.J, Osoba, D., Murphy, K., Tannock, I.F., Armitage, A., Findlay, B., *et al.*, (1994). Use of palliative end points to evaluate the effects of mitoxantrone and low-dose prednisone in patients with hormonally resistant prostate cancer. *J. Clin. Oncol.*, **12**, 689–694.

8. De Vita, V.T, Hellman, S. and Rosenberg, S.A. (1993). *Cancer: Principles and Practice of Oncology*, 4th edn. Philadelphia: J.B. Lippincott.

9. Frei III, E. (1985). Curative cancer chemotherapy. *Cancer Res.*, **45**, 6523.

10. Frei III, E. and Canellos, GP. (1980). Dose: a critical factor in cancer chemotherapy. *Amer. J. Med.*, **69**, 585.

11. Williams, S.D., Birch, R., Einhorn, L.H., Irwin, L., Greco, F.A. and Loehrer, P.J. (1987). Treatment of disseminated germ-cell tumors with cisplatin, bleomycin, and either vin-blastine or etoposide. *N. Engl. J. Med.*, **316**, 1435–1440.

12. Advanced Colorectal Cancer Meta-Analysis Project. (1992). Modulation of fluorouracil by leucovorin in patients with advanced colorectal cancer: evidence in terms of response rate. *J. Clin. Oncol.*, **10**, 896–903.

13. Goldie, J.H. and Coldman, A.J. (1988). Mathematic modeling of drug resistance. In *Mechanisms of drug resistance in neoplastic cells*, edited by P.V. Wooley, K.D. Tew, pp. 13–28. San Diego: Academic Press.

14. Sirotnak, F.M., Moccio, D.M., Kelleher, L.E. and Goutsas. L.J. (1981). Relative frequency and kinetic properties of transport defective phenotypes among methotrexate resistant L1210 cloncal cell lines derived *in vivo. Cancer Res.*, **41**, 4447.

15. Goldenberg, G, J., Vanstone, C.L., Israels. L.G., Isle, D. and Bihler, D. (1970). Evidence for a transport carrier of nitrogen mustard in nitrogen mustard-sensitive and resistant L5178Y lymphoblasts. *Cancer Res.*, **30**, 2285.

16. Endicott, J, A. and Ling, V. (1989). The biochemistry of P-glycoprotein-mediated multidrug resistance. *Ann. Rev. Biochem.*, **57**, 137–171.

17. Dalton, W.S., Crowley, J.J., Salmon, S.S., Grogan, T.M., Laufman, L.R., Weiss, G.R., *et al.* (1995). A phase III randomized study of oral verapamil as a chemosensitizer to reverse drug resistance in patients with refractory myeloma. A Southwest Oncology Group study. *Cancer*, **75**, 815–820.

18. Bodey, G.P., Buckley, M., Sathe, Y.S., Freireich, E.J. (1966). Quantitative relationships between circulating leukocytes and infection in patients with acute leukemia. *Ann. Intern. Med.*, **64**, 328–340.

19. Hughes, W.T., Armstrong, D., Bodey, G.P., Feld, R., Mandell, G.L., Meyers, J.D., *et al.* (1990). Guidelines for the use of antimicrobial agents in neutropenic patients with unexplained fever. *J. Infect. Dis.*, **161**, 381–396.

20. Crawford, J., Ozer, H., Stoller, R., Johnson, D., Lyman, G., Tabbara, I., *et al.* (1991). Reduction by granulocyte colony-stimulating factor of fever and neutropenia induced by chemotherapy in patients with small-cell lung cancer. *N. Engl. J. Med.*, **325**, 164–170.

21. De Mulder, P.H.M., Seynaeve, C., Vermorken, J.B., van Liessum, P.A., Mols-Jevdevic, S., Allman, E.L., *et al.* (1990). Ondansetron compared with high dose metoclopramide in prophylaxis of acute and delayed cisplatin induced nausea and vomiting. *Ann. Intern. Med.*, **113**, 834–840.

22. Marty, M., Pouillart, P., Scholl, S., Droz, J.P., Azab, M., Brion, N., *et al.* (1990). Comparison of the 5-hydroxy-tryptamine3 (serotonin) antagonist ondansetron (GR 38032F) with high dose metoclopramide in the control of cisplatin-induced emesis. *N. Engl. J. Med.*, **322**, 816–821.

7. Aspects of Palliative Care

CAROL L. DAVIS

Macmillan Senior Lecturer in Palliative Medicine, Countess Mountbatten House, Southampton, UK

INTRODUCTION

Palliative care has been defined as "the active, total care of patients whose disease is not responsive to curative treatment". Control of pain, of other symptoms and of psychological, social and spiritual problems is paramount. The goal of palliative care is achievement of the best quality of life for patients and their families. Many aspects of palliative care are also applicable earlier in the course of the illness in conjunction with anti-cancer treatments (WHO, 1990). The primary aim of palliative care is not to prolong life, but to make the life that remains as comfortable and meaningful as possible. It encompasses attention to detail in several domains:

- physical
- psychological
- social
- cultural
- spiritual

As such, palliative care is practiced, to a varying extent at any given time, by all health care professionals in a wide range of health care settings. The principles of palliative care are an integral part of good clinical practice.

THE SCOPE OF PALLIATIVE CARE

Optimal control of physical and psychological problems are vital aspects of palliative care, but they are not the only ones. Palliative care aims to allow the patient and their family to focus on issues that are important to them which may include coping with changing roles, emotional adjustment to progressive disease and death and dealing with "unfinished business" as well as best possible relief of their symptoms. Issues around sexuality should not be forgotten.

Many lay people and some doctors regard palliative care and terminal care as synonymous. This is not the case; terminal care is one part, albeit an important one, of palliative care, which may also include bereavement support if necessary. Most adults (but not children) with cancer will die of this disease. It has been argued, therefore, that in some patients, palliative care should begin at diagnosis. In general as the role of specific anticancer treatments diminishes that of palliative care increases, but this relationship is not linear and can vary at different stages of the disease process (Figure 7.1).

Although it is easy for a patient to see their need for palliative care in a negative light, it frequently engenders hope; hope for relief of pain, hope for

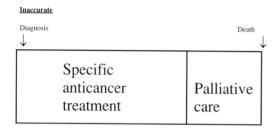

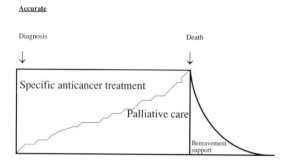

Figure 7.1. Inaccurate and accurate depictions of the relationship between palliative care and specific anticancer treatment.

adequate relief of other symptoms, and hope for a peaceful death. Furthermore rehabilitation is an important aspect of palliative care. It is viewed much more widely than physical rehabilitation and also encompasses psychological, spiritual and social rehabilitation of the patient and their family and friends.

ORGANIZATIONAL ASPECTS

Specialist palliative care services are those services with palliative care as their core specialty, whose staff have developed a specific interest and expertise in the subject and have additional qualifications relevant to the specialty. Such services provide care for patients with advanced cancer. Many also care for patients with HIV disease and motor neurone disease, while some provide a service that extends to those with other chronic, life-threatening diseases such as end-stage chronic renal failure and chronic non-malignant lung diseases. Worldwide, there is an increasing groundswell of opinion that specialist palliative care should not be restricted to patients with malignant disease, but should be available, when appropriate, to patients with any

potentially life-threatening disease and earlier in the course of the disease. The general principles of palliative care apply to all these patients, but the detail and choice of therapeutic interventions vary. For specialists in palliative care, the challenge is to facilitate the provision of appropriate palliative care for all who need it without becoming "Jacks of all trades and masters of none". This chapter considers palliative care in the context of patients with advanced malignant disease.

There is no single model for the provision of specialist palliative care services which may include some or all of the following aspects:

- specialist domiciliary care/advice
  — nursing
  — medical
  — other — occupational therapy, physiotherapy, social-work
- inpatient care
  — hospice
  — designated beds/ward within a general/specialist cancer hospital
- outpatient clinics
- day care
- hospital palliative care team providing advice/support for in-patients, and occasionally outpatients, in general/specialist hospitals
- support groups for carers
- bereavement support
- education
- research

These services are provided by a multi-disciplinary team often supplemented by trained volunteers. A multi-disciplinary specialist palliative care team usually includes nurses, doctors, physiotherapists, occupational therapists, chaplains and social workers. People with advanced cancer are usually based at home and so the focus of care must be in the community. The patient remains under the care of their general practitioner/family doctor and the rest of the primary health care team. The palliative care team provides advice and support for the patient, their family and the primary health care team.

PSYCHOLOGICAL FACTORS

It is almost impossible to separate the psychological aspects of cancer from the physical, social,

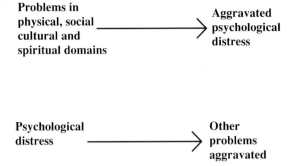

Figure 7.2. The inter-relationship of psychological and other factors in patients with advanced cancer.

cultural and spiritual aspects, even in the same person. They are closely inter-related and influence each other (Figure 7.2).

Receiving bad news can generate a wide range of feelings including fear, sadness, horror and anger. Uncertainty fuels anxiety.

A person can react to the news of a diagnosis of cancer, recurrence, incurable disease or impending death and to living with cancer in more than one way and the balance of feelings and reactions varies across time. It is important to remember that, in general, there is no right or wrong way to face up to these situations.

A simple question such as, "How does this leave you feeling?" encourages a person to ventilate their feelings. The old adage, "A problem shared, is a problem halved", often holds true; feelings do not need answers, they need listening to.

A wide range of coping strategies might be employed by a patient. Different patients employ different coping strategies at different times and so do their families and close friends. It is important, although not always easy, to recognize when such coping mechanisms become maladaptive. Persistent anger, pathological anxiety or depression must be addressed. It can be particularly difficult to delineate appropriate sadness from clinical depression.

Assessment of psychological problems and psychological care must be an integral part of the overall care of patients with malignant disease. Such psychological care should always be individualized and should be aimed at facilitating and strengthening that person's adaptive and coping mechanisms. To achieve this, those involved in the delivery of cancer care need to:

- Think of the patient as a person within a family unit
- Employ good listening skills
- Communicate openly and honestly
- Have a caring attitude and be alongside the patient and their problems
- Adequately assess problems in all the domains of care
- Set realistic goals with the patient
- Recognize that a patient's problems and their needs change over time and review and revise plans and goals accordingly.

Some patients will require more formal psychological intervention, for example relaxation therapy, counselling or psychotherapy.

SOCIAL FACTORS

A basic tenet of palliative care philosophy is that the patient is regarded as part of a unit which also includes his or her family, friends and carers. These people are linked by a series of complex relationships, which may be strengthened, weakened and/or changed by the challenge of incurable disease. The response of an individual to the knowledge that, say, their partner is going to die will, in turn, affect that partner. Problems encountered include not only the distress and anxiety that such news will cause, but also the need to change roles and to adopt new ones. The patient is often distressed for their partner. Palliative care extends beyond the patient and includes all those close to them.

Caring for a terminally ill family member can be both physically and psychologically exhausting. Provision of some form of "respite" in the form of a day or nightsitter or a short admission of the patient to a hospital or hospice can be invaluable for both the patient and their carer. It is not unusual for one or both parties to feel guilty that such support is needed and they may need reassurance that this is a common problem and not one that just pertains to them.

Financial and legal worries can have a devastating effect on the ability of a patient and their family to cope with terminal illness. These can be easily overlooked particularly as people may be embarrassed to raise this topic themselves. Once a possible problem has been identified, input from a medical social-worker can be invaluable.

Risk factors for abnormal grief in bereavement include the sudden, unexpected loss of a loved one and the loss of a partner with whom the bereaved had an ambivalent relationship. These and other risk factors can often be identified before the patient dies and this facilitates the design of a proactive, individualized counselling program for the bereaved person aimed at preventing abnormal grief.

Consideration of and attention to social factors and needs is another crucial component of good palliative care and part of the doctor's role.

CULTURAL FACTORS

Many societies are increasingly multi-cultural. Cultural factors may exert a very marked influence on an individual's attitude to illness, pain, other disease-related problems, treatment measures, death and bereavement. They must be considered and respected. Assessment of any symptom or problem in a patient with cancer should include consideration of the effect of culture. Such information is not always volunteered and it is often necessary to ask a person about their culture and related beliefs and needs.

In the United Kingdom, it is recognized that patients from ethnic minorities are under-represented in the hospice population. The reasons for this are probably complex, but cultural issues must be a factor. Some cultural groups may not agree with the philosophy of palliative care or be wary of it for other reasons. Problems may arise if a health care professional and a patient are from different cultural backgrounds. In modern societies, which are increasingly mobile, views about cultural norms vary within any one cultural group particularly across different generations. There may be no easy solution to these dilemmas, but awareness of cultural differences together with a sensitive and flexible approach to care will help to prevent and resolve problems.

SPIRITUAL CARE

Even in some modern dictionaries, the terms spirituality and religion are defined in very similar ways. These words have often been used interchangeably, but they are now increasingly distinguished from each other. Spirituality encompasses

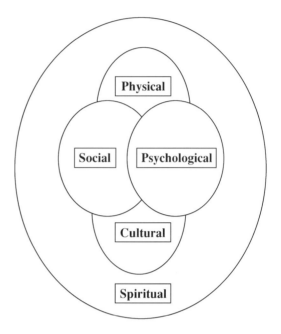

Figure 7.3. The importance of spirituality to the concept of total care.

the purpose and meaning of one's life and is the basis for an individual's attitudes, values, beliefs and actions. It is usually grounded in cultural, religious and family traditions, but is influenced by life experience; spiritual beliefs may change with time particularly when a person is faced with a life crisis. Religion is a system of faith and worship, often of god or god-like figures, characterized by specific rites, rituals and texts. Followers of a certain religious faith often do not form a homogenous group. It is important to make no assumptions about the meaning of a declared religious faith to a person, but to explore what it means to them, as an individual.

Everyone faced with a life-threatening disease will have spiritual needs and spiritual issues will influence the way that they cope with the problems of having that disease. In some people, but not all, religious beliefs will be central to their spirituality. Spiritual needs are very individual and questions about spirituality do not, usually, have clear-cut answers. The recognition that a person has spiritual needs and, perhaps, spiritual distress can be very comforting to them. One should not, however, impose one's own spiritual beliefs on others. Signs of spiritual distress can vary greatly, but may include persistent severe pain, hopelessness, fear of sleep, recurrent dreams and questions like, "Why me?", "What have I done to deserve this?". In many ways, the spiritual dimension brings together the physical, psychological, social and cultural dimensions of suffering (Figure 7.3).

Any professional involved in patient care can address spiritual issues with the patient and their family. Chaplains have special expertise and are often regarded by the patient as being separate from the clinical team. Their input is not restricted to patients with strong religious beliefs.

PHYSICAL PROBLEMS

Many physical problems and symptoms can be caused by malignant disease. They are best treated by curing the cancer, or at least achieving a clinical remission, but even if this is achieved some problems persist. The pain caused by vertebral collapse in a patient with multiple myeloma, for example, is long-standing whether or not disease remission is achieved. Most patients with advanced cancer have multiple symptoms, some of which are amenable to intervention. Unfortunately, the common symptoms of weakness and poor appetite often persist and inevitably worsen as the disease progresses. Ill patients, however, do not always regard these symptoms as major problems.

It is impossible to cover the range of physical problems encountered by patients with advanced cancer in this chapter. Instead, some general principles of symptom management are suggested and then the management of two common symptoms, pain and constipation, is discussed.

General principles of symptom management

- Good communication with the patient and their family as well as with all professionals involved in their care is essential for effective symptom management and palliative care.
- Thorough assessment of the problem is required with attention to detail so that an appropriate plan can be formulated, instigated, monitored and evaluated (Figure 7.4).
- Reassurance and explanation are always appropriate.
- An individualized approach is essential.
- Effective symptom management usually requires both pharmacological and non-pharmacological

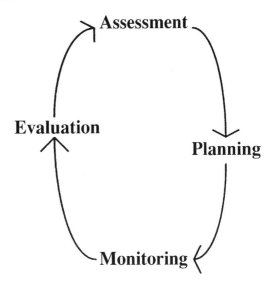

Figure 7.4. The crucial role of assessment in formulating the approach to a specific problem.

intervention.
- Treatment should be as simple as possible.
- Avoid polypharmacy whenever possible.
- Persistent symptoms warrant regular medication.
- Recognize that advanced cancer is a dynamic changing situation: review effectiveness and appropriateness of intervention frequently and revise management accordingly.

Pain

Pain is one of the most common and most feared symptoms of cancer. Most lay, and indeed professional, people have a particular fear of dying in pain. One-third of patients with cancer have pain at diagnosis and over two-thirds of those with advanced cancer suffer pain. Worldwide, it has been estimated that several million people with cancer die in pain every year.

The physical component of the suffering caused by cancer pain and other symptoms is undoubtedly important but, nonetheless, it is only one component. Psychological, social, cultural and spiritual factors also contribute to the totality of cancer pain.

Approach to the management of cancer pain

Good communication with the patient, their family and other health care professionals is vital to good pain control. Attention to detail, a collaborative interdisciplinary approach to assessment and management and frequent review of the situation and revision of the management plan are essential.

Pain needs to be recognized and assessed promptly in patients with cancer. Adequate assessment requires skills in taking a history from both the patient and their carers, physical examination, psychosocial assessment and the appropriate use of carefully selected diagnostic investigations. Blood tests, plain X-rays, radioisotopic bone scans, ultrasound scans, CT and MRI scans can all be invaluable in some instances. Their use must be governed, however, by the physical condition and likely prognosis of the patient as well as consideration of whether the result of the investigation is likely to affect management.

Causes of pain in a patient with cancer include:

- Direct effect of primary or secondary tumor
- Treatment-related
- Related to the debility caused by cancer
- Unrelated to cancer (e.g. ostearthritis)

Approaches to management include:

- Modification of disease process
- Elevation of pain threshold
  - pharmacological
  - non-pharmacological
- Interruption of pain pathways
- Modification of way of life and environment

Frequently, more than one approach is employed at any one time, but they should be used in a systematic, consistent way. All of these interventions should be carried out within a patient-centered framework with explanation and reassurance and due attention to the contribution of other, non-physical factors to the pain.

It is well established that cancer pain can be controlled in the majority of patients by simple, cheap pharmacological intervention. Such treatment should be based on the World Health Organization guidelines, which advocate a step-wise or ladder approach to the pharmacological management of cancer pain (Figure 7.5). If pain is not controlled at maximum dosage at one step, then a move up to the next step is required. There is no maximal dose of strong opioid. Variations to this model are sometimes employed, but they are all grounded in the same principles:

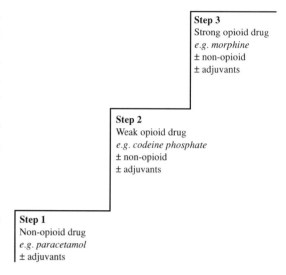

Figure 7.5. The World Health Organisation analgesic ladder (WHO, 1986).

- "By the mouth" (the oral route is the preferred route of administration)
- "By the clock" (chronic cancer pain requires treatment with regularly administered analgesics)
- "By the ladder" (treatment should be approached in a logical, stepwise manner)

Every medical student should have an understanding and working knowledge of non-opioid and opioid drugs. Readers are referred to any basic pharmacology text and the bibliography. Nociceptive pain, such as caused by bone or liver metastases, usually responds well to opioid drugs either alone or in combination with adjuvant drugs such as non-steroidal anti-inflammatory drugs or corticosteroids. On the other hand, neuropathic pain often responds less well to opioids and usually requires the addition of adjuvant analgesics such as anti-depressant or anti-convulsant drugs.

Pain can often lead to decreased mobility and abnormal position and careful positioning, simple exercises and physiotherapy can all be helpful. Other non-pharmacological measures include transcutaneous electrical nerve stimulation (TENS) and acupuncture. The use of appropriate appliances and aids can reduce pain and minimize disability. Psychological, social, cultural and spiritual factors should be considered and addressed.

In some patients with cancer, pain is particularly difficult to control. The reasons for this can be complex and include problems in all the domains of care.

Mary, a fifty-year-old, married nurse with advanced metastatic breast cancer involving her bones (lumbo-sacral spine) and liver was admitted to hospital with a short history of increasing lower back and bilateral leg pain. She had already received a range of anticancer therapies including maximal radiotherapy to her lumbo-sacral spine. She was distressed and had signs of nerve root compression at L4-S1. Her pain took several days to control. Measures used initially included reassurance, explanation, oral opioids, a non-steroidal anti-inflammatory drug, an anti-depressant as an adjuvant analgesic, high dose corticosteroids and, eventually, an epidural infusion of local anesthetic and morphine. Her pain and distress improved considerably, but not totally. She was now well enough to talk freely and explore the components of her pain and distress, which included fear of dying in pain, worry about her children and recognition that her nursing expertise raised specific fears of spinal cord compression with paralysis, incontinence and pressure sores. A multi-disciplinary approach to her care included input from not only nurses and doctors, but also the chaplain, physiotherapist and pharmacist. A pressure relieving mattress was used. She became pain-free and, once the amount of local anesthetic in the epidural was reduced, more mobile. Mary was discharged home with an epidural infusion and was supported in the community by her family, friends, the primary health care team, the local palliative care team and her minister. She remained pain-free until her death, six weeks later.

A multi-faceted, interdisciplinary approach to the management of cancer pain is essential. The appropriateness of different interventions varies with time.

Constipation

Constipation can be defined as the infrequent and difficult passage of small hard feces. There is no such thing as normal bowel habit for a population of patients. Patients' symptoms need to be rated

Table 7.1. Causes of constipation in patients with advanced cancer.

General	Specific
Anorexia	Gastro-intestinal and gynecological malignancy
Dehydration	Spinal cord compression
Shortness of breath	Metabolic (e.g. hypercalcemia, uraemia)
Reduced mobility	Iatrogenic (e.g. vincristine, opioids, iron, tryclic antidepressants) antimuscarinics such as hyoscine

against their own definition of constipation and what they consider to be a normal or acceptable bowel habit for them. It is a common and important symptom in patients with advanced cancer. Causative factors are shown in Table 7.1.

Constipation can cause other symptoms including anorexia, nausea and vomiting, abdominal pain, confusion and diarrhea. In addition, it can exacerbate other symptoms such as breathlessness or back pain. It can have a marked adverse effect on quality of life and some patients find it as distressing as pain. Many patients find constipation embarrassing, whether at home or in hospital. Treatment can cause urgency and incontinence, which can be particularly distressing for patients from some cultural groups. The economic consequences of constipation include the cost of nursing and medical time as well as of oral and rectal laxatives.

General principles of management

1. Take a detailed history and establish normal bowel habit for that patient and use of laxatives.
2. Palpate abdomen and check bowel sounds.
3. Perform rectal examination.
4. Identify and treat any underlying correctable cause(s) if appropriate.
5. Encourage fluid intake.
6. Increase dietary fiber in fitter patients unless bowel obstruction present. Patients with advanced cancer are unlikely to be able to tolerate enough fiber and fluid to make any significant difference to the problem.
7. Consider use of regular oral laxatives, choose laxative according to individual circumstances including age, urinary continence and cause of constipation.

Table 7.2.   Classification of laxatives.

Type	Action	Example
Bulk forming agents	Increase mass and water content of stool and thus stimulate peristalsis. Need to maintain/ increase fluid intake. Avoid if risk of intestinal obstruction.	Increased dietary fiber intake. Ispaghula husk (e.g. fybogel) Methylcellulose Stercula (e.g. normacol)
Osmotic laxatives	Attract water into the bowel lumen and thus increase stool output. Some also have a stimulant action (e.g. magnesium salts).	Magnesium hydroxide Magnesium sulphate Lactulose syrup Liquid paraffin and magnesium hydroxide
Stimulant laxatives	Stimulate the colon, increase peristaltic movement and reduce water absorption from gastrointestinal tract. May cause abdominal cramps. Avoid in patients with intestinal obstruction.	Senna Danthron-containing laxatives, e.g. codanthramer suspension, codanthrusate capsules. Bisacodyl Sodium picosulphate (tends to cause fecal urgency)

8. Consider rectal intervention if oral measures ineffective or hard stool in rectum.
9. Nurses are usually more expert in the management of constipation than doctors.

Laxative Drugs

A classification of laxative drugs is shown in Table 7.2. Bulk laxatives are used infrequently in palliative care because patients are often unable to maintain the necessary high fluid intake. Danthron-containing laxatives should be avoided in patients with urinary or fecal incontinence and those with a urinary catheter (in case of leakage around catheter) because danthron can cause superficial skin burns. Patients and carers should be warned that danthron-containing laxatives cause discolored (red/ brown) urine.

Rectal interventions (shown in Table 7.3) are indicated if there is hard stool in the rectum and/

Table 7.3.   Rectal measures for constipation.

Predominant softening action
Glycerine suppository
Sodium docusate suppository
Arachis oil enema

Predominant stimulant action
Bisacodyl suppository
High phosphate enema
Sodium citrate micro-enema

Manual evacuation with sedative cover

or appropriate oral measures have been ineffective. The first choice rectal intervention for uncomplicated constipation is glycerine suppositories. If these are ineffective, then a stimulant enema such as a high phosphate enema should be administered.

Oral and rectal stimulant laxatives should be avoided in patients with possible or proven bowel obstruction. Gentle rectal measures can sometimes be effective in emptying the rectum and lower colon (e.g. glycerine suppository, sodium docusate suppository, arachis oil enema). Oral softening agents are useful if the obstruction is incomplete. It should be remembered that constipation can cause bowel obstruction.

Opioid induced constipation

Opioids cause constipation through several different effects on the gastrointestinal tract, namely:

- Increased water absorption from gut (they also cause dry mouth for this reason)
- Decreased gastric, biliary and pancreatic secretions
- Decreased gastrointestinal mobility
- Decreased rectal sensitivity to fecal load

Thus a combination of a stool softener and a stimulant laxative is usually required for the prevention and treatment of opioid induced constipation. Regular prophylactic laxatives should be prescribed for almost all patients on strong opioids, the exception being those with profuse diarrhea such as caused by a carcinoid tumor. There is no evidence that constipation is proportional to opioid dose. The most commonly prescribed regimes in the United Kingdom are either a combination of lactulose or magnesium hydroxide and senna or single agent codanthrusate or codanthramer (a combination of danthron and polyxamer).

Opioid induced constipation should be managed by adhering to the general principles detailed above. Laxative drugs will need to be used in higher doses than when used propylactically. The regimen should be reviewed regularly, at least every few days, and be adjusted if necessary. If ineffective, then rectal interventions should be added and a change in the regimen or choice of oral laxatives should be considered.

PALLIATIVE CARE AND CHILDREN

The philosophy and principles of palliative care pertain to children as well as adults and they apply whether the child is the patient or has an ill sibling, parent or other close relative or friend. Children have unique needs, many of which are determined by their age, and they require specialized services.

If a child is dying of cancer, they are usually best cared for at home if at all possible. The principles of palliative care and symptom control will be the same as in adults, but the detail will differ.

Bereaved children form a special group. The value of helping children express their feelings in a variety of ways, including through drawing and painting, is now well recognized. Specialized program for bereaved children have been developed in several countries and many are employing innovative techniques for helping children cope with bereavement.

ETHICAL ISSUES IN PALLIATIVE CARE

Ethical dilemmas can arise at any stage of a patient's disease process and in any healthcare setting. Particular dilemmas that may arise in palliative care include issues around nutrition and hydration, patient autonomy and the role of the patient's relatives in decision-making and requests for euthanasia. Another potential ethical dilemma is the fact that the dose of strong opioid drug required to control

an individual's pain may sometimes contribute to respiratory depression and directly or indirectly, to death. This is known as double effect. Further detailed discussion of these issues is outside the remit of this chapter, but interested readers are referred to the bibliography.

It is important to remember that dilemmas arise when a situation or plan is not "black and white". There is never a perfect answer to a dilemma. An ethical dilemma must be considered from the patient's point of view, preferably alongside the patient, within an ethical and legal frame-work. Decisions need to be balanced and to achieve this it is usually necessary both to think widely and to discuss the issue widely, but appropriately. The patient, family and other health-care professionals, particularly nurses, should all contribute to this process. Others' views must be respected. Ethical decision-making should always be individualized and relate to the individual circumstances of that patient.

We are required always to act in the patient's best interests. Relatives' contribution to a discussion aimed at identifying what is in the patient's best interests is always important. Nonetheless, consideration of their views needs to be tempered by the fact that the agenda of the relatives may be different from that of the patient. In the United Kingdom, the relatives should not be asked to make proxy decisions for the patient unless the patient has signed an enduring power of attorney.

CONCLUSION

This chapter will have achieved its aim if it has acquainted the reader with the philosophy and basic principles of palliative care and the correct approach to the management of constipation! The bibliography is purposely scanty, but selective reading of it will provide a wealth of further information and food for thought.

Bibliography

ABC of Palliative Care. British Medical Journal, in press. (Up-to-date series of articles on many aspects of palliative care due to be published late 1997).

Doyle, D., Hanks, G.W.C., MacDonald, N. (1994). *Oxford Textbook of Palliative Medicine*. Oxford. Oxford University Press. (Large definitive textbook; second edition due to be published in late 1997).

Randall, F. and Downie, R.S. (1996). *Palliative Care Ethics*. Oxford: Oxford University Press.

Saunders, S. and Sykes, N. (1993). *The Management of Terminal Malignant Disease*. London: Edward Arnold Ltd.

Stedeford, A. (1996). *Facing Death*, 2nd edn. Oxford: Sobell Publications.

Twycross, R. (1994). *Pain relief in advanced cancer*. Edinburgh: Churchill Livingstone.

Twycross, R. (1995). *Introducing Palliative Care*. Oxford: Rodcliffe Medical Press Ltd. (small book, written in lecture-note style).

Wall, P.D. and Melzack, R. (1994). *Textbook of pain*, 3rd ed. Edinburgh: Churchill Livingstone. (Definitive textbook on pain, emphasis on non-malignant pain).

WHO (1990). *Cancer Pain Relief and Palliative Care*. Report of WHO Expert Committee; Technical Report Series 804. Geneva: World Health Organization.

8. Nursing Care of the Cancer Patient and Family

JOANNE LESTER

6360 Rising Sun Road, Grove City, Ohio 43123, USA

INTRODUCTION

The care of oncology patients has clearly developed into a specialized field, especially over the past two decades. With technologic advances, expanded knowledge of the cancer disease process, and improved oncologic patient management, professionals caring for oncology patients are challenged to gain knowledge and apply innovative techniques. As the number of patients increases, due in part to early detection, improved survival rates, and an aging population, the array of professionals with oncology expertise must also increase. An interdisciplinary team approach, utilizing professionals from various disciplines, will offer oncology patients the most comprehensive care.

Interdisciplinary team/rehabilitation plan

Depending on the specific cancer diagnosis, the interdisciplinary team should include the family physician/practitioner, surgeon, medical/radiation/surgical oncologist(s), nurse(s), social worker, physical/occupational therapist(s), nutritionist, ministry, and any other applicable disciplines.

Interdisciplinary comprehensive care can very effectively be delivered via a cancer rehabilitation plan. This plan should be initiated with the patient and their family at the time of diagnosis, and extend throughout the patient's lifetime. In cancer rehabilitation, the interdisciplinary team is focused on the whole patient and family, including physical, emotional and spiritual needs.

At the very least, the rehabilitation plan should include events surrounding the cancer diagnosis and initial treatment, financial concerns, psychosocial adjustments, management of side effects of treatment, long-term care issues, preventative health care maintenance and a healthy lifestyle. The focus of the rehabilitation plan is to maximize effectiveness of cancer treatment and minimize the side effects and long-term sequelae of the cancer experience. Quality of life during this period should always be of concern.

The members of the interdisciplinary rehabilitation team may change over time, depending on the needs of the patient and family, and the course of the cancer disease process. It is very important for the patient and family to sense there is one primary person overseeing the entire plan, although this person may vary depending on the circumstances. Nursing is a vital component of this team.

Nursing

Nursing, through its evolution over the past century, has amassed professionals from a variety of educational programs and levels of expertise, depending on what state, province, or country she/he has practiced in. At times, this creates much confusion regarding roles, degree of responsibility, and scope of practice. In short all levels of nursing are important when dealing with oncology patients and their families. Each level requires additional education pertaining to oncology practice, whether through classes, seminars, or formal degree programs.

Many oncology physician practices and hospitals are utilizing advanced practice nurses, also known as clinical nurse specialists and nurse practitioners. These nurses are vital in providing continuity of care and symptom management for oncology patients and their families. Through collaborative or independent practices with physicians, comprehensive specialized care can be provided in a cost-effective manner. This is particularly true in rural or socio-economically-deprived populations. Ideally, a combination of surgical, medical and radiation oncologists are available to the patient. But in situations where this is not so, advanced practice oncology nurses can provide an important link.

This chapter will focus on nursing management of oncology patients and their families. Many of the concepts require collaboration with the interdisciplinary team, especially the physician. The following topics will be discussed: symptom management for the side effects of surgery, chemotherapy, radiation, biotherapy, and progressive cancer, including education of the patient, family and interdisciplinary team, and supportive psychosocial care.

SURGICAL MANAGEMENT

Most oncology patients will have some type of surgical procedure during their cancer experience. This may range from a simple biopsy, line placement, or palliative relief of symptoms, to primary surgical treatment of a cancer. It is important for nurses to be familiar with basic surgical techniques and procedures as a baseline for care. This should include, but is not limited to, sterile technique, sterile dressings, drainage tube placement, irrigation and management, wound and incision care, suture/staple removal, ostomy care, etc.

Many of these surgical nursing care needs are basic and learned in fundamental nursing, but others may require additional training: central venous access devices (i.e. single- and double-lumen external catheters, and implantable ports), intra-arterial hepatic lines and pumps, and intraventricular fluid access devices.

Central venous access devices

Central venous access devices (CVADs) are catheters inserted in a central vein leading to the right atrium which then exits via a subcutaneous tunnel through the chest wall skin. The skin acts as a barrier to avoid infection. CVADs have made the administration of chemotherapy, blood products, antibiotics, hydration fluids, nutritional components and intravenous pain medications easier and safer for the cancer patient. CVADs offer a relatively painless and easy way to draw blood and can relieve the patient's anxiety level knowing that multiple venipunctures are unnecessary. In addition, CVADs potentially offer a safer mechanism than peripheral access when administering vesicant antineoplastic agents. When used properly, a CVAD virtually eliminates the incidence of extravasation. Prior to initiating chemotherapy, all patients should be screened as to their viable venous access and the possible need for a CVAD.

CVADs have provided multiple opportunities for treating inpatients and outpatients throughout the entire cancer experience. This includes patients who are ambulatory, active and working as well as those homebound or terminal. It has enabled many patients to have more control of their environment as well as personal time, and for terminal patients to comfortably live their last months or days at home. CVADs have enabled the use of innovative drug protocols, utilizing programmable pumps for intermittent or continuous infusions of chemotherapy and other necessary drugs.

All too often, the issue of venous access is not discussed until the patient has endured much pain and frustration regarding unsuccessful venipunctures. Even the most skilled phlebotomists and chemotherapy nurses cannot access certain patients due to excess subcutaneous tissue resulting in poor visualization of veins, scarred veins secondary to medications and chemotherapy, limited access possibilities due to specific cancer (i.e. avoiding affected arm of breast cancer patients who have had an axillary node dissection), or fear. No patient, young or old, should have to endure such pain, or compromise the safety of chemotherapy administration, when CVADs are available. Often, a CVAD can be inserted during the primary cancer surgery if chemotherapy administration is anticipated as part of the treatment plan.

There are three basic types of CVADs, each offering different advantages, but also with some disadvantages. It is very important to educate the patient and family on the different types of catheters, as well as the pros and cons of each. Ideally, a model should be available as a visual example, as well as written materials. Many patients benefit from talking one-to-one with other patients, in order to determine the best type of catheter for their lifestyle.

Silastic atrial catheters

Silastic atrial catheters are inserted as an outpatient with a local anesthetic agent and intravenous sedation. There are several brand names, but generally, either a single- or double-lumen catheter is inserted, tunneled under the chest wall, with the catheter exiting the chest wall above the breast.

Advantages	Disadvantages
Easy access without needle sticks	External device
Easily visualized by caregiver	Increased potential for infection
Capability of double lumen	Increased maintenance, requiring at least weekly (and up to daily) flushing with saline and/ or heparin
Access needles can "lock" onto caps	Alterations in bathing, requiring protection of exit site
Easily removed in office with local anesthetic	No swimming
	Viability approximately 6–12 months
	Require physician placement

Subcutaneous implanted port

Subcutaneous implanted ports are also inserted as an outpatient with a local anesthetic agent and intravenous sedation. Again, there are several brand names, with both single- and double-lumen ports; generally, a single-lumen port is inserted. The atrial catheter is tunneled under the chest wall and attached to an implanted port in a subcutaneous pocket above the breast.

Advantages	Disadvantages
No external tubing when catheter not accessed	2–3 cm incision required to make port pocket
No dressing when catheter not accessed	Most generally removed in outpatient surgery with local anesthetic and/or intravenous sedation
Viability of catheter potentially lifetime, which is excellent for high-recurrence patients	Must be accessed with a needle, which is not the best option if patient is afraid of needles
Allows bathing, swimming, etc. without danger to catheter	Potential for needle dislodgement with continuous infusions
Easy maintenance, requiring heparin instillation every 4–6 weeks	Potentially more difficult to obtain blood, depending on catheter placement and anatomy of patient
	Requires physician placement
	Must be accessed with a Huber, non-coring needle

Peripherally placed catheter

Peripherally-placed central venous catheters can be inserted at the bedside, office or at home by a specially trained RN. A 14- to 16-gauge peripheral catheter is threaded several inches through a large peripheral vein, allowing long-term use without multiple venipunctures. The catheter exits from the insertion site, generally the lower forearm or antecubitus.

Advantages	Disadvantages
Can be placed by specially trained RN	Often placed in antecubital space, limiting wide range of motion of affected arm
Excellent for short-term use	Questionable safety for administration of vesicant antineoplastic agents
Placed at bedside with local anesthetic agents only	External device, more visible than centrally-placed catheters
Cost-effective	Easily infected

Easily removed at bedside or office by RN	Increased maintenance, requiring daily flushing with saline and/or heparin
Can be inserted at home	Three times a week, and up to daily, dressing changes
	Alteration in bathing, requiring protection of exit site
	No swimming
	Viability approximately 3–6 months
	Can migrate

Care of CVADs

CVAD maintenance is dependent on the type of catheter inserted, the disease process, and individual idiosyncrasies. The two most common complications are infection and occlusion of the catheter. Prevention of these complications is very important and must be reinforced to the patient and caregiver.

Dressing

External catheters all require a dressing, which may vary from a 4 × 4 gauze pad or transparent occlusive dressing, to a 2 × 2 gauze pad, or bandaid. A newly-inserted catheter should be sterilely prepped with Betadine and alcohol swabs daily and redressed sterilely with an occlusive dressing. Once the internal cuff has adhered (approximately 1–2 weeks), a 2–3 times per week schedule can be assumed, using clean technique rather than sterile. Sterile technique should always be used during periods of neutropenia and post-bone marrow transplant. Many patients are allergic to various tapes and occlusive dressings; therefore it is important to ascertain good skin integrity and prevent problems. Occasionally, especially during warm weather, a topical fungal rash may appear, requiring application of a dry, loose dressing and 1% antifungal ointment.

Heparinization

External catheters should be flushed at least weekly, but may require daily irrigation with saline and/or heparin. There is a wide variance among institutions regarding these practices, and the literature supports both ends of the spectrum. One should consider the number of times a catheter is entered and the potential for infection. If a catheter is well-maintained with weekly heparinization, then that schedule is very appropriate for that patient.

A Groshong-brand catheter, which has a distal pressure-sensitive valve, is typically irrigated with 3–5 cc normal saline after each use, or at least weekly (and up to daily), in each port. Other external catheters should be irrigated with 2.5–3 ml of 10 units/ml of heparin after each use, or at least weekly, in each port.

Implantable ports should be irrigated with 5 ml of 100 units/ml heparin after each use, or at least every 4–6 weeks. Again, the frequency is dependent on the institutional practice, as well as the behavior of the catheter.

Occlusion

There are several hints to prevent occlusion of a catheter: limit the number of different caregivers accessing catheter; flush with 10–20 ml of normal saline after using catheter prior to heparinization; flush with 40–50 ml of normal saline after platelet infusions, prior to heparinization; flush with brisk motion to prevent accumulation of fibrin on distal tip; consider using clot dissolving medication if catheter is sluggish; administer Coumadin 1 mg daily if repeated problems. If a catheter is occluded it is extremely important to avoid forcing irrigation, as the catheter could rupture internally, or force a clot into the patient's circulatory system. When attempting to flush an occluded catheter, using a 10 ml syringe or larger may prevent undue pressure internally.

Once complete occlusion has been established, one of the known clot dissolving agents should be gently instilled in an attempt to declot the catheter. If two attempts of a clot dissolving agent are ineffective, mechanical catheter occlusion should be considered and the patient should be sent for a radiographic dye study. In any occlusion situation, the patient should always be assessed for superior vena cava syndrome.

Infection

Preventing infection in CVADs is very important but the occurrence is not uncommon due to the nature of the cancer disease process and the frequent occurrence of neutropenia. If an infection is suspected either around the catheter, or septicemia, appropriate intravenous antibiotics should be given via the catheter. If a patient has a double-lumen catheter, the antibiotics should be infused via the catheter, alternating ports. Very often, the first impulse is to remove the catheter or implantable port. Most generally, the infection will resolve with appropriate treatment, thus saving the catheter and a lot of frustration for the patient.

Intra-arterial line and pumps

In recent years, there has been a resurgence of the administration of intra-arterial chemotherapy via arterial lines and implantable pumps. This delivery system allows a high concentration of antineoplastic agent(s) to be delivered to the tumor, maximizing effectiveness, while minimizing systemic side effects. This approach often is utilized in primary brain cancers, primary liver tumors, or other primaries with metastatic disease confined to a specific area, such as the liver.

These approaches can be utilized with intra-arterial administration of chemotherapy: (1) Radiographic placement of intra-arterial line via the femoral, brachial or carotid access. This line is generally in place for 3–5 days during intense chemotherapy administration and subsequently removed. It requires hospitalization for the 3–5 days, with complete bedrest in a supine position to prevent occlusion or migration of the catheter. If at least two courses of chemotherapy are given with a notable response, often a more permanent catheter is inserted. (2) A central venous access implantable port can be inserted at the time of surgery when primary resection of the tumor is not complete, or confined metastases are identified, i.e. hepatic. This placement allows outpatient administration of chemotherapy via bolus push or an external pump device. The care is similar to CVADs, although since the catheter is placed in the artery, once accessed, positive pressure must be used at all times to prevent an arterial bleed. If the patient is sent home with a pump, detailed instructions must be reviewed with the patient and caregiver to prevent arterial backflow. This approach is not the safest way to administer intra-arterial chemotherapy, and ideally, a more permanent access device would be inserted. (3) An implantable arterial pump is inserted surgically and placed in a subcutaneous pocket generally in the abdomen or chest. Most implantable arterial

pumps have two delivery system options: utilizing a sideport access for bolus pushes and/or a central access with a bellows pump reservoir for continuous delivery of chemotherapy. These ports should be accessed only by personnel who have been adequately trained as faulty filling and/or emptying of the bellows pump could result in permanent damage to the pump.

The patient and family must be taught to observe the surrounding skin for evidence of irritation, infection, or edema. Prolonged hot baths, showers, saunas or hot tubs should be avoided as they may increase the pump delivery rate. Changes in altitude related to geographic locations or air travel should be reported as they may also increase the pump delivery rate, and adjustments may be necessary for the chemotherapy dosage. The pumps require heparinization after use, and at least every 15–20 days for the central pump reservoir. Failure to maintain heparinization may result in permanent occlusion of the central bellows pump.

Intraventricular fluid access device

Intraventricular fluid access devices, or cerebrospinal fluid reservoirs, are surgically implanted devices that allow access to the cerebral spinal space. Better known as an Ommaya reservoir, this device is used primarily to administer ongoing or periodic intrathecal chemotherapy, eliminating the need for multiple lumbar punctures. In addition, the reservoir can be used to administer appropriate intravenous drugs or antibiotics, cerebrospinal fluid sampling and ventricular peritoneal shunting.

Nursing care includes education of the patient and family about the device, mental status assessment and prevention of side effects, specifically infection. Prior to accessing or caring for an intraventricular fluid access device, the nurse must be familiar with the chemotherapeutic agents used and potential side effects, as well as complications with the catheter, such as cerebrospinal fluid and/or drug leakage, hemorrhagic oozing, or catheter blockage. It is important to remember that this device directly accesses the pathways in the brain and epidural space; therefore, strict sterile technique is imperative to avoid life-threatening infections. In addition, all medications or fluids administered via an intraventricular fluid administered must be free of any preservatives to avoid neurotoxic side effects. A patient's mental status should be assessed frequently to note any changes related to the device or medications.

CHEMOTHERAPY MANAGEMENT

The administration of chemotherapy and management of potential and actual side effects are areas that nursing can significantly impact with positive outcomes for the patient and family. Numerous texts have been devoted to these topics; therefore, only broad concepts will be discussed in this chapter.

Administration of chemotherapy

Only those persons with specialized training should administer chemotherapeutic agents, due to the multiple potential side effects, as well as necessary precautions and preventative measures required. Specifically, chemotherapeutic agents that are given by intravenous push, and all vesicant agents should be limited to those nurses and physicians with experience and training. Many institutions have a chemotherapy administration course and require successful completion of this course prior to administering antineoplastic drugs.

Many of the side effects of chemotherapy can be prevented, or at least minimized, with appropriate and timely interventions. The unpreventable side effects can be made more tolerable with agressive interventions, education and understanding. Nursing plays a very important role in patient and family education, prevention, ongoing symptom management, psychosocial support and sexuality.

Patient and family education

Prior to initiating chemotherapy, an education packet should be given and thoroughly explained to the patient and family. This should include information on chemotherapy in general, the specific agents being given, the immune system, alopecia, bone marrow suppression (with emphasis on neutrapenia and thrombocytopenia precautions), prevention of nausea, vomiting, diarrhea, constipation, mouth sores, and management of fatigue. Depending on the specific agents given and regimen, these are the most commonly encountered side effects of chemotherapy. There are innumerable potential side effects that may never occur, but should be assessed

for with each visit. If adequate time is spent with the patient and family, many side effects can be minimized or prevented.

Prevention — extravasation, neutrapenia sepsis, nausea and vomiting

Extravation

One cannot emphasize enough the importance of prevention complications from chemotherapy. An excellent example is extravasation of vesicant or irritant agents, which is leakage of the drug into surrounding tissue. On a rare occasion, extravasation may occur, but it should be a very rare event. Skilled personnel are familiar with venous assessment, accurate venous access, and maintenance of access throughout administration. The maxim "if in doubt, pull it out" should always be practiced if there is any doubt in patency of a blood vessel. With the availability of central venous access devices (CVADs), painful, compromised or dangerous conditions should rarely occur. Insertion of a CVAD early in a patient's chemotherapy course will prevent many problems if venous access is in question.

Neutrapenia sepsis

Another frequently preventable side effect is infection or sepsis as a result of neutrapenia. Nearly all chemotherapeutic agents cause neutrapenia at varying degrees throughout a patient's treatment course. Frequent, thorough handwashing with an antibacterial soap in a pump dispenser by the patient and all family members is the best preventative action.

Patients should be made aware of their absolute neutrapenia count (ANC) when interval serum studies are performed. Once the ANC is below 1000–1500, neutraprenia precautions should be instituted, with more intense precautions if the ANC is below 500. Instructions should be reinforced frequently regarding avoidance of crowds, confined spaces, betadine scrubs prior to venipunctures, immediate reporting of oral temperatures > 100.5 degrees F, and any evidence of local or systemic infection. Patients on steroids should be carefully monitored as their response to infectious agents may be diminished from the immunosuppressive properties of steroids. In addition, patients with a low ANC may not exhibit as high a fever due to the immunosuppression, so all signs of infection should be assessed and treated, regardless of actual temperature. Depending on the patient and disease process, some institutions may prophylactically treat with oral broad-spectrum antibiotics when the ANC is below 500. Also, granulocyte colony stimulating factors (GCSF) may be administered to hasten bone marrow recovery or to prevent an ANC of less than 1000 during subsequent courses.

Nausea and vomitting

Even though most chemotherapeutic agents are emetogenic, persistent nausea and vomiting can be prevented in many cases. Attention should be given to the emetogenic potential of the specific agents being administered, the patient's dietary habits, rest patterns, and the level of anxiety regarding anticipated nausea and vomiting. Medications can be administered that affect the chemoreceptor trigger zone and the true vomiting center. Combinations of various antiemetic drugs should be used to block both of these areas, thus preventing nausea and vomiting. Ongoing assessment is important in order to improve outcomes, as well as manage cumulative effects of the drug.

Anticipatory nausea and vomiting is a known phenomenon and should be addressed with the patient when it occurs. The presence of certain oncology personnel or equipment, olfactory sensations, or just arriving at the office or hospital may induce profound nausea and vomiting. Certain medications can be utilized the night and morning prior to chemotherapy, as well as relaxation techniques and ongoing psychosocial support. The patient and family need to realize this phenomenon is real and potentially treatable.

Ongoing symptom management

Symptoms experienced as a result of cancer and chemotherapy should be assessed on a regular basis and addressed appropriately. Continuity of personnel caring for each patient is very important, as the nursing and medical personnel are familiar with the patient and vice versa. It is difficult for the patient and family to interact with new personnel with each visit and telephone conversation. Nursing provides an invaluable role in ongoing symptom management and reassurance for the patient. Many institutions have standing orders or protocols that can be followed for the most common side effects, without directly involving the physician. There is always some intervention(s) that can be implemented, no matter how small. This allows the patient and family to feel as though you care and understand their symptoms and frustrations.

Symptoms as a result of chemotherapy should be assessed at each visit and via the telephone in-between. Management of these symptoms should be altered in order to provide the maximum benefit with the minimum negative side effects possible. This requires documentation of progression and changes in the plan of care, so all involved personnel can review past interventions and assist the patient.

Psychosocial support

Ongoing care and concern are integral components of psychosocial support of the patient and family. Most patients experience a myriad of emotions when undergoing chemotherapy treatments as a result of the disease process, lack of control, self-image changes, fears and frustrations, changes in work or home environment, financial challenges, etc. It is important to acknowledge these feelings with patients and their families, and to enable verbalization, as well as interactions with others. The nurse is in a perfect position to address these situations, especially during the long and frequent periods of chemotherapy administration.

Sexuality

The impact the cancer disease process and treatment modalities have on a patient's and partner's sexuality is an area often not discussed. This lack of discussion is due in part to a knowledge deficit among professionals, lack of prioritization of the problem and hesitation on everyone's part to engage in such a personal matter. Whether a patient is young or old, single or married, heterosexual or homosexual, free of disease or dying, sexuality is an issue that should be availed to the patient.

The discussions regarding sexuality may include birth control, loss of fertility, estrogen replacement therapy, loss of libido, impotence, alterations in function or anatomy secondary to treatment, etc. As an example, in breast cancer patients, it is important to discuss the deleterious role of hormones, specifically estrogen. Many women experience moderate to severe side effects upon immediately discontinuing their estrogen replacement therapy, which often gives them more symptoms than the breast cancer treatment itself. Pre-menopausal women with breast cancer receiving adjuvant chemotherapy must be informed that menses may permanently cease with resulting chemical menopause and permanent sterilization. Young men, for example, with testicular cancer should be informed of potential sperm banking, prior to undergoing treatment.

The potential sexual implications are limitless and should be discussed openly with patients and their partners. Nursing, by virtue of their empathetic nature, and continuity of care providing a trusting relationship, is in an ideal position to explore these topics with patients. Nurses can explain etiologies of symptoms and possible solutions, offer reassurance and understanding, and potentially improve the sexual impact of cancer.

RADIATION THERAPY MANAGEMENT

Radiation therapy is a treatment modality used at varying stages of the cancer experience, ranging from prevention to active treatment to palliation. It can be given as a single treatment modality or in combination with others, such as surgery, chemotherapy or immunotherapy. Radiation is most often delivered in fractionated doses, requiring daily trips to the radiation facility. When considering the potential and real side effects of radiation therapy, one must understand that radiation can have immediate, delayed (up to six months) and long-term (after six months) side effects.

Often patients are managed by radiation oncologists and technicians, without the added benefit of nurses. Studies have shown that patients benefit from specially trained nurses in the field of radiation oncology. Ongoing assessment, education of the patient and family, and preventative symptom management are integral components of nursing care of the radiation patient. All radiation therapy facilities should consider employing at least one nurse or advanced practice nurse to augment the continuity of care.

Many patients confuse localized radiation with systemic chemotherapy. It is important to explain that radiation is a localized treatment that works where it is directed; therefore, the side effects are related to where the radiation beam is directed. The most common side effects are skin changes, fatigue, bone marrow suppression, tissue damage relevant to the area radiated, and psychosocial concerns. As

in chemotherapy, side effects may vary from patient to patient; therefore, each patient must be individually assessed and managed.

Patient and family education

Similar to chemotherapy, education for the patient and family should include information regarding the disease process, reason for radiation, treatment regimen, potential side effects and preventative measures. As in chemotherapy, there are several probable side effects and innumerable potential side effects. Continual reinforcement of symptom management can lessen the discomfort patients experience, and ultimately improve the time necessary to complete the course of radiation.

Skin changes

Changes in the epidermal layers of the skin are the most frequent side effect of radiation. These changes can range from slight erythema to diffuse, painful erythema and edema, to dry desquamation, and finally, to wet desquamation. As a result of technologically advanced equipment and techniques, patients are very rarely deeply burned with radiation.

Prevention of epidermal changes is the primary goal and prevention of complications deeper in the skin is secondary. Once skin changes have begun to occur, care must be taken to protect the area from direct sun exposure, irritating chemicals or lotions, infection, extreme hot or cold, tight clothing, adhesive tape or dressings, and undue moisture. It is imperative that radiation personnel direct preventative measures in order to minimize complications and maximize results of treatment. With the exception of epidermal thickening and hyperpigmentation changes (especially in the black or African-American population), most radiation skin changes completely resolve.

Most often, a light dusting of cornstarch is successful in treating slight changes to the skin. It is soothing and also prevents the accumulation of body moisture, which may in turn lead to more pronounced skin changes. A thin layer of petroleum-based ointment is often used in areas of wet desquamation to promote healing. This must be removed if radiation treatments are restarted. Then, a non-oily-based cream should be applied sparingly daily after bathing and removed prior to radiation.

Fatigue

Prolonged fatigue, or a lack of energy, is a commonly experienced side effect even during well-tolerated radiation treatments. Most treatment regimens require daily trips (Monday through Friday) to a radiation facility for 4–6 weeks. Depending on the geographical location of a facility, a patient could spend several hours per day just driving. Patients should be reassured that their energy level will increase and return to near normal levels up to several months after radiation treatments are completed, providing no other complications of the cancer disease process occur.

Bone marrow suppression

Depending on the area(s) of the body receiving radiation, bone marrow suppression may or may not be experienced. All efforts are made to shield areas of bone marrow exposure, but at times, these areas must be included in the radiation field. Most commonly, the long bones, including the humerus, femur, sternum and pelvis are the most common generators of adult bone marrow. Therefore, when these areas are directly radiated, mild to moderate myelosuppression can be experienced. This can progress to severe myelosuppression depending on cancer involvement of the marrow and concomitant use of chemotherapeutic agents.

Management of bone marrow suppression is similar to that of chemotherapy. At least weekly blood counts are done to assess the degree of myelosuppression, and the resulting necessary precautions.

Tissue damage

There is a wide variety of deep tissue damage syndromes that can occur relative to the area being radiated. These can include nausea and vomiting, esophagitis, stomatitis, xerostomia, diarrhea, pneumonitis, cystitis, and tenesmus. Treatment of these side effects is dependent on the cancer disease process, concomitant use of chemotherapy, and timing within the radiation treatment regimen. Once again, prevention of these side effects is imperative, as well as aggressive intervention once the side effects are identified. Prolonged deep tissue side effects with treatment result in irreversible tissue damage, as well as a rapid decline of the patient.

Psychosocial concerns

As in chemotherapy, many psychosocial concerns may arise related to the cancer disease process and resulting side effects of radiation. Again, it is important for patients to discuss their feelings openly and to resolve ongoing concerns. The required daily visit to the radiation facility can be overwhelming for some patients and families, regarding time consumption, finances for transportation, alterations in work schedules, transportation alternatives, etc. Often, social services is able to assist the patient and family in solving these issues through outside services and aid. It is important to discuss transportation and time issues when radiation is initiated to prevent frustration and barriers to completion of the prescribed regimen.

Another frequent frustration for cancer patients receiving radiation is disease recurrence or progression. Often, patients will recur or progress outside the radiation field; this can sometimes occur during the current treatment regimen. Again, it is important to emphasize that radiation works only where it is directed, not systemically. Nothing is more frustrating to a patient and family than to complete six weeks of active or palliative radiation, only to need to restart another series, focused on another area of active cancer.

BIOTHERAPY MANAGEMENT

Biotherapy, or immunotherapy, with the use of biologic response modifiers (BRMs) is an emerging field in cancer care. It is clear that the more common treatment modalities of surgery, chemotherapy, and radiation therapy are not controlling or curing all cases of cancer. Studies have turned to investigating the role of the immune system in both preventing and controlling cancer growth.

BRMs are being studied regarding their roles in the human immune response, tumor lysis, and the ability to work with other agents in eradicating or modulating the replication of tumor cells. These agents are classified as tumor necrosis factor (TNF), interferon (IFN), interleukin (ILK), colony stimulating factors (CSF), and monoclonal antibodies.

The role of nursing in biotherapy is limitless, as current and future research progresses. The nurse as an educator for the patient and family is invaluable, as there is little published lay literature to read, and the scientific literature is often too complex. As patients embark on experimental protocol regimens, the nurse is often the direct liaison to explain and reiterate the purpose of treatment, expected results and potential side effects. Much of this territory is still unknown and thus requires a strong trusting relationship between the patient and family and interdisciplinary team.

Collectively, the most common side effects of BRMs are myelosuppression, muscle pain and flu-like symtoms. As in other treatment modalities, these are best managed in a preventative manner with prophylactic acetaminophen, steroids, dephenhydramine, heat or ice, relaxation and imagery techniques, etc. To discuss all of the potential side effects of BRMs is futile, depending on the specific agent, use of that agent, dosage, duration, etc. Comprehensive articles and texts are now being published, specific to each BRM and their use. Nurses must educate themselves through seminars, published materials, as well as direct involvement in clinical trials.

PROGRESSIVE CANCER

Recurrent or progressive cancer is devastating to all concerned, regardless of when it occurs in the cancer continuum. In some patients, a recurrence or progression may evoke an increased will to fight, and in others, it may elicit futile thoughts and a sense of hopelessness. It is necessary for the patient and family to understand the pathophysiology of the disease process, the potential treatment options and side effects, the potential benefit of further treatment and the potential results of no treatment.

Often, when a cancer recurs, treatment is reserved until the patient is symptomatic or developing complications. This concept is quite different from when a cancer is diagnosed and the urgency to begin treatment is stressed. Helping a patient to understand this difference, to understand the role of palliative care, and to help guide a patient towards an appropriate treatment plan, can be very challenging. Frequently, the primary nurse who has been involved with the patient's care from the begining is turned to for support and advice. This nurse is in a pivotal position to help the patient and family through a very difficult time.

When cancer recurs or progresses, the discussions regarding quality of life versus quantity of life typically emerge. Patients and their families must explore their own feelings, thoughts and philosophies regarding life, death, relationships, long-term goals, etc. It is a very emotional time when a constant resource to the patient and family is needed. The primary nurse may often be in this role, along with the primary physician. Many times, the facts must be reiterated and explained, as people struggle through this portion of their cancer experience.

Another common concern and fear is potential pain and the ability to control it. Patients need to be assured that pain can be effectively managed, allowing them to live, and die, comfortably. With the multitude of agents available today, no patient should experience moderate to severe pain for an extended period of time.

Although in most situations, pain medications and narcotics need to be initiated by a physician, the nurse is in an ideal position to help the patient manage their pain on an ongoing basis. As with any treatment regimen, additional side effects may occur, including nausea, constipation, safety issues, etc. The nurse can very effectively manage these side effects and ensure a positive outcome with excellent pain control.

SUMMARY

Throughout this chapter, the value of nursing involvement in the care of oncology patients and their families has been discussed. Nurses are an integral member of the interdisciplinary team, and are often the common link between services, providing continuity of care, and a sense of wholeness.

As patients recover from their cancer experience and return to a normal lifestyle, nurses are in an excellent position to educate patients on healthy lifestyle behaviors, such as stress reduction, exercises, protective dietary habits, preventative health care maintenance, smoking cessation and ongoing surveillance of their cancer. In many situations. advanced practice nurses assist the physician in providing this link for patients as they strive to remain free of disease. Maybe some day, all of us will be teaching patients how to prevent cancer instead of treating it.

References

Brown, J.K. and Hogan C.M. (1992). Chemotherapy. In *Cancer Nursing: Principles and Practice*, edited by S.L. Groenwald *et al.*, pp. 230–273. Boston: Jones and Barlett Publishers.

Clark, J.C. and McCee, R.F. (1992). *Core Curriculum for Oncology Nursing*, 2nd edn. Philadelphia: W.B. Saunders Company.

Foltz, A.T., Faines. G. and Gullate, M. (1996). Recalled Side Effects and Self-Care Actions of Patients Receiving Inpatient Chemotherapy, *Oncology Nursing Forum*, **23**(4), 679–683.

Groenwaid. S.L., Frogge, M.H., Goodman, M. and Yarbro, C.H. (1992). *Cancer Nursing: Principles and Practice*, 2nd edn. Boston: Jones and Bartlett Publishers.

Hilderly, L.J. (1992). Radiotherapy. In *Cancer Nursing: Principles and Practice*, edited by S.L. Groenwald *et al.*, pp. 199–299. Boston: Jones and Bartlett Publishers.

Hilton, B.A. (1996). Getting Back To Normal: The Family Experience During Early Stage Breast Cancer. *Oncology Nursing Forum*, **23**(4), 605–614.

Jassak, P.F. (1992). Biotherapy. In *Cancer Nursing: Principles and Practice*, edited by S.L. Groenwald *et al.*, pp. 284–306. Boston: Jones and Bartlett Publishers.

McCaffrey-Boyle, D. (1995). Documentation and Outcomes of Advanced Nursing Practice. *Oncology Nursing Forum*, **22**(8), 11–17.

Murphy, G.P., Lawrence, W. and Lenhard, R.E. (1995). *American Cancer Society Textbook of Clinical Oncology*, 2nd edn. Atlanta: The American Cancer Society.

Rhodes. V.A., McDaniel. R.W., Simms, S.G. and Johnson, M. (1995). Nurses' Perceptions of Antiemetic Effectiveness. *Oncology Nursing Forum*, **22**(8), 1243–1252.

9. Quality of Life of Cancer Patients and their Relatives

PETER MAGUIRE

CRC Psychological Medicine Group, Stanley House, Christie Hospital, Manchester, UK

INTRODUCTION

Individuals who experience adverse events in life (for example, bereavement) or chronic difficulties (for example, financial, housing, occupational or relationship problems) are more likely to develop an anxiety disorder or major depressive illness than those who do not (Brown and Harris, 1978). Events which threaten or cause a major loss are especially potent in this respect.

When patients learn that they have cancer they are faced with the reality that their disease could progress or recur, cause much suffering and a premature death. Moreover, treatment may cause the loss of a crucial body part or function. If the cancer progresses or recurs the patient's ability to fulfill his or her social, occupational and personal roles will be compromised. Such role changes are especially likely if the treatment given for cancer causes serious side effects. Cancer patients are more likely to develop an affective disorder, body image or sexual problems than individuals who are free from the disease. These affective disorders, body image problems and sexual difficulties markedly impair their quality of life unless they are recognized and treated appropriately.

Similarly, it has been found (Haddad *et al.*, 1996) that close relatives of cancer patients are also at higher risk for affective disorder and impairment of the quality of their lives.

PROBLEMS ASSOCIATED WITH DIAGNOSIS

Patients and relatives have to come to terms with several hurdles if they are to cope psychologically. These include the uncertainty of prognosis and whether or not the cancer will return and cause premature death. Doctors can only make general estimates about the likelihood of survival in individual patients. Patients have, therefore, to try to adapt to this uncertainty. Attempts to do so may be undermined by frequent references in newspapers and television to their particular cancer or cancers in general and by raising controversial issues about the value of treatment. If their treatment has left them with residual evidence of their predicament (for example, an empty chest wall after mastectomy) this can trigger worries about survival every time they catch sight of themselves.

Most patients and relatives cope better with a crisis if they can explain why it has happened. The problem with having cancer is that there are few established reasons why a given individual develops cancer. This creates a psychological vacuum into which patients and relatives can project their own concerns. These include the view that the cancer was caused by their own behavior (an inability to cope with stress, or problems in expressing feelings). Alternatively, they may believe that their cancer developed because of cruelty or stress caused by others.

Cancer patients and their families face the problem of how to be open with others because of the stigma associated with the disease. Those who are able to be open with friends and family about diagnosis and treatment are more likely to cope psychologically than those who keep it secret. However, if they are open about their disease and treatment this may lead other people to avoid them because they find it hard to discuss their predicament. When other people respond adversely and withdraw their support this can seriously interfere with the patients' and relatives' attempts to adjust psychologically.

Most people facing adverse events expect other people to be supportive and help them through their traumas. Similarly, cancer patients and relatives fare much better if they perceive that other people, including those involved in their medical and nursing care, are supportive practically and emotionally. When they perceive that such support is lacking they are more likely to develop an affective disorder and experience an impaired quality of life.

Patients who face adversity and feel there is something they can do to combat the threat to survival or complications of diagnosis and treatment cope much better than those who feel helpless. Those patients who appraise their situation and have a greater number and severity of concerns about it are more likely to develop anxiety and depression (Parle *et al.*, 1996). Those who respond to such negative appraisals by feeling helpless are also at considerable risk of an affective disorder. Patients with four or more major concerns about their predicament are especially likely to develop anxiety and depression. So, it is important to check how they are trying to cope with these various hurdles.

ASSESSING ADAPTATION

Newly diagnosed patients should, therefore, be asked "How do you see your disease working out?". Those who are plagued by uncertainty should be asked questions to elicit whether or not they have developed an anxiety state or depression. Patients should also be asked "Have you any idea why you should have developed cancer?". Those who blame themselves or others are much more likely to have later problems. They should also be asked the extent to which they perceive they are getting practical and emotional support from their friends, relatives, doctors and nurses. They should be asked how much they feel they can contribute to their survival whether it be by joining a volunteer group or adopting a more healthy diet. Patients who feel there is nothing they can do should be monitored closely.

Generally any patient who is struggling to adapt to two or more of these major hurdles is at major risk of anxiety and depression.

PSYCHOLOGICAL MORBIDITY RESULTING FROM SURGERY

Up to 25% of those who undergo mastectomy for breast cancer develop an anxiety state and/or depressive illness because they cannot come to terms with the diagnosis and/or breast loss (Maguire, 1992). This represents an increased relative risk three to four times higher than that which would be found in the general population. Sexual problems are also more common and are strongly related to women being unable to accept the loss of a breast and developing body image problems.

These body image problems may be evident in three ways. First, the woman may feel unable to accept that she is less than whole. This may lead to a profound loss of self-esteem and a greater vulnerability to adverse life events. Second, she may feel increasingly self-conscious and worried, albeit wrongly, that other people notice she has lost a breast. This can lead to social phobias where the woman actually avoids meeting new people. Third, the woman may experience a loss of femininity and attractiveness. This may cause her to believe that her partner no longer finds her attractive and does not want to continue the relationship.

The loss of important bodily functions through surgery such as the ability to evacuate the bowels or speak normally (after colostomy and larangectomy respectively) also increases the risk of psychiatric morbidity. A substantial minority of patients (25–32%) are unable to come to terms with these changes. They become self-conscious and excessively pre-occupied with their disability. These body image problems can lead to sexual problems which can also result from surgical destruction of the nerves supplying the genital organs.

Surgery for cancer may cause complications like pain and swelling of the affected arm because of lymph node clearance after mastectomy. Such pain can hinder movement of the arm and trigger worries that cancer is still present. This can have an adverse impact on the woman's personal relationships and her ability to function within the home and work.

Treating breast cancer by wide local excision and radiotherapy results in a similar incidence of affective disorder and sexual problems (Fallowfield *et al.*, 1990). The reduction in body image problems in those treated with mastectomy is offset by greater worries that the cancer has not been fully removed and that radiotherapy is only given to mop up remaining cancer cells.

It is, therefore, important when patients have undergone surgery which results in the loss of an important body part or function that they are asked how they felt about losing that part or function and whether or not that has caused any relationship problems, impairment of daily function or mood disturbance.

EFFECTS OF OTHER TREATMENTS

The risk of anxiety, depression and impairment of quality of life increases when treatments like radiotherapy or chemotherapy are given and cause adverse effects, particularly in the gastrointestinal tract (Devlen *et al.*, 1987). These effects are mediated in three ways. There is the strain of enduring unpleasant side effects. Patients become increasingly worried about these as treatment progresses. They may misattribute side effects to disease progression or recurrence. Finally, treatment may have a direct biological effect on mood by causing chemical changes in the brain, as for example, after an infusion of chemotherapy.

It has been established that the use of chemotherapy, especially in combination, causes conditioned responses in 25% of patients (Morrow, 1982). Any smell, sight or sound which reminds patients of chemotherapy causes them to feel nauseous and to vomit. This can provoke avoidance of treatment and lead to an anxiety state and/or depressive illness. Chemotherapy may also cause a loss of libido, infertility or sterility through adversely affecting hormone production. Ablation of the ovaries by radiotherapy has similar effects.

Even when there are compelling psychological and treatment-related explanations for impaired quality of life, anxiety and/or depression it is important to consider disease-related factors. These include disease spread or recurrence, the use of drugs (like steroids) and metabolic changes such as hypercalcemia. It is important that these psychological disorders are recognized early and patients offered help. Unfortunately, there are major barriers to this and their quality of life often remains seriously impaired.

BARRIERS TO DETECTION

Patient-led reasons

Patients assume that the problems they develop are an inevitable consequence of cancer and its treatments. They believe, therefore, that they cannot be alleviated and there is no point in mentioning them to anyone involved in their care. They fear that if they complain they will be labelled as ungrateful or inadequate and this will disadvantage their subsequent treatment. Consequently, many patients strive to maintain a "brave front." This can mislead the doctor and nurse into thinking that they are coping well.

Paradoxically, the more patients come to respect and like the health professionals caring for them the more they tend to protect them from their worries. They know the staff are busy and they do not wish to burden them unnecessarily. They worry that if they spend time talking about any social and psychological problems this might detract from the attention paid to ensuring their physical survival from the cancer. They also believe, albeit wrongly, that it is not legitimate to mention concerns which are not obviously related to physical aspects of their disease or treatment. They do so because they claim that they are rarely asked questions which indicate that the health professional is interested in these areas.

Patients also claim that when they are faced with this lack of questions they try to give verbal or nonverbal cues which indicate they have worries. They say that it is rare for their cues to be acknowledged and explored by the doctor or nurse. Instead, they report that carers block their cues by using tactics designed to maintain a safe emotional distance from their problems. The key question, therefore, is whether these claims by patients are valid.

Objective studies of consultations between cancer patients and doctors or nurses found that appropriate questions are asked infrequently (Rosser and Maguire, 1982) and that distancing tactics are used commonly (Wilkinson, 1991; Maguire *et al.*, 1996). Consequently, few data are obtained about the quality of patients' lives.

A common distancing tactic is to normalize any distress. Thus, the patient or relative is told that it is normal to worry in this situation and the worry will dissipate. Doctors and nurses are keen to make the patient feel better for genuine reasons. They are tempted to provide reassurance the moment they hear a problem. This can result in them providing reassurance before they have understood the basis of the concern. For example, a patient explained that he was very upset about having had a colostomy. He was told "there is no need to be upset. We have such good bags these days and I am sure we can help you." This reassurance is premature because no attempt had been made to establish why he was upset. He was a homosexual and worried about the effects of the stoma on future relationships.

This bid to reassure patients may include false reassurance. Here the health professional realizes that the patient's fear is correct but wishes to protect the patient from a harsh reality as in the following example.

Patient   I am going to die, aren't I?
Doctor   You are being unduly pessimistic at this stage. I am pretty sure we can control things. I don't think you should be thinking that way.

When potentially distressing topics are raised suddenly by a patient it is tempting for the health professional to switch the topic to safer waters. Sometimes this switching is done automatically so that the health professional does not realize it has happened.

Doctor   How have you been feeling since your operation?
Patient   I am continuing to get pain and I feel so exhausted. I am beginning to think I am not going to make it.
Doctor   How much pain are you getting?
Patient   It's there all the time. It doesn't seem to be getting easier. It makes me think I am not going to make it.
Doctor   I think we better discuss how we can better control your pain.

These distancing tactics serve to prevent the patient disclosing important problems which may provoke distress whether they are from a physical, social or psychological domain.

Reasons for distancing

In-depth interviews with doctors and nurses established that they fear that direct enquiry about how a patient is coping will cause serious psychological problems. They worry that they will unleash strong feelings of anger or despair which cannot be contained or resolved. If they show interest in patients' concerns this could make heavy demands on their time. It might also encourage patients to ask difficult questions such as "Am I dying?" or "Why didn't you diagnose it sooner?". If they were to explore patients' concerns more effectively this would bring them face to face with the reality of their predicaments and suffering. This might cause them to doubt the value of their own work in treating patients with cancer and reinforce doubts about the ability of medicine in general to relieve suffering and cure disease. Doctors and nurses are also aware that if they identify the reality of their patients' suffering this may put them under emotional strain and affect their ability to function. Thus, if a surgeon were to establish how each woman felt after mastectomy he might get to the point of wondering about the wisdom of doing a mastectomy because of the adverse emotional sequelae. So, for all these reasons it is best not to routinely enquire about patients' concerns other than those which are volunteered spontaneously.

Recent research has established two other reasons for distancing. Health professionals involved in cancer care feel they have not been equipped by their undergraduate and postgraduate training with the skills necessary to promote patient disclosure and deal with key tasks like breaking bad news and handling difficult questions. Second, they fear that they would be unsupported if they tried to get a more holistic notion of how their patients were coping. They worry that they might be criticized if they presented data on a ward round about patients having problems in psychological and social areas as opposed to reporting the latest test results concerning disease and disease progression.

Improving the detection of patients' concerns

The major task for medical and nursing staff is to show patients and relatives from the first consultation that they are genuinely interested in how the cancer and its treatment is affecting the quality of their lives. The addition of directive questions to routine history taking facilitates this. Questions about how a woman reacted when she found a breast lump will educate her that the doctor is interested in her feelings. If she is also asked what she thought the lump might be due to, this indicates an interest in her perceptions. These questions will result in her giving more cues about underlying concerns whether they are physical, social or psychological in nature (Maguire *et al.*, 1996). They make her feel that the doctor or nurse is empathic and interested in her as a person and will promote disclosure of her thoughts and feelings about her predicament.

When patients give a history they give important cues about problem areas. If the doctor or nurse pauses to acknowledge these cues ("You say you felt upset when you had a colostomy?") and invites the patient to clarify them ("Would you like to tell me in what way you are upset?") it reinforces the notion that the doctor or nurse is interested in the patient as a person.

Patients are not used to being asked about the impact of the diagnosis or treatment on them and their lives. But, specific enquiry leads them to be more honest about the impact of the diagnosis and treatments on their daily lives, personal relationships, sexual adjustment and mood. The nature, intensity and duration of any problems so revealed can then be explored and attempts made to resolve them.

Summarizing what the patient has said at various points in the consultation is also helpful. It lets patients know that the interviewer has heard what they have been saying. It also gives them a chance to qualify or correct what the interviewer has understood, or elaborate on a complaint. Once the health professional has established the key problems it is important to check which the patient most wants help with and work through the patient's priority list unless there is a medical imperative like severe pain. Once a patient's concerns have been dealt with then the health professional can cover his or her agenda by asking relevant questions (for example, the presence of key symptoms).

Although health professionals often suspect intuitively that a patient or relative is depressed, angry, distressed and having difficulty coping they tend to keep these intuitions private. They fear that if they voice them and are wrong this will spoil their relationship with the patient. The making public of these intuitions (the use of educated guesses) informs patients that the health professional is making a real effort to get alongside the patient's experiences. Such guesses lead to elaboration (the patient tells the interviewer more about the problem), refutation (where the patient corrects the interviewer and educates them as to the real problem) or confirmation (where the patient admits the guess is right but does not elaborate).

Unfortunately, health professionals use as many interviewing behaviors that inhibit disclosure (distancing tactics) as those that promote disclosure. Fortunately, training health professionals can help them acquire the key skills and relinquish the distancing tactics.

Management of problems

It is important that health professionals involved in cancer care maximize the chances that patients and relatives disclose their concerns so that these can be resolved as soon as possible, otherwise they are at much greater risk of anxiety and depression. Even so, some patients will still develop major problems and require psychological help. The management of the more common conditions is now considered.

Anxiety state

Patients who cannot cope because of a severe anxiety state require a low dose of a major tranquilizer such as Thioridazine. Those with a moderately severe anxiety state benefit from a Benzodiazepine such as Lorazepam or Diazepam taken only as required for no longer than three to four weeks in order to avoid dependence. They should also be taught anxiety management techniques including progressive muscular relaxation and positive imaging. When patients develop conditioned responses Lorazepam should be taken as required in the 48 hours before each treatment. Most patients will then complete their course of chemotherapy. Propanalol is of use when somatic symptoms of anxiety predominate.

Depressive illness

Depression should not be dismissed as an understandable reaction providing there are sufficient signs and symptoms to justify an objective diagnosis. Most patients respond to a four to six month course of antidepressant medication. A drug such as Dothiepin in a dose of 75 to 150 mgs at night is usually effective. The new serotonergic uptake inhibitors are also effective and are to be preferred if there are risks of cardiovascular complications, problems with glaucoma, prostatism and sedation. Thus, Prozac may be started in a dose of 20 mgs daily increasing to 40 mgs if there is no response at the lower dose.

Compliance with medication will be high if the patient is informed that the antidepressant is not a tranquilizer, will not cause dependence and will aleviate the depression by correcting an underlying chemical imbalance caused by the diagnosis of cancer and its treatment. It should also be impressed on the patient that medication is not being used merely to suppress the patient's worries. Once there is a lift in mood any remaining problems will be tackled systematically.

Body image problems

Avoidance of looking at the affected part of the body can be helped by relaxation and graded exposure. The patient is first taught relaxation and then asked to imagine looking at the affected part for only a short time. Then he or she is asked to look at the affected part in reality. The exercise is repeated with an increasing length of time being spent on imaging and looking.

However, body image problems can lead to irrational beliefs. Thus, a man might believe that because he cannot accept his colostomy his wife will not be able to do so. Since his wife can't accept his colostomy she no longer loves him. Here, cognitive therapy is worth trying. This involves establishing which of the man's beliefs are irrational (his wife can't accept him as he is and no longer loves him) and challenge these in a systematic way.

In cases where surgical reconstruction is possible this should be considered. Patients need to know the possible benefits and disadvantages, to see photographs of good and bad outcomes and have a chance to talk to somebody familiar with the procedures before they agree to undergo it.

Sexual problems

The treatment of sexual problems depends on the cause. If sexual functioning has been destroyed by surgery the couple can be taught alternative modes of pleasuring. Psychologically based sexual problems usually respond to conjoint Masters and Johnston therapy. Once the couple's problems have been explored a ban is put on intercourse. They are encouraged to find different ways to pleasure each other in order to take the tension out of their sexual relationship. As they build up confidence they can begin to consider re-establishing sexual intercourse.

Hormone-related problems respond to replacement therapy but this cannot be used if the tumor is hormone dependent. Sexual problems that arise from anxiety, depression or body image problems usually resolve when these problems are treated appropriately.

Prevention

Specialist nurses and social workers have been appointed in the hope that counselling before and after cancer treatment prevents psychological problems and improves the quality of life. However, there is no conclusive evidence that such approaches do so. Encouraging patients to discuss treatment options in the short term and following their preferences appears to reduce problems. Similarly, taking care to tailor information about their diagnosis to their need for information rather than assuming they want all the relevant information or little of it enhances psychological adjustment. Making efforts to identify patients' concerns early and resolve them is also likely to reduce psychological morbidity and improve the quality of life (Parle et al., 1996).

Identifying those at risk

Ideally, those at risk should be offered help before problems develop. However, those judged to be at risk may not accept they need help and comply with the offered intervention. It is probably more productive to monitor those who have difficulty surmounting key hurdles. Thus, those who feel plagued by uncertainty, feel helpless, blame themselves or others for their disease, feel stigmatized, are secretive about their illness or feel unsupported merit close monitoring since they are likely to develop an anxiety state and/or depressive illness and suffer a major impairment in their quality of life. A past history of psychiatric morbidity is another predictor. Those patients who have more than three concerns are worth assessing closely.

Self-help

Self-help groups can reduce the sense of stigma and isolation as well as provide practical advice and emotional support. However, they must be led by people with a sound knowledge of groups and group dynamics who are willing to use health care professionals as a resource. Volunteers also have a place, provided they are selected carefully, trained in basic listening and responding skills and are willing to have their performance audited.

References

Brown, G.W. and Harris, T.O. (1978). *Social origins of depression. A study of psychiatric disorder in women*. London: Tavistock Publications.

Devlen, J., Maguire, P., Phillips, P., Crowther, D. and Chambers, H. (1987). Psychological problems associated with diagnosis and treatment of lymphoma. II A prospective study. *BMJ*, **295**, 985–987.

Fallowfield, L.J., Hall, A., Maguire, G.P. and Baum, M. (1990). Psychological outcomes of different treatment policies in women with early breast cancer outside a clinical trial. *BMJ*, **301**, 575–580.

Haddad, P., Pitceathly, C. and Maguire, P. (1996). Psychological morbidity in the partners of cancer patients, In *Cancer and the Family*, edited by L. Baider, C.L. Cooper and A. Kaplan de Nour, pp. 257–270. Chichester: John Wiley.

Maguire, P. (1992). Improving the recognition and treatment of affective disorders in cancer patients, In *Recent Advances in Clinical Psychiatry*, edited by K. Granville-Grossman, pp. 15–30. Edinburgh: Churchill Livingstone.

Maguire, P., Faulkner, A., Booth, K., Elliott, C. and Hillier, V. Helping cancer patients disclose their concerns. *Eur. J. Ca.*, in press.

Maguire, P., Booth, K., Elliott, C. and Hillier, V. Helping health professionals involved in cancer care acquire key skills. *Eur J Ca.*, in press.

Morrow, G. (1982). Prevalence and cohorts of anticipatory nausea and vomiting in chemotherapy patients. *J. Natl. Cancer Inst.*, **68**, 585–588.

Parle, M., Jones, B. and Maguire, P. Maladaptive coping and affective disorders among cancer patients. *Psychological Medicine*, **26**, in press.

Rosser, J. and Maguire, P. (1982). Dilemmas in general practice: The care of the cancer patient. *Psy. Med.*, **16**, 315–322.

Wilkinson, S. (1991). Factors which influence how nurses communicate with cancer patients. *J. Adv. Nursing*, **16**, 677–688.

10. Squamous Cell Carcinoma, Basal Cell Carcinoma and Merkel Cell Carcinoma

MICHAEL POULSEN

Queensland Radium Institute, Herston, Australia

Cancer of the skin is by far the most common cancer in men and women and makes up about a third of all cancers diagnosed. Although cure rates are high, it is important to remember that deaths still occur despite widespread public awareness of the importance of early diagnosis. This chapter reviews the common non-melanoma skin cancers (NMSC) which are squamous cell carcinoma (SCC), basal cell carcinoma (BCC) and also discusses the most aggressive of all skin cancers — a rare tumor called merkel cell carcinoma (MCC).

EPIDEMIOLOGY

The epidemiological data for SCC, BCC and MCC are similar. These are diseases of fair skin populations and those of Celtic origins seem to be more prone.[1] The risk of NMSC steadily rises the closer one gets to the equator. More than 90% of NMSC develop in exposed areas of skin such as the head, neck and limbs.

Incidence

BCCs are four times as common as SCCs.[2] By comparison, MCCs are rare but the true incidence is yet to be determined as there is an increasing awareness on the part of clinicians and pathologists as to the diagnosis.

Accurate data on the incidence is difficult to obtain as these tumors are treated by a wide variety of specialists and general practitioners, sometimes without histologic confirmation. Population-based studies have shown an incidence in the USA of 232.6 per 100,000 for whites, 3.4 per 100,000 for blacks and in Australia, almost 1000 per 100,000. Increases of 15–20% have been reported from 1971 to 1977.[3]

Age

The median age for BCCs and SCCs is 68 years.[1] With increased recreational sun exposure and the movement of fair skin people to sunnier climates, it has become increasingly common to see NMSCs in younger people. MCC has a median age of 74 years[4] although it has occurred in people as young as 30.

Sex

The male to female ratio for BCCs and SCCs is 4:1[2] and this probably relates to relative exposure. The data on the ratio in MCC is equivocal.[4]

Predisposing and risk factors

The major risk factors for skin cancer are skin color and exposure to ultraviolet light.[5] Those who tan with sun exposure are at one-third the risk of those who say that they never tan and only burn. The presence of solar keratoses is also an important risk factor for NMSC.[3] Sun exposure in childhood is critically important in determining the risk in later life. There is considerable concern about the depletion of the ozone layer and the impact this will have on skin cancers in the future.

Rare genetic conditions predisposing to skin cancer include xeroderma pigmentosum and Gorlin's syndrome while prolonged immunosuppression for organ transplantation results in a 20-fold increase in NMSC.[1]

Other uncommon predisposing factors include exposure to chemicals such as arsenic, tar, nitrogen mustard and ionizing radiation. Sites of trauma from burns or smallpox vaccination scars are also more prone to skin cancers.

PATHOLOGY

BCC

They are characterized by nests of pallisading small basal type cells with relatively large and basophilic nuclei. The stroma is rich in mucopolysaccharides which imparts a mucinous appearance. The morphologic types found are (1) solid, (2) cystic, (3) adenoid, (4) keratotic, (5) pigmented, (6) multifocal superficial, (7) sclerosing or morphoea-like (8) infiltrating, (9) basosquamous, (10) the premalignant fibroepithelial tumor of Pinkus.[6]

Although rich in mitotic figures, BCCs are very slow growing and this is thought to be due to a high rate of apoptosis or programmed cell death.[1] BCCs are locally destructive and nodal spread is exceedingly rare (0.002%).

SCC

These tumors arise from epidermal keratinocytes and are typified by invasive nests of prickle cells showing variable central keratinization and horn pearl formation. Unlike BCCs, intercellular bridges are seen.[6]

SCCs (particularly the ulcerative type) tend to be more aggressive than BCCs. The major mode of spread is by local extension. Nodal metastases are infrequent. Invasion into perineural spaces uncommonly occurs.

MCC

This is a neuroendocrine tumor which was first described in 1972. The presumed cell of origin lies in the basal layer of epithelium, particularly around hair follicles. The tumor is composed of sheets of small cells, sometimes arranged in a trabecular pattern. The diagnosis can be confirmed by immunoperoxidase stains for neurone-specific enolase or demonstrating neurosecretory granules on electron microscopy. It is a highly malignant tumor with a high propensity for local recurrence (33–77%), nodal spread (62%) and distant spread (54%).[7] Spontaneous regression has been documented.

PROTECTIVE FACTORS

Skin cancer prevention has been mainly in the form of education programs aimed at altering attitudes about sunlight and suntans. In Australia, this has resulted in increased hat wearing, avoidance of the sun around the middle of the day and the increased use of sun screens.[3] Recent data demonstrating that regular use of sunscreens can prevent the development of new solar keratoses and hasten the remission of existing ones show that these products have the potential to reduce the long-term risk of NMSC.[8]

SCREENING

Because of the accessibility of the skin, screening for malignant skin conditions should be carried out at every opportunity in patients at high risk. Formal mass screening is uncommon but the American Academy of Dermatologists initiated the National Melanoma/Skin Cancer Prevention Program in 1985 which reached over 600,000 people and diagnosed more than 35,000 NMSCs and 3500 melanomas.[9]

CLINICAL PRESENTATION

BCC

This usually presents as a slowly growing, well-circumscribed papule with a pearly surface and telangiectasia on the surface (Figure 10.1). Larger lesions may ulcerate and be difficult to distinguish from SCCs. Central regression may occur, typically

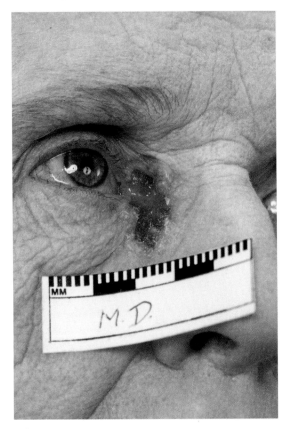

Figure 10.1.   This ulcerating BCC of the inner canthus of the eye displays some of the features of BCC with a pearly edge, telangiectasia and a central ulcer. This contrasts with SCC which tend to have a scaly surface which may later ulcerate with a rolled edge.

with the sclerosing type of BCC which has an indistinct border.

SCC

They typically present as a scaly nodular lesion, subsequently ulcerating with a rolled edge. Growth is more rapid than BCCs, particularly the more undifferentiated type. Half the patients were present with multiple lesions.

MCC

The diagnosis is usually made on the pathological specimen and is rarely made clinically. The cutaneous nodule is usually rapidly growing, painless, shiny with a bluish red color. The overlying skin is usually intact.[5] Presentation with nodal disease occurs in a third of cases, sometimes without an obvious primary.[4]

INVESTIGATIONS

Examination should be undertaken in good light with the aid of magnification. Lesions should be measured in size and depth of infiltration and documented with diagrams. The relevant lymphatic drainage should be examined. Suspicious lesions should be biopsied with a shave excision or a 4 mm punch biopsy under local anaesthetic. The patient's spectacles should be removed to inspect the eyelids and obscure areas such as the ala nasi and post-auricular groove should be specifically examined. All dressings should be removed to allow full inspection of the skin.

Advanced lesions may need further evaluation to establish the true extent of disease. Lesions adjacent to the orbit, attached to bone or with perineural spread associated with symptoms or signs should have a CT or MRI of the relevent area.

MCCs have a high metastatic potential and require a baseline workup with full blood count, liver function tests and chest X-ray.

The TNM staging system[11] defines the primary tumor by size but ignores important prognostic variables such as site. The majority will fall into the T1 and this tends to limit its application and sensitivity.

PROGNOSTIC FACTORS

Certain clinical and pathological factors should alert the doctor to an increased risk of local recurrence. Tumors of the eyelids, nose and ears are at increased risk.[12] These are areas where repairs are more difficult and where inadequate excisions are more common. Should recurrence occur at these sites, further treatment is difficult and sometimes unsuccessful leading to eventual death. Other poor prognostic factors are cartilage or bone involvement, poorly differentiated histology and recurrent lesions.[2] The presence of perineural infiltration in the pathology specimen is an adverse finding and post-operative irradiation should be considered in these cases.[13]

Table 10.1. Treatment options.

Treatment	Advantages	Disadvantages
Curettage and cautery	Good cure rates, quick, inexpensive, good cosmesis widely available.	Restricted to low risk lesions, no histologic control. Not for SCC.
Cryotherapy	Good cure rates in experienced hands. No cutting. Relative sparing of dermis and cartilage.	Requires specialized equipment and training. No histologic control. Requires visual estimation of margins and depth. Post-op. care needed. Not for SCC.
Resection	Good cure rates. Rapid. Widely available. Histologic control. Cost-effective. Good cosmesis.	Complicated around eyes, ears and nose. Requires visual estimation of margins. May need GA. Post-op. care needed.
Moh's surgery	Very high cure rates. Complete histologic control. Spares normal tissue. Local anesthesia. Allows for confident reconstrucion.	Slow, multistage. Expensive. Not widely available. May need reconstruction.
Radiotherapy	Good cure rates. No pain or cutting. Effective in difficult areas (eye, ear, nose). Good cosmesis. Ideal in frail and elderly.	Multiple visits. Specialized staff and equipment. Visual estimation of depth and margins. Scars get worse with time. Carcinogenesis.

TREATMENT

The aim of treatment should be to cure the tumor with the best cosmetic result. This is readily achievable in early lesions but in advanced lesions, cure becomes increasingly difficult and cosmesis becomes relatively less important.

Table 10.1 summarizes the pros and cons of the major treatment modalities available.

BCCs and SCCs

Early lesions

The majority of early lesions will be suitable for local excision. The extent of the excision should never be compromised to make the repair easy. If the tumor is in a difficult area, then the patient should be referred on. Margins will from 2–4 mm for a nodular BCC to 6–9 mm for a sclerosing BCC or recurrent lesion.[1] Margin of 5–15 mm are required for SCCs but this will vary according to the site and size of the lesion.[10] Tumors with positive margins should be re-excised or, if this is difficult, referred for post-operative irradiation.

Where there are multiple early BCCs in low risk areas, cryotherapy or curette and cautery may be attempted. The concern is that an infiltrating tumor may be undertreated and this should be avoided in critical areas, e.g. adjacent to the eye. These techniques should never be used to treat SCC.

Superficial X-ray therapy is appropriate if the patient is elderly or frail, or where surgery will result in major deformity, e.g. lower eyelid, nose and ears. Radiation should be avoided in areas of poor blood supply or areas which will be exposed to friction, trauma or excessive sunlight. A favorable response is less likely to occur with infiltration of bone or cartilage.

Advanced lesion

Large, extensively infiltrating lesions are best managed in a multi-disciplinary clinic with sur-

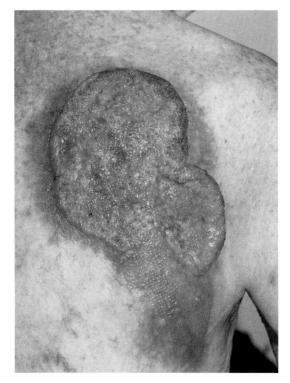

Figure 10.2a. This 70-year-old man presented with a fixed 14 by 20 cm SCC on his back. It was treated with radical radiotherapy.

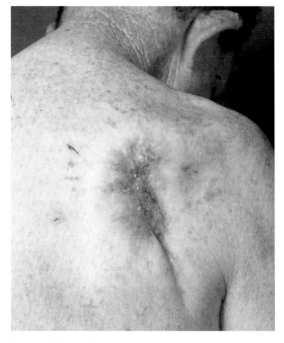

Figure 10.2b. This photo was taken 2 years later. Biopsy showed no evidence of malignancy. He died of an intercurrent illness five years following treatment.

geons and radiation oncologists. The decision to treat with surgery or radiation will depend on the patient's general condition and the likely cosmetic deficit to be caused by surgery (Figure 10.2). On many occasions, combined treatment is undertaken to minimize the morbidity of the surgery (e.g., sacrifice of the facial nerve or exenteration of the eye) and still provide acceptable tumor control. Postoperative irradiation is indicated for advanced or recurrent lesions, positive margins, tumor spill, perineural spread or lymphovascular invasion. When the tumor is inoperable, radiation may be given to relieve bleeding, infections, odor and pain.

Elective nodal treatment is not required for BCCs and SCCs as the incidence of nodal spread is so low. Clinically involved nodes should be therapeutically dissected after confirmation with cytology. Postoperative radiotherapy is indicated if there are multiple nodes involved or extracapsular spread. Nodes less than 2–3 cm in size may be controlled with radiation alone.

Lesions with poorly defined margins or recurrent lesions can be treated with Moh's micrographic surgery which involves progressive horizontal resections with histologic mapping using cryosectioning. This can be accomplished in multiple outpatient visits under local anesthesia and reconstructed at a late date.[12]

MCC

This requires specialist treatment. The primary tumor should be resected with a 3 cm margin if practical.[7] Given the high recurrence rate locally and nodally, this should be followed by wide field irradiation to the primary site and relevant nodal areas with coverage of the intransit areas[4] (Figure 10.3). As well as being radiosensitive, the tumor is moderately chemosensitive. Metastatic disease may respond to adriamycin containing regimens such as CHOP (Cyclophosphamide, adriamycin, vincristine, prednisone), carboplatin or etopiside.[14] However, the role of adjuvent chemotherapy is yet to be determined.

Risks of treatment

Treatment-related mortality is extremely low for all modalities of treatment. Surgical scars will improve with time but radiation scars may deteriorate with increased telaiigiectasia, altered pigmentation and

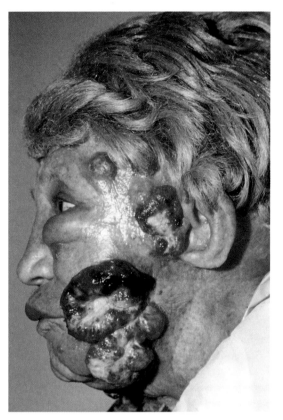

Figure 10.3. This 62-year-old woman had advanced Merkel Cell Carcinoma which recurred in the primary site on the forehead, parotid and cervical nodes, in transit areas and later developed liver secondaries. The primary lesion presented as a small red lump on the forehead which was initially thought to be a BCC.

dermatitis. For external irradiation, an excellent or good cosmetic result occurs in 92% of patients and the overall complication rate is 5.5%.[15] The risks of treatment will increase with the size of the tumor.

Results of treatment

BCCs and SCCs

The five-year disease-free survival for BCCs treated with Moh's micrographic surgery, surgical excision and radiotherapy is 99%, 89% and 91.3% respectively.[12] Eighty-four percent of recurrences will occur in the first two years and 97% with five years of treatment.[16] Results for SCC are marginally inferior with a 4-year disease-free survival of 92.3% treated with radiation.[17]

MCC

The three-year overall and disease-free survival for the group of 80 patients treated at the Queensland Radium Institute is 68% and 29% respectively.[4] The median time to recurrence is 5.5 months and about half of the relapses are systemic.

FOLLOW-UP

Follow-up is an integral part of the patient's care. The purpose should be to diagnose recurrent disease as early as possible as well as to detect new skin lesions. Patients should be encouraged at all times to continue preventive strategies. For BCCs, intervals of six months are reasonable but closer surveillance is required for high risk lesions. The visits for SCCs should be monthly initially and should include examination of the draining lymph nodes. Follow-up should continue until the patient has been disease-free for five years.

MCCs require assessment every 2–3 months as relapses occur early. This includes assessment of the primary, nodal and distant sites.

References

1. Emmett, A. (1991). Basal cell carcinoma. In *Maglinant Skin Tumors*, edited by A.J. Emmett and M.G. O'Rourke, pp. 109–127. Churchill Livingstone.
2. Ashby, M.A. and McEwan, L. (1990). Treatment of non-melanomatous skin cancer: A review of recent trends with special reference to the Australian scene. *Clincal Oncology*, **2**, 284–289.
3. Marks, R. (1995). An overview of skin cancer. *Cancer*, **75**, 607–612.
4. Meeuwissen, J.A., Bourne, R.G. and Kearsley, J.H. (1995). The importance of postoperative radiation therapy in the treatment of merkel cell carcinoma. *Int. J. Radiation Oncology Biol. Phys.*, **31**, 325–321.
5. Safai, B. (1993). Cancers of the skin. In *Cancer: Principles and Practice of Oncology, 4th edn*, edited by V. De Vita and S. Hellman, p. 1567. Philadephia: J.B. Lippincott Co.
6. Weedon, D. (1991). Pathology. In *Malignant Skin Tumours*, edited by A.J. Emmett and M.G. O'Rouke, p. 27. Churchill Livingstone.
7. O'Rourke, M.G. (1991). Merkel cell or neuroendocrine tumour of skin. In *Malignant Skin Tumors*, edited by A.J. Emmett and M.G. O'Rouke, pp. 157–159. Churchill Livingstone.
8. Thompson, S., Jolley, D and Marks, R. (1993). Reduction in solar keratoses regular sunscreen use. *N. Engl. J. Med.*, **329**, 1147–51.

9. McDonald, C. (1995). Status of screening for skin cancer. *Cancer*, **72**, 1066–70.

10. Harris, T.J. (1991). Squamous cell carcinoma. In *Malignant Skin Tumours*, edited by A.J. Emmett and M.G. O'Rouke, pp. 143–51. Churchill Livingstone.

11. International union against cancer (UICC) (1988). *TNM classification of malignant tumours*, 3rd edition. Geneva.

12. Fleming, I.D., Amonette, R., Monaghan, T. and Fleming, M.D. (1995). Principles of management of basal and squamous cell carcinoma of the skin. *Cancer*, **75**, 699–704.

13. Bourne, R.G. (1991). Radiation treatment. In *Malignant Skin Tumours*, edited by A.J. Emmett and M.G. O'Rouke, pp. 217–226. Churchill Livingstone.

14. Boyle, F., Pendlebury, S. and Bell, D. (1995). Further insights into the natural history and management of primary cutaneous neuroendocrine (merkel cell) carcinoma. *Int. J. Radiation Oncology Biol. Phys.*, **31**, 315–323.

15. Lovett, R., Perez, C.A., Shapiro, S.J. and Garcia, D.M. (1990). External irradiation of epithelal skin cancer. *Int. J. Radiation Oncology, Biol. Phys.*, **19**, 235–242.

16. Mendenhall, W.M., Parsons, J.T., Mendenhall, N.P. and Million, R.R. (1987). T2-T4 carcinoma of the skin of the head and neck treated with radical irradiation. *Int. J. Radiation Oncology Biol. Phys.*, **13**, 975–981.

17. Brady, L., Binnink, S. and Fitzpatrick, P. (1987). Skin Cancer. In *Principles and Practice of Radiation Oncology*, edited by C. Perez and L. Brady, pp. 377–394.

11. Malignant Melanoma

W.H. McCARTHY

Sydney Melanoma Unit, Royal Prince Alfred Hospital, Camperdown, Australia

EPIDEMIOLOGY

Melanoma is one of the most rapidly increasing major cancers in the world. In all countries where white skin predominates, incidence has been increasing by 3–8% each year from the early 1960s until 1995.* Increases have been particularly obvious in Scotland, New Zealand and the Australian populations. In non-white populations the increases have generally been small. Mortality has increased generally in the same period but at a much lower rate than these incidence rises. Melanoma now comprises approximately 1.2% of all new cancers worldwide and between 7–8% of new cancers in men and women in developed countries. In Australia where the incidence of melanoma is the highest in the world, it is now the third most common cancer overall and the commonest cancer in the heavily sun exposed state of Queensland. Worldwide, more than 92,000 new cases of melanoma were reported in 1985. Melanoma is the major cause of death in young adult populations, i.e. between 20 and 50, in higher sun exposure countries such as Australia and New Zealand.

PREDISPOSING AND RISK FACTORS

Only two risk factors have been definitely determined as etiologically important for melanoma.

These are sunlight exposure and genetic inheritance. A genetic phenotype which includes light colored hair and eyes, a tendency to freckling, an inability to tan easily and the early development of multiple nevi predisposes to melanoma.

Sunlight exposure is the dominant etiological factor for melanoma and is variously estimated as being responsible for 70–80% of human melanoma. Exposure patterns are important in that intermittent exposure is more closely correlated with melanoma than with non-melanoma skin cancer but in high incidence areas such as Queensland, Australia, this effect is not noted, suggesting that cumulative exposure also plays a significant role in the development of melanoma.

Melanoma has been attributed to other environmental carcinogens such as air pollution from motor vehicles, chemical exposure, stress and diet but none of these factors has been validated as major causes of melanoma. It is not known how sun exposure and genetic susceptibility interact. Early exposure, i.e. before the age of 20, is clearly important and to a large extent determines the number of nevi a person will develop. The number of nevi is a significant indicator of propensity to develop melanoma in later life. While ultraviolet B is known to be a major component in the development of melanoma, recent studies have suggested that ultraviolet A may also play a significant role in the genesis of this cancer. Melanoma is not highly associated with other cancers but an increased incidence of lymphoma and breast cancer has been reported in people who have had melanoma.

---

*Recent data suggests the upward trends in incidence have now ceased in Australia, New Zealand and Scotland.

PATHOLOGY

For many years melanoma was classified according to its morphology, i.e. its clinical appearance and mode of development on the skin. The classification system generally in use describes four basic types of melanoma — superficial spreading melanoma, nodular melanoma, Hutchinson's melanotic freckle melanoma (Lentigo maligna melanoma) and acral lentiginous melanoma. In recent years a fifth category, the desmoplastic neurotropic melanoma was added in some classification systems. The desmoplastic neurotropic melanoma has the propensity to spread along nerves and is more likely to recur locally after apparently adequate excision.

This morphological classification system has now been superseded by the Breslow tumor thickness classification system. Breslow determined that the prognosis for melanoma was closely related to the vertical diameter of the most nodular part of the tumor. Breslow's tumor thickness is measured from the granular cell layer of the epidermis to the deepest malignant cell detected by the pathologist, excluding extension down hair follicles. The Breslow thickness measurement has superseded the Clark McGovern classification in which the depth of the tumor was measured according to the level of the tumor in the skin, i.e. *Level 1 — in situ* lesions at the basement membrane, *Level 2 —* with penetration into the upper papillary dermis, *Level 3 —* reaching the papillary reticular interface, *Level 4 —* reaching into the reticular dermis level, *Level 5 —* the subcutaneous fat. The level is also usually reported by pathologists and does retain a marginal effect on prognosis, i.e. a thin melanoma which reaches level 4 has a slightly worse prognosis than the same lesion at level 2.

The Breslow tumor thickness has now been adopted by the UICC (International Union against Cancer) and the AJCC (American Joint Committee on Cancer) and entered into the TNM (International tumor classification system): T = Tumor, N = Nodes, M = Metastases.

The TNM system uses Breslow thickness to delineate the T stages. The system is as follows:

TIS — tumors confined to the basement membrane (melanoma *in situ*)

T1 — melanoma $\leq$ 0.75 mm in tumor thickness

T2 — melanoma 0.76 mm – 1.5 mm in tumor thickness

T3a — melanoma > 1.5 mm – 3.0 mm in tumor thickness

T3b — melanoma > 3.0 mm – 4.0 mm in tumor thickness

T4 — melanoma > 4.0 mm in tumor thickness

N1 — metastasis $\leq$ 3 cm in diameter

N2 — metastasis > 3 cm in diameter and or in-transit metastases

M — metastatic disease beyond the draining lymph node field

The previous clinical staging system has also been altered to include four stages of melanoma development.

Stage 1 — primary tumor only, tumor thickness $\leq$ 1.5 mm

Stage 2 — primary tumor only, tumor thickness > 1.5 mm

Stage 3 — positive metastatic lymph node involvement regardless of tumor thickness

Stage 4 — metastasis beyond regional lymph nodes

Figure 11.1 shows survival related to tumor thickness. There is a fall off in survival, parallel to increasing tumor thickness.

Histopathology

Clearly the histopathology report is the basic tool for optimal therapy for melanoma. It is important that the clinician provides the appropriate clinical information to assist the pathologist to provide the best possible report. Clinical information on the request form must include the age and gender of the patient, the exact site of the lesion, its size and color and the duration of symptoms. A previous history of melanoma is important as is a family history and the presence of other skin lesions, particularly the dysplastic nevus syndrome. A diagram of the excision specimen with markers for orientation should be provided. It is very important that specimens be carefully placed in separate, accurately labeled containers particularly when more than one lesion is excised. The pathologist must then provide for the clinician all of the histopathological parameters which are necessary for determining therapy and prognosis. An adequate pathology report should include the following clinical and pathological features:

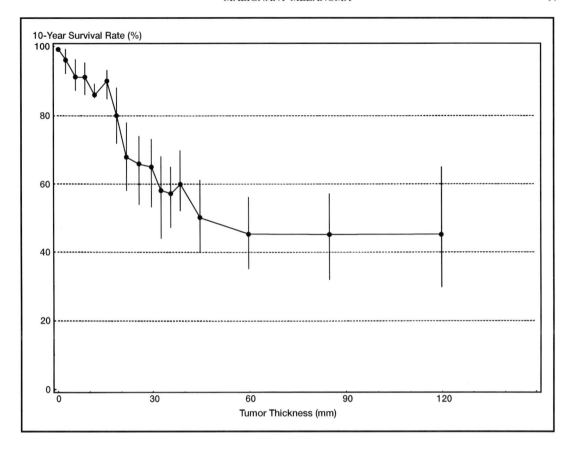

Figure 11.1. Relationship between tumor thickness and 10-year survival rates in primary cutaneous melanoma. The solid curve represents an estimation of the observed relationship. The vertical bars indicate the 95% confidence intervals. Buttner *et al.* (1995). *Cancer*, **75**, 2499–2506.

1. The site and size of the macroscopic lesion in relation to the size and shape of the total biopsy specimen.
2. The physical characteristics of the lesion, i.e. color, shape, nodularity, areas of regression.
3. The margin of excision from the visible edge of the tumor.
4. The presence of other important prognostic features such as satellites, surgical scar and ulceration.

The histopathological report should include:

1. The type of melanoma, i.e. SSM, nodular, acral lentiginous etc.
2. The tumor thickness
3. The Clark level
4. The mitotic rate
5. The presence of regression

6. The presence or absence of ulceration
7. The presence and site of satellites
8. The presence or absence of lymphatic or vascular invasion
9. The characteristics of any lymphocytic infiltration detected
10. The presence or absence of pigment
11. The presence of desmoplasia and/or neurotropism
12. The excision margins as measured microscopically

It is advisable that the clinician consults with the pathologist if the pathology report does not accord with the clinician's diagnosis of the tumor. In cases of doubt, a second opinion should be sought.

The histopathology report on lymph nodes should report on the size of the lymph nodes, the number of lymph nodes resected, the size of any lymph node which contains melanoma, the degree to which an individual lymph node is replaced by melanoma and the number of involved nodes. Extranodal spread should also be reported as should the involvement or otherwise of the apical lymph nodes in node dissection. All these factors determine the risk of local recurrence in the operative area and the overall prognosis for the patient.

PROTECTIVE FACTORS

The only known protective factor against melanoma is sunlight avoidance. While sunscreens are useful in the prevention of melanoma, the most effective way to avoid sunlight damage to the skin is restriction of exposure to sunlight during the peak intensity periods, i.e. between 11.00 a.m. and 3.00 p.m., particularly in the summer months. Additional benefit can be gained by the wearing of a hat and appropriate clothing with high protective factors, such as colored fabrics, fabrics impregnated with ultraviolet absorbers, and loosely fitted clothing which covers the limbs as well as the trunk. The provision of shade structures for recreational activity is also important in the prevention of sunlight damage to the skin.

Sunscreens should be seen as complementary to general sun avoidance. High protection factor sunscreens should be chosen especially by those with the risk factors noted above. Water resistant sunscreens are needed for swimmers. Broad spectrum sunscreens with UVB and some UVA protection are recommended.

SCREENING

Population screening for melanoma is not considered to be cost-effective. However, opportunistic screening, i.e. case finding, by an informed community and trained health professionals has achieved a substantial reduction in mortality from melanoma in high incidence countries such as Australia. The median tumor thickness in Australia in the past 20 years has fallen from 2.0 mm to 0.75 mm suggesting the success of public education programs relating to early diagnosis and opportunistic screening by the population themselves, as well as by medical and health professional practitioners.

In Australia a single television program undertaken by the 60 Minutes television team and the Melanoma Foundation of the University of Sydney, resulted directly in the diagnosis of 1000 new melanomas in the three months following the television program, attesting to the power of television as a public education medium and an effective method of encouraging self-screening for melanoma.

CLINICAL PRESENTATION

Although melanoma is still classified morphologically as superficial spreading melanoma (SMM), nodular melanoma (NM), lentigo maligna melanoma (LMM, Hutchinson's melanotic freckle melanoma) and acral lentiginous melanoma (ALM), Breslow thickness has become the important descriptor to determine prognosis and therapy. The clinical history is important, particularly the role of change of the lesion. Inflammatory and traumatized skin lesions develop in days or weeks, melanoma change is measured in months and benign pigmented lesions such as seborrhoeic keratoses and pigmented basal cell carcinomas have a very long history with very little change having been noted. However, these characteristics are not immutable and many melanomas have been reported to have been present and slowly changing for as long as 20 years while still remaining superficial on histopathological criteria. The changes indicative of melanoma are variation in color, increase in size, irregularity of the borders and elevation of part or all of the lesion. Intermittent itch is often noted. Melanoma can occur from a pre-existing nevus or from unblemished skin.

The clinical diagnosis of melanoma is assisted by the ABCDE classification of descriptors.

A — Asymmetry: Asymmetry is also sometimes described as point and axial asymmetry in that one quadrant of the lesion does not resemble the same area on the opposite quadrant (Figure 11.2).

B — Border: The border description is that of a "coastline" with an irregular border which is often well defined at least in one area of the circumference (Figure 11.3).

C — Color: The color descriptor refers to the variegation of the color, not specifically a blue black color which is often said to be characteristic of melanoma, but a multiplicity of colors which in-

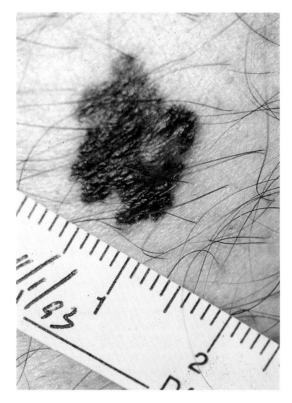

Figure 11.2. Melanoma — asymmetry.

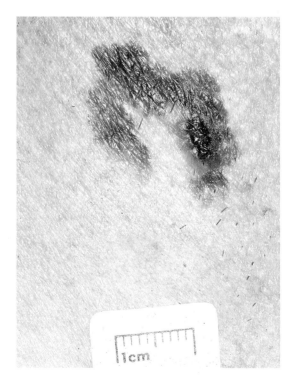

Figure 11.3. Melanoma — "coastline" border.

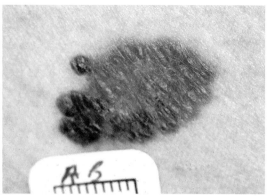

Figure 11.4. Melanoma — multiple colors.

cludes blues, black, red, gray and even total depigmentation resembling normal skin in some areas of the lesion (Figure 11.4).

D — Diameter: Diameter refers to the fact that most melanomas when they first present will be greater than 6 mm, although it is now possible to diagnose these lesions as small as 2 mm.

E — Elevation: Elevation in recent years has been replaced by "**Examination**" as attempts are now made to ensure that diagnosis is made before a nodular component develops. **E** is therefore used to alert the clinician to compare the suspicious lesion with the patient's other nevi, i.e. EXAMINE all the patient's nevi.

Other clinical findings useful in the diagnosis of melanoma are the development of a fine keratin scale on the surface of the lesion, a loss of skin lines giving an amorphous glassy appearance (Figure 11.5), the development of a small red halo around the lesion, loss of hair as the lesion develops, lack of extensive keratinization making the lesion feel

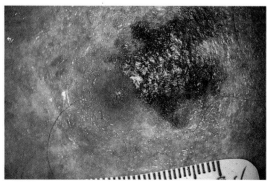

Figure 11.5. Melanoma — amorphous surface.

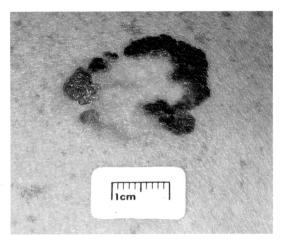

Figure 11.6. Melanoma — regression.

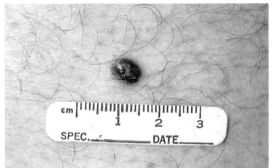

Figure 11.7a. Hemangioma — clinical appearance.

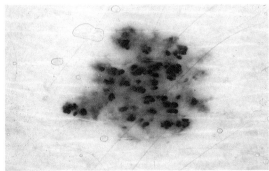

Figure 11.7b. Hemangioma — surface microscopy.

relatively soft to the touch in relation to other skin lesions, and the presence of depigmented areas (regression) (Figure 11.6).

Primary malignant melanoma may develop from a pre-existing nevus, particularly of the dysplastic type, or may develop from normal skin. Superficial spreading melanoma is more likely to derive from a pre-existing nevus while nodular melanoma may arise from a nevus or the normal skin. The degree to which melanoma can be attributed to pre-existing nevi is contentious with estimations ranging from 30–70%.

DIFFERENTIAL DIAGNOSES

Melanoma can be diagnosed by direct observation and surface microscopy but it is useful to consider the differential diagnoses and confirm the diagnosis by exclusion of the other common pigmented lesions. The lesions most commonly mistaken for melanoma are dysplastic nevus, blue nevus, hemangioma, pigmented basal cell carcinoma and pigmented seborrhoeic keratosis. Each of these lesions has characteristic clinical and dermatoscopic appearances (Figures 11.7–11.10).

Dysplastic nevi

Dysplastic nevi are diagnosed by size, shape and color. Dysplastic nevi tend to be larger than normal nevi, usually greater than 6.0 mm, in maximum diameter irregular in outline, although usually oval

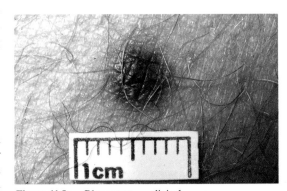

Figure 11.8a. Blue nevus — clinical.

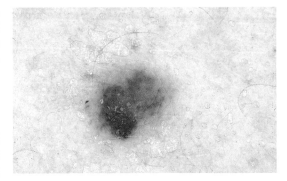

Figure 11.8b. Blue nevus — surface microscopy.

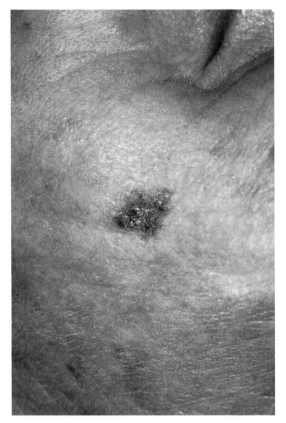

Figure 11.9a. Pigmented basal cell carcinoma (BCC) — clinical.

Figure 11.9b. Pigmented BCC — surface microscopy.

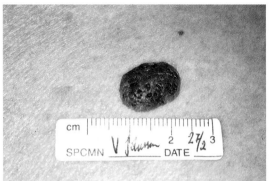

Figure 11.10a. Seborrhoeic keratosis — clinical.

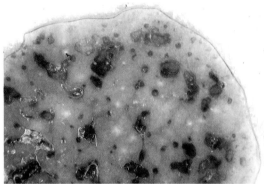

Figure 11.10b. Seborrhoeic keratosis — surface microscopy.

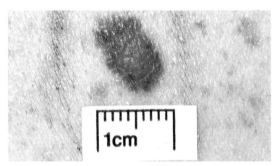

Figure 11.11a. Dysplastic nevus — clinical.

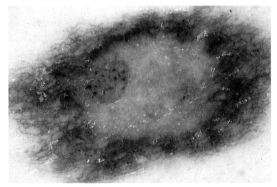

Figure 11.11b. Dysplastic nevus — surface microscopy.

or round (Figures 11.11a,b). The pigmentation within the nevus varies in intensity but shades of brown predominate with the occasional area of redness and partial depigmentation. The edge of the lesion is indefinite and fades off into the surrounding tissue, sometimes called a "shoulder." Dysplastic nevi are often multiple and in some cases a hereditary tendency exists. Where multiple nevi of this type occur, with more than 50 dysplastic nevi being present on the patient's skin, with nevi on non-

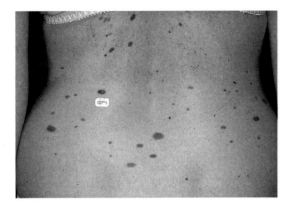

Figure 11.12a.   Dysplastic nevus syndrome.

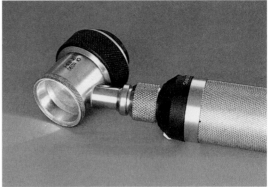

Figure 11.13.   Surface microscope (dermatoscope).

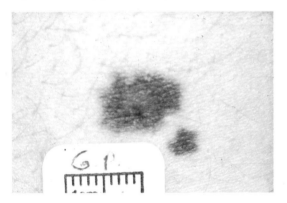

Figure 11.12b.   Dysplastic naevi — variation in size.

exposed areas, i.e. below the waist, in the axilla or in the scalp, the condition is referred to as the dysplastic nevus syndrome (DNS) or the atypical mole syndrome (AMS) (Figures 11.12a,b). Patients with these syndromes are more likely to develop malignant melanoma and this predisposition is particularly apparent in patients where the DNS phenotype has a clear hereditary component. If melanoma has occurred in a family with the DNS phenotype, the person with DNS has a very high likelihood of developing a melanoma and must be placed on a lifetime skin surveillance program.

Surface microscopy

Surface microscopy (dermatoscopy, epiluminescence surface microscopy) is now gaining a place in the clinical diagnosis of melanoma and pigmented tumors of the skin. The cumbersome epiluminescence microscope has been replaced by a simple hand-held instrument, the dermatoscope (Figure 11.13). This instrument provides for the clinician a

10-times magnification of the lesion and the use of microscope oil on the skin renders the keratin layer of the skin translucent, allowing a range of features in the epidermis and dermis to be visualized. Many pigmented lesions which formerly were confused with melanoma have characteristic dermatoscopic appearances, e.g. hemangioma, seborrhoeic keratosis, pigmented basal cell carcinoma and blue nevus (Figures 11.8b, 11.9b, 11.10b, 11.11b, 11.12b). Training in the use of the dermatoscope is essential to achieve its maximum benefit but all clinicians can improve their diagnostic accuracy for pigmented lesions of the skin with the use of dermatoscopic atlases and experience with the instrument. A number of features which indicate that a lesion is likely to be malignant have been developed. The main fea-

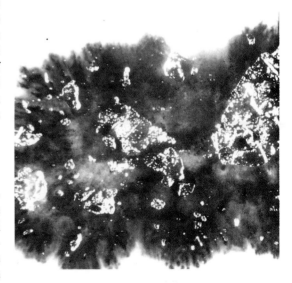

Figure 11.14.   Melanoma — radial streaming and pseudopods.

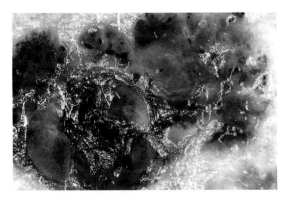

Figure 11.15. Melanoma — Peripheral black dots and globules.

tures which delineate a melanoma from a dysplastic nevus and other benign pigmented lesions are radial streaming and pseudopods (Figure 11.14), peripheral black dots (Figure 11.15), a blue/gray veil (Figure 11.16) and a multiplicity of colors (Figure 11.17).

Biopsy of pigmented lesions

Careful clinical examination and the use of the

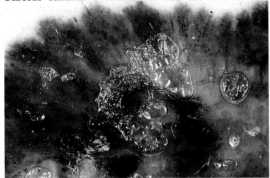

Figure 11.16. Melanoma — blue gray veil.

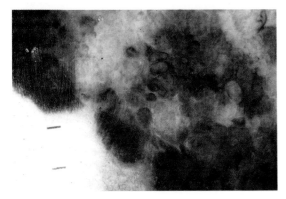

Figure 11.17. Melanoma — multiple colors.

dermatoscope will delineate at least 90% of pigmented tumors of the skin. However, there will remain a small number of pigmented lesions where the clinical and dermatoscopic features are not diagnostic and in these cases clinical excision/biopsy must be undertaken to determine the exact histopathology of the lesions. Shave and punch biopsies should only be undertaken when the lesion is too large for excision biopsy. Shaves and punch biopsies may fail to obtain the necessary histological features to adequately plan the subsequent definitive therapy. A biopsy margin of 2 mm is recommended.

Occult primary melanoma

Occult primary melanoma comprises at least 4% of the presentation of melanoma in the community. Occult melanoma indicates that the patient presents with secondary tumors, usually in the lymph nodes, but sometimes systemically, without any primary tumor being detected on the skin. In Australia, melanoma is now the commonest cause of the presentation of an asymptomatic lymph node in a patient between the age of 20 and 50.

Secondary melanoma (metastases)

Secondary melanoma, apart from metastases in the lymph nodes, characteristically metastasizes to four main areas — the brain, the lung, the liver and the subcutaneous tissues, but melanoma has the propensity to metastasize to virtually every organ in the body.

Paraneoplastic syndromes

Paraneoplastic syndromes are extremely rare in melanoma but hypercalcemia and dermatomyositis have been reported.

INVESTIGATIONS

Systemic investigation of patients with primary melanoma is not cost-effective for stages 1 and 2. In some centers systemic investigation is undertaken for stage 3 patients with chest X-ray, FBC and LFTs including LDH, and whole body CT scanning. However, there is no indication that these staging procedures are cost-effective for most of the melanoma patients. It is quite rare to detect systemic dissemination at the time of primary diagnosis. Most recent investigative methods such as MRI and PET (positron emission tomography) scanning have little or no place in the clinical staging of melanoma patients at the time of the first presentation.

PROGNOSTIC FACTORS

The prognosis of primary melanoma is almost entirely dependent on the tumor thickness measurement. The finding of ulceration of the lesion and a high mitotic rate has some independent prognostic value but at the present time all other features have little or no independent prognostic significance. Age, gender and site of the tumor have been declared to have some independent prognostic value but these studies have not been confirmed appropriately. Prognostic indicators such as nuclear volume, total tumor volume, T cell infiltrate have as yet no proven independent value. The survival rate from melanoma closely parallels the tumor thickness measurement (Figure 11.1).

TREATMENT

The treatment of a primary melanoma and lymph node involvement is entirely surgical. The recommended margins of excision of a primary melanoma are as follows:

1. **TIS** — excision with a minimum margin of 5 mm
2. **TI to T3 tumors** — excision with a minimum margin of 1 cm
3. **T4 tumors** — excision with a minimum margin of 2 cm

In no instance is a margin greater than 3 cm necessary for the adequate treatment of primary melanoma. For T1, T2 and T3 tumors it is difficult to justify a margin greater than 2 cm. In most instances primary closure can be achieved but in some areas of the body, flap repair may provide a better cosmetic outcome.

Elective lymph node dissection

At the present time no evidence exists that elective lymph node dissection offers any benefit for tumors < 1.5 mm. The question of elective lymph node dissection for thicker melanoma, i.e. T3 and T4 tumors, has been addressed recently by two randomized controlled trials. Both of these trials show no benefit for elective lymph node dissection for melanoma of the limbs. However, subset analyses of these studies have suggested a benefit may continue to exist for trunk melanoma, particularly in males. A final decision relating to this matter awaits the final publication of these international trials.

In recent years a new technique known as sentinel node biopsy and selective lymphadenectomy has been developed as an alternative to elective lymph node dissection and for staging of patients with primary melanoma. In this technique the "sentinel" node is detected by lymphoscintigraphy and marked on the skin. At the subsequent operation patent blue dye is injected around the biopsy site and an incision is made over the previously marked sentinel node. The node which is then blue is removed and submitted to histopathology, including immunohistochemistry. Should the node be found to contain melanoma an elective lymph node dissection is performed. This technique is currently being validated by a major international controlled clinical trial. Prior to the results of this trial being reported, this technique cannot be recommended for general use. Without excellent lymphoscintigraphy and specific training in the surgical technique, the management of the melanoma patient can be compromised by inadequate identification and biopsy of non-sentinel nodes.

RISKS OF TREATMENT

The treatment for primary melanoma is virtually without morbidity, apart from the usual surgical complications of wound infection and wound dehiscence, both of which are rare complications. Node dissection may lead to persistent lymphodema, particularly in the leg, and subsequent development of repeated attacks of cellulitis. Lymphodema is treated by compression stockings and antibiotics are used to control the cellulitis which is usually streptococcal in origin and responds well to the appropriate antibiotics such as penicillin and flucloxacillin.

Treatment of metastatic melanoma

Metastatic melanoma confined to the lymph nodes is treated by radical lymph node dissection. Metastasis beyond the lymph nodes, i.e. in the lung, brain and sometimes in the abdomen, may be treated surgically by excision if the metastasis is found to be solitary at that time. Surgical excision of secondary melanoma provides good palliation but seldom results in long-term cure. It must therefore be considered in the context of overall treatment for the patient which may include other forms of therapy such as chemotherapy, radiotherapy and experimental protocols such as immunotherapy. The standard chemotherapeutic agent for melanoma is DTIC (dimethyl triazeno imidazole carboxamide) but complete remissions of only 5% and partial remissions up to 20% only can be expected. Currently less than 5% of patients with disseminated melanoma survive longer than two years and only 1% survive longer than five years. Most melanoma chemotherapy at the present time thus involves the patient in controlled clinical trials of newer agents or combination regimens.

RESULTS OF TREATMENT

The overall results of treatment of primary melanoma are excellent at the present time especially in countries of high incidence such as Australia. Early diagnosis of thin tumors has led to an overall survival in excess of 80%. The survival figures for melanoma are approximately as follows:

T1S tumors — 100% survival
T1 tumors — 97% survival
T2 tumors — 90% survival
T3 tumors — 75% survival
T4 tumors — 45% survival

With lymph nodes involved, the outcome is related to the number of lymph nodes involved. With only one lymph node involved the 10-year survival is around 40% but if five or more lymph nodes are involved it is rare for survival to exceed 10%.

ADJUVANT THERAPY

To date no adjuvant therapy has been developed which has a survival benefit. Chemotherapy, immunotherapy with vaccines and interferon have been shown to prolong survival but do not at the present time influence overall survival. It is thus important that patients with high risk melanoma be offered entry into clinical trials of new therapies if the prognosis for these patients is to be improved in the future.

FOLLOW-UP

Follow-up protocols are based on tumor thickness. Little benefit is to be gained by continuous follow-up of patients with thin melanomas, i.e. < 1.5 mm unless the person has a family history of melanoma or one of the atypical mole syndromes. An acceptable protocol for T1 and T2 tumors is a six-monthly review for two years and a skin surveillance examination on a yearly basis where the number of moles justifies such an approach. For T3 and T4 tumors a more extensive follow-up protocol may be appropriate with a four-monthly review for two years, six-monthly review for two years and thereafter yearly for 10 years. For stage 3 melanoma (i.e. node positive) a similar protocol is appropriate but systemic investigation on a regular basis, initially at six months, again at eighteen months and thereafter yearly for five years may be appropriate. Systemic investigation is currently best achieved with a CT scan of the brain, lung and abdomen as well as a general clinical examination.

At all follow-up visits the clinical examination includes careful inspection and palpation of the primary site, palpation of the draining lymph nodes, examination of any subcutaneous masses indicated by the patient and a general skin surveillance to check the other nevi.

References
1. Balch, C.M., Houghton, A.N., Milton, G.W., Sober, A.J. and Soong S.J. (1992). *Cutaneous Melanoma*. J.B. Lippincott Company.
2. Lejeune, F.J., Chaudhuri, P.K. and Das Gupta, T.K. (1994). *Malignant Melanoma: Medical and Surgical Management*. McGraw-Hill.
3. Gallagher, R.P. and Elwood, J.M. (1994). *Epidemiological Aspects of Cutaneous Malignant Melanoma*. Kluwer Academic Publishers.
4. Cascinelli, N., Santinami, M. and Veronesi, U. (1990).

Cutaneous Melanoma Biology and Management. Masson.

5. Menzies, S.W., Crotty, K.A., Ingvar, C. and McCarthy, W.H. (1996). *An Atlas of Surface Microscopy of Pigmented Skin Lesions*. McGraw-Hill.

6. Stolz, W., Braun-Falco, O., Bilek, P., Landthaler, M. and Cognetta, A.B. (1994). *Color Atlas of Dermatoscopy*. Blackwell Science.

7. Barnhill, R.L., Fitzpatrick, T.B., Fandrey, K., Kenet, R.O., Mihm, M.C. and Sober, A.J. (1995). *Color Atlas and Synopsis of Pigmented Lesions*. McGraw-Hill.

8. McCarthy, W.H. and Shaw, H.M. (1992). Progress Symposium on Melanoma. *World J Surg*, **16**, 155–286.

9. Guidelines for the Management of Cutaneous Melanoma (1997). Australian Cancer Network.

Melanoma of Skin

Rapid recent increases in white populations

Lifetime risk
in USA whites:
 M 1 in 85
 F 1 in 100

in New South Wales:
 M 1 in 26
 F 1 in 41

Relative five-year survival in 1983–87
in USA whites:
 M 80.1%
 F 88.8%

Risk factors
Exposure to sunlight, especially in childhood
Fair skin, fair hair, blue eyes
Dysplastic nevus syndrome
Family history of melanoma

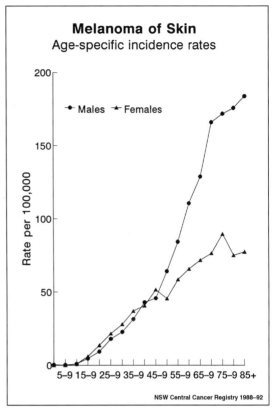

Melanoma of Skin
Age-specific incidence rates

NSW Central Cancer Registry 1988–92

Geographical variation in 1995
Highest rate
M. 46.2 per 100,000 in NSW, Australia
F: 28.8 per 100,000 in NSW, Australia

Lowest rate
M: 0.2 per 100,000 in India, Bombay
F: 0.2 per 100,000 in India, Bombay

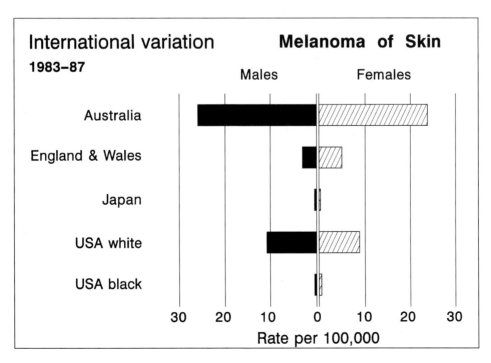

International variation 1983–87
Melanoma of Skin
Males   Females
Australia
England & Wales
Japan
USA white
USA black
Rate per 100,000

12. Central Nervous System Tumors

GEOFFREY SHARPE and MICHAEL BRADA

Neuro-oncology Unit & Academic Unit of Radiotherapy & Oncology, The Institute of Cancer Research & The Royal Marsden NHS Trust, Downs Road, Sutton, Surrey SM2 5PT UK

EPIDEMIOLOGY

Primary tumors of the central nervous system are uncommon with an age adjusted annual incidence ranging from 6–12 per 100,000 population. They represent less than 5% of all primary tumors in adults, but are the commonest non-hematological group of tumors in childhood. The brain and spinal cord are also a frequent site of metastatic disease.

Primary brain tumors have specific age predilection, with most adult tumors arising within the cerebral hemispheres, whereas in childhood the majority occur within the posterior cranial fossa. Primitive neuro-ectodermal tumors (PNETs), pilocytic astrocytomas, craniopharyngiomas and optic nerve gliomas occur most frequently in childhood, intracranial germ cell tumors present in the teens and early twenties while the incidence of most glial and meningeal tumors is highest in adults and increases with age. Gliomas constitute the largest histological group of primary brain tumors.

ETIOLOGY

The mechanisms involved in the causation and progression of primary brain tumors remain unclear and the majority of patients have no discernible predisposing factors.

Table 12.1. Familial disorders predisposing to a higher risk of primary CNS neoplasm.

Familial predisposition	Associated brain neoplasms
Peripheral neurofibromatosis (von Recklinghausen's disease, NF1)	Optic nerve glioma Astrocytoma Ependymoma
Central neurofibromatosis (Bilateral acoustic neurofibroma, NF2)	Meningioma
Gorlin's syndrome	Medulloblastoma
Tuberous sclerosis	Giant cell astrocytoma
Turcot's syndrome (Familial adenomatous polyposis and brain tumor)	Medulloblastoma Astrocytoma
von Hippel–Lindau syndrome	Hemangioblastoma

Inherited predisposition

Type I neurofibromatosis (von Recklinghausen's disease, NF1) predisposes to the development of optic nerve/chiasma glioma as well as meningioma and other glial tumors. Type 2 neurofibromatosis (NF2) (bilateral acoustic neuroma) is associated with increased incidence of meningiomas which are often multiple. Other genetic predispositions are shown in Table 12.1.

Acquired

Immune deficiency following organ transplantation and with HIV infection is associated with increased incidence of primary cerebral lymphoma. Cranial irradiation in childhood is associated with an increased risk of development of glioma and meningioma. Similar tumors have also been described following radiotherapy for benign tumors such as pituitary adenoma and craniopharyngioma. Exposure to low dose irradiation within the nuclear industry or in atomic bomb survivors has not been associated with higher risk.

PATHOLOGY

Primary intracranial tumors may arise from any intracranial tissue. A simplified version of the WHO classification[1] which defines tumor type on the basis of the putative cell of origin is shown in Table 12.2. The commonest brain tumors are of neuro-epithelial origin and include low and high grade astrocytomas. Based on cellular and tissue features many of the brain tumors can be graded according to the degree of malignancy, although the distinction into benign and malignant neoplasms is not as clear as in systemic tumors. Apparently histologically benign tumors can show invasion and simply the presence of a space occupying lesion within the cranial cavity may be fatal. The majority of intracranial tumors do not metastasize but spread locally within the CNS. Germ cell tumors may disseminate systemically via surgical shunts while medulloblastomas and primary cerebral lymphomas may relapse outside the CNS in the absence of shunting.

CLINICAL MANIFESTATION AND DIAGNOSIS OF BRAIN TUMORS

Patients with a brain tumor present with a combination of features of increased intracranial pressure, epilepsy and focal or global neurological deficit. The classical features of raised intracranial pressure are morning headache, vomiting and papilloedema. Focal or generalized convulsions first appearing in adults normally indicate a structural brain lesion and may be the first or only presenting feature of a brain tumor. Neurological deficit commonly relates to site of tumor (Table 12.3), although some

Table 12.2. WHO classification of CNS tumors.

I	TUMORS OF NEUROEPITHELIAL TISSUE
	A. ASTROCYTIC TUMORS including
	Astrocytoma
	Anaplastic (malignant) astrocytoma
	Glioblastoma
	Pilocytic astrocytoma
	Pleomorphic xanthoastrocytoma
	Subependymal giant cell astrocytoma
	B. OLIGODENDROGLIAL TUMORS
	C. EPENDYMAL TUMORS
	D. MIXED GLIOMAS
	E. CHOROID PLEXUS TUMORS
	F. NEUROEPITHELIAL TUMORS OF UNCERTAIN ORIGIN
	G. NEURONAL AND MIXED NEURONAL-GLIAL TUMORS
	including ganglioma, Central neurocytoma, Olfactory neuroblastoma
	H. PINEAL TUMORS
	pineocytoma and pineoblastoma
	G. EMBRYONAL TUMOR
	including Neuroblastoma, Ependymoblastoma, Retinoblastoma and Primitive neuroectodermal tumors (PNETs) especially Medulloblastoma
II	TUMORS OF CRANIAL AND SPINAL NERVES SCHWANNOMA AND NEUROFIBROMA
III	TUMORS OF THE MENINGES
	A. TUMORS OF MENINGOTHELIAL CELLS
	Meningioma (bening, atypical and malignant)
	B. MESENCHYMAL, NON-MENINGOTHELIAL TUMORS
	Benign or malignant (e.g. meningeal sarcoma)
	C. PRIMARY MELANOCYTIC LESIONS
	Melanosis, Melanocytoma and Malignant melanoma
	D. TUMORS OF UNCERTAIN ORIGIN
	Hemangiopericytoma and Haemangioblastoma
IV	HAEMOPOETIC NEOPLASMS
	including Primary cerebral lymphoma and Plasmacytoma
V	GERM CELL TUMORS
	Germinoma and Teratoma
VI	CYSTS AND TUMOR-LIKE LESIONS
VII	TUMORS OF THE ANTERIOR PITUITARY
	Pituitary adenoma
VIII	MALFORMATIONS AND LOCAL EXTENSIONS OF REGIONAL TUMORS
	Craniopharyngioma
	Chordoma, Chondroma and Chondrosarcoma
IX	METASTATIC TUMORS

Table 12.3. Specific clinical syndromes.

Frontal lobe
   Changes in personality and intellectual impairment
   Epilepsy
   Dysphasia (dominant hemisphere)
   Weakness of facial muscles or hemiparesis
   Disturbance of gait ("frontal ataxia")
   Physical signs include abnormal grasp and pouting
     responses

Pariental lobe
   Sensory and visual inattention
   Dysphasia (dominant hemisphere)
   Lower homonymous quadrantinopia
   Apraxia/Agnosia (non-dominant hemisphere)
   Finger Agnosia/Acalculia/Agraphia (dominant lobe –
     Gerstmann's Syndrome)

Temporal lobe
   Epilepsy with auditory, olfactory or gustatory features
   Hemiparesis
   Dysphasia (dominant hemisphere)
   Upper homonymous quadrantinopia

Occipital lobe
   Visual disturbance
   Homonymous hemianopia

Cerebellum
   Ataxic gait
   Intention tremor
   Dysmetria
   Dysarthria
   Nystagmus

apparently focal features such as sixth cranial nerve palsy may be misleading and can be a described as "false localizing sign."

The investigation of choice in patients with suspected brain tumor is computerized tomography (CT) scan or magnetic resonance imaging (MRI). CT scan usually demonstrates distortion of normal brain architecture and the presence of space occupying lesion of varying radiological density. The degree of enhancement following intravenous contrast is characteristic for each tumor type. Enhancing lesions have to be distinguished from abscess, multiple sclerosis, infection, sarcoid, vascular abnormalities and hemorrhage. Low density unenhancing lesions have to be differentiated from localized encephalitis, multiple sclerosis or infarction.

MRI provides similar information to CT scan with better contrast discrimination. It is superior in demonstrating lesions in the posterior and temporal fossi as it is free of bone artefacts although calcification and bone changes are more difficult to demonstrate. Cerebral angiography may help to distinguish vascular lesions (arteriovenous malformations and aneurysms) from neoplasia and demonstrate the details of circulation proir to surgical intervention. MR angiography demonstrates larger vessels without the need for contrast angiography, but currently cannot reliably demonstrate low-flow vascular lesions.

Positron emission tomography (PET) has currently little primary diagnostic role, but may complement other imaging modalities especially in the distinction of radiation necrosis from recurrent tumor.

In the diagnosis of spinal tumors MRI with and without contrast (gadolinium EDTA) is the investigation of choice. If not available, plain X-ray myelography and CT myelography are used although the enhancement characteristics of intrinsic cord lesions cannot be demonstrated.

TREATMENT OF BRAIN TUMORS

Medical management

Prior to definitive diagnosis and before specific anti-tumor therapy patients with features of raised intracranial pressure are treated empirically with corticosteriods (initial oral Dexamethasone 4 mg 3–4 times daily) and occasionally with osmotic diuresis (10–20% mannitol, 100–200 mls, given two or three times a day). This provides symptomatic relief and may also produce a transient improvement in focal neurological deficit. Corticosteroid dose should be reduced and titrated against symptoms to the lowest effective level. In patients who derive little or no benefit they should be withdrawn. Once definitive anti-tumor therapy has started it is important to monitor the dose closely and discontinue corticosteroids at the earliest opportunity to avoid potentially disabling long-term side effects. Epilepsy is treated with appropriate anticonvulsants.

Surgery

Neurosurgical intervention as in other oncological surgery aims to obtain tissue for histological diagnosis and remove tumor with curative or palliative intent. However, direct tumor involvement of eloquent regions in the brain increases the hazards of any surgical procedure often with unacceptable consequences.

Neurosurgical techniques and morbidity have seen great advances. Image directed stereotactic methods allow three-dimensional (3D) localization and visualization of intracranial lesions. Stereotactically guided needle biopsy can obtain small tissue samples with high precision. It carries minimal morbidity and obviates the need for craniotomy. Surgical resection can also be aided by 3D image reconstruction from CT and MRI in the plane of resection and by intraoperative ultrasound and endoscopy. Awake craniotomy with electrophysiological mapping also allows for more controlled tumor resection with diminished morbidity.

Traditional neuro-surgical approaches involve a craniotomy with the lifting of a skull flap which permits biopsy or resection under direct vision. Sites previously inaccessible to conventional craniotomy such as the region of the skull base can now be reached through novel trans-oral, facial or orbital approaches. However, deep-seated hemispheric or brain stem tumors which are closely involved with functionally critical structures cannot normally be removed without unacceptable neurological morbidity.

Malignant tumors are usually widely infiltrating and complete excision is rarely if ever possible. Tumor resection provides effective relief of symptoms but in most malignant tumors the influence of extent of resection on tumor control and survival is not clear. In patients with suspected malignant tumors surgery is frequently limited to a biopsy. Radical resection is an essential component of management in some malignant tumors such as medulloblastoma and ependymoma.

Palliative surgical procedures such as shunting and cyst drainage are important components of treatment and palliative tumor resection may be useful in patients with symptomatic poorly chemo and radioresponsive tumours.

Radiotherapy

Radiotherapy is one of the most effective treatment modalities in the management of patients with intracranial tumors. In some rare malignant brain tumors such as germinoma, radiotherapy is curative. The excellent disease control following conservative surgery and radiotherapy in the more benign tumors such as optic nerve glioma, pituitary adenoma and craniopharyngioma has established radiotherapy as the essential component of treatment. Radical radiotherapy is also a potentially curative treatment in medulloblastoma and other PNETs. In high grade gliomas radiotherapy achieves prolongation of disease-free survival and survival. In low grade glioma and meningioma the role of radiotherapy is not yet clear and the suggestion of its effectiveness is based on selected series of patients receiving radiotherapy following incomplete tumor excision. Radiotherapy is also an effective palliative treatment in patients with brain metastases.

The amount of radiation which can be delivered to CNS tumors is limited by the normal radiation tolerance of the brain and spinal cord. Radiation damage can be classified according to time of appearance into early and late. Late radiation damage to the CNS is due to depletion of oligodendrocytes and endothelial cells leading to demyelination and necrosis and consequent neurological deficit specific to the damaged site. Late damage to the spine is expressed as progressive radiation myelopathy causing paraparesis. The risk of late injury is highly dependent upon dose-fractionation parameters, with the highest risk of damage following large doses given in few fractions. Neurological sequelae of radiation may also be enhanced by chemotherapy (e.g. methotrexate), given either within a short time of radiation or concurrently.

The developing brain is particularly sensitive to injury and brain irradiation in young children may result in severe neuropsychological impairment. Cranial irradiation is best avoided for children under 3–4 years of age. The likelihood of global damage diminishes with full myelination and beyond the age of seven years the neurotoxicity is similar to that in adults. The pituitary gland is also sensitive to radiation with delayed pituitary failure which is dose dependent.

The precision of cranial irradiation has improved with the use of neurosurgically derived stereotactic technology. Small lesions can be treated by highly localized radiation which achieves better sparing of normal tissue and this is described as stereotactic external beam radiotherapy (SRT) or by stereotactically guided interstitial radiotherapy. (SRT) can be either fractionated or single fraction treatment (described as "radiosurgery").

Radiosurgery is also used for the eradication of small inoperable arteriovenous malformations and is being investigated in the treatment of solitary brain metastases.

Chemotherapy

Within a tumor, the blood-tumor barrier (BTB) is usually permeable and the main determinant of the effectiveness of chemotherapy is most likely the primary chemosensitivity of the individual tumor types. Cranial germ cell tumors, PNETs and primary cerebral lymphoma are chemosensitive intracranial tumors and chemotherapy is being used with increasing frequency, although the precise role in the management of these tumors is not yet fully defined. Although the overall effectiveness of chemotherapy in gliomas is poor it occasionally achieves palliation in recurrent tumors and in an adjuvant setting produces a marginal survival advantage.

Rehabilitation and continuing care

Patients with CNS tumors frequently have major neurological deficits with physical disability as well as cognitive impairment, communication difficulties and personality change. All those with reasonable life expectancy need active rehabilitation managed by a multidisciplinary rehabilitation team. Rehabilitation should not await the completion of specific therapy but should be started shortly after diagnosis as an integral part of management.

The diagnosis of a brain tumor and the accompanying disability often have a devastating effect on the patient, the family and friends and all require sympathetic and practical support.

SPECIFIC BRAIN TUMORS

Gliomas

Gliomas are neuro-epithelial tumors arising from supporting glial tissue and are classified as astrocytomas, oligodendrogliomas and ependymomas. Astrocytomas constitute two thirds of all gliomas and are graded on the basis of cytological and tissue features into three grades of increasing malignancy as astrocytoma, anaplastic astrocytoma and glioblastoma (WHO) or four grades (I–IV) under the Kernohan grading system. Pilocytic astrocytoma and giant cell astrocytoma are localized low grade gliomas and are classified separately.

High grade astrocytomas

High grade astrocytomas are the most common primary malignant brain tumors and are classified into anaplastic astrocytoma and glioblastoma. The incidence increases with age with a peak in the sixth and seventh decade. Anaplastic astrocytoma and glioblastoma are distinguished by the degree of cellular anaplasia, pleomorphism, necrosis, and the presence of endothelial proliferation and hemorrhage. On CT scan high grade gliomas are usually inhomogeneous hyperdense masses enhancing after IV contrast and surrounded by oedema.

Management and prognosis

Clinical suspicion of diagnosis requires histological confirmation usually by stereotactic biopsy. Surgical tumor debulking may follow or replace biopsy. It relieves raised intracranial pressure and may improve neurological deficit. More extensive resection is associated with prolonged survival, but it is likely that it is the resectability of the tumor rather than the debulking itself which is the determinate of outcome as only accessible, moderately sized tumors in relatively fit patients are considered for surgery.

Radiotherapy is the mainstay of treatment and is effective in prolonging survival but is not curative and long-term tumor control and survival remain poor. If effective, it leads to improvements in neurological deficits with a reduction in steroid requirements. The current radiotherapy practice is to treat patients with daily fractions over a period of six weeks to a dose of 55–60 Gy to the tumor and a margin of suspected infiltration. An acceptable alternative is a twice daily accelerated treatment which effectively halves the treatment time. Older or more disabled patients may receive a short course of palliative radiotherapy.

Lower doses of radiation result in worse survival[2] while increasing the dose of localized irradiation with stereotactic external beam radiotherapy or with brachytherapy may improve tumor control and is currently being tested in randomized trials. However, it carries a risk of radiation damage with consequent morbidity and this may require surgical intervention.

Nitrosoureas (BCNU, CCNU) are at present the most effective chemotherapeutic agents in the treatment of high grade gliomas. In randomized studies of adjuvant chemotherapy, the overall survival advantage is 9% at one year and 3% at two years with no increase in long-term survival.[3] The value of adjuvant chemotherapy to an individual patient with high grade glioma is therefore debatable and it is reasonable not to offer routine adjuvant chemotherapy as the small potential benefit may be outweighed by treatment toxicity. However, the poor overall results should encourage clinicians to enter patients into randomized trials testing new treatment approaches.

Considerable research effort is directed to finding new ways of controlling malignant gliomas. This includes optimization of conventional treatment modalities and evaluation of novel treatments such as new chemotherapeutic agents, antibody-directed therapy and gene therapy.

The median survival of patients with high grade glioma treated with conservative surgery and radiotherapy is 40 to 50 weeks with only 10–20% of patients surviving two years. Older age, high histological grade and poor performance status are the most important adverse determinants of survival.[4] Short history of symptoms, the absence of convulsions and limited resection are additional poor prognostic features of lesser significance. The current treatment recommendation is biopsy or tumor debulking followed by radiotherapy. The treatment, however, has to be tailored, to the patient's age and general condition. In severely disabled and elderly patients with short life expectancy it may be appropriate not to offer active treatment. In addition to continuing care, and specific anti-tumor treatment, patients and families require sympathetic care and intensive support from many professionals within a neuro-oncology team.

Low grade gliomas

Low grade gliomas include low grade astrocytomas (defined as astrocytomas on WHO classification), oligodendrogliomas, mixed oligo-astrocytomas and low grade ependymomas as well as a subgroup of localized gliomas such as pilocytic astrocytoma. They present with a long history of features of intracranial tumor and presentation with convulsions is particularly common. On CT scanning they tend to be of low density without enhancement and are occasionally associated with calcification. The MR features are equivalent with low signal intensity on T1 and high intensity on T2-weighted images and they do not enhance with contrast.

Astrocytomas are usually infiltrating tumors occurring in all age groups while pilocytic astrocytomas are well localized and present predominantly in childhood in the posterior fossa. Oligodendrogliomas and mixed oligoastrocytomas which consist of both astrocytic and oligodendroglial components occur in all age groups with a peak incidence between 40 and 60 years.

Ependymomas project from ependymal surfaces, most commonly the floor of the fourth ventricle, and less frequently from the canal of the spinal cord, or the lateral and third ventricles and may also arise in the brain parenchyma. Ependymomas are graded into low and high grade variants.

Management and prognosis

Posterior fossa pilocytic astrocytomas, particularly of cystic type, and low grade ependymomas of the fourth ventricle are best treated with radical resection. Other low grade gliomas often diffusely involve cerebral parenchyma and are not fully excisable. Debulking surgery has a role here as in high grade tumors although the role of more radical procedures is being evaluated. The role of radiotherapy in the treatment of low grade gliomas is controversial and is currently being assessed in prospective randomized studies. However, retrospective studies of incompletely excised tumors suggest a survival advantage for irradiation[5] and radiotherapy is an effective symptomatic treatment and can stabilize or improve the neurological deficit caused by the tumor. The current practice is to treat a localized volume including the radiologically abnormal region with a margin to a dose of 55 Gy over a period of $6\frac{1}{2}$ weeks.

The prognosis in low grade gliomas is determined by age and performance status and to a lesser extent the histology and extent of resection. The five-year survival rate for patients with pilocytic astrocytoma is 80–90% and for patients with astrocytoma, oligodendroglioma, mixed oligo-astrocytoma and low grade ependymomas 40–60%.

Brain stem gliomas

Glial tumours may involve any region of the brain including the thalamus, hypothalamus and the brain stem from mid brain to pons and medulla. Patients with brain stem tumors are mainly children who present with a variety of cranial nerve palsies and posterior fossa signs often causing severe disability. Excision of brain stem tumors is often not possible and frequently even surgical biopsy is considered hazardous. Radiotherapy is the mainstay of treatment and frequently results in neurological improvement. The dose fractionation schedules are similar to low grade gliomas. The prognosis of patients with low grade gliomas is poor with less than 20% becoming long-term survivors.

Optic nerve glioma

Optic glioma is an indolent low grade astrocytoma of the optic pathways which occurs predominantly in childhood and is frequently associated with NF1. Visual disturbance with restriction of visual field and acuity is the commonest presenting feature with occasional headache. The tumor may also compress surrounding structures and cause hydrocephalus. Imaging with MR or CT shows enhancing tumor of the optic chiasm or optic nerves. A biopsy is rarely required, particularly in patients with neurofibromatosis. However, in cases of doubt, histological confirmation can be sought with stereotactic biopsy.

Management and prognosis

The overall management has to take into account age, visual impairment and other disabilities as well as the apparent natural history of the tumor. The majority of patients with slowly progressive or stable tumors do not require immediate therapy. They should be carefully followed with clinical and opthalmological examination and interval scanning. Intervention in the form of radiotherapy, surgery or chemotherapy should be reserved for patients with progressive or symptomatic disease.

Localized radiotherapy is effective at arresting further tumor growth with excellent long-term survival.[6] It also improves or stabilizes vision in the majority.[7] The risk of radiation-induced damage to normal brain can be reduced if the treatment is delayed beyond 4 years of age or more. Progressive tumors in young children can be treated initially with chemotherapy to delay more definitive treatment. Tumors anterior to the chiasma and large exophytic tumors may be resected.

Craniopharyngiomas

Craniopharyngiomas are benign neoplasms arising from epithelial rests in the suprasellar region and commonly have a cystic component. They mostly present in childhood, although may occur at all ages with apparent second peak at 50 to 60 years.

The enlarging suprasellar mass may compress and adhere to adjacent structures which include the optic nerves and chiasma, the pituitary, hypothalamus and the third ventricle. Presenting features depend on the structures affected and include endocrine, visual, or mental disturbances and hydrocephalus. CT or MR scans are frequently diagnostic and show partly cystic and solid suprasellar mass with calcification in the cyst wall.

Management and prognosis

Hydrocephalus requires urgent shunting, tumor decompression or both. Total excision is curative treatment in selected patients, particularly young children, although it carries high morbidity and mortality. The wall of the craniopharyngioma is firmly adherent to surrounding structures and attempts at complete removal may lead to damage which includes severe endocrine deficiency and hypothalamic damage with altered temperature control, fluctuating level of consciousness and uncontrolled obesity. Following incomplete surgery alone, the risk of recurrence is high (65–75%). Radiotherapy is highly effective in controlling the growth of craniopharyngioma and therefore the recommended treatment policy is conservative surgery (aspiration or partial resection) followed by radical local radiotherapy. The recommended dose is 50 Gy in 30 to 33 daily fractions. Following this treatment approach the recurrence rate is 10–20% with 80–100% five-year and 70–90% 10-year survival.[8] Radiation may result in unacceptable damage in young children and these should be treated with radical or limited excision with radiotherapy reserved for the time of recurrence thus allowing the child to reach an age when radiation can be given more safely.

Primitive neuro-ectodermal tumors (PNETs)

PNETs have a common histological appearance of densely cellular masses of uniform small oval or round cells. They include the medulloblastoma of the posterior cranial fossa and histologically similar tumors arising elsewhere in the CNS. They all have a tendency to seed through the subarachnoid space to the spinal cord and distant intracranial sites.

The medulloblastoma is the most common PNET and patients typically present with the signs of cerebellar infiltration and raised intracranial pressure.

Management and prognosis

Patients with medulloblastoma require radical surgery and craniospinal irradiation. Full staging investigations include CSF cytology for the presence of malignant cells and spinal MRI to detect occult spinal seeding. Post-operative radiotherapy is indicated in all patients regardless of the extent of tumor resection. Whole craniospinal axis is irradiated to a dose of 35 Gy and this is followed by a boost to the posterior fossa to a total dose of 55 Gy. Isolated spinal seeding is treated with a local boost.

PNETs are chemosensitive tumors and the role of adjuvant chemotherapy is being assessed in large randomized trials.

With present treatment strategies the five-year survival of patients with medulloblastoma is 50–60%.

Meningiomas

Meningiomas comprise 10–20% of intracranial tumors and their frequency increases with age. They arise in the arachnoid villi of the meninges in the cerebral convexity, the falx and less frequently the sphenoid and suprasellar region, posterior fossa and the tentorium. Most meningiomas are encapsulated solitary tumors attached to the dura. In patients with NF2 they may be multiple. Invasion of the brain parenchyma in benign meningiomas is rare but tumors may invade adjacent skull eliciting an osteoblastic reaction which can be seen on skull X-ray.

Meningiomas present in an indolent fashion with gradual development of focal deficit and occasionally deterioration in intellectual function and personality, which may pass unnoticed. The characteristic CT appearance of a meningioma is a well-defined extra-axial mass with attachment to the meningeal surface. It is usually uniformly hyperdense showing homogenous enhancement with contrast.

There are a number of histological variants of benign meningioma describing the predominant cell pattern. The histological subgroups have no prognostic significance except hemangiopericytic and angioblastic forms which are considered to have

worse prognosis. More aggressive behavior is also associated with higher mitotic rate, necrosis and cellular atypia. Malignant meningeal sarcoma has the appearance of a spindle cell sarcoma and is an invasive malignant tumor.

Management and prognosis
The primary treatment of benign meningioma is complete surgical resection. Tumours which are poorly accessible through conventional craniotomy (e.g. sphenoid) can be approached through skull base techniques, which improve access and may allow for complete tumor excision. Radiotherapy is reserved for patients with incompletely excised or recurrent meningioma. Retrospective studies suggest that high dose local irradiation halves the risk of recurrence.[9] Radiotherapy has also been recommended as adjuvant treatment following incomplete excision of malignant meningioma although the effectiveness is not proven.

The prognosis in patients with meningioma is determined by extent of surgery, tumor histology and neurological performance status. The recurrence rate following complete excision of benign meningioma is less than 3%. Incompletely excised benign tumors following radiotherapy have a five-year progression-free survival of 80–85%. Prognosis in patients with incompletely excised malignant meningioma/sarcoma is poor with a median survival of less than one year.

Pineal tumors

Germ cell tumors (GCTs) including germinoma and non-germinomatous GCTs arise in the suprasellar or pineal regions, and represent more than 60% of the primary tumors at these sites. Germinomas which are histologically equivalent to testicular seminomas are the commonest type.

Pineal region tumors usually present with hydrocephalus and features of compression of the quadrigeminal plate with failure of upward gaze and pupils unresponsive to light or accommodation (Parinaud's syndrome).

Cranial germ cell tumors like their testicular and ovarian counterparts may secrete alphafetoprotein (AFP) or human chorionic gonadotrophin (HCG). The detection of AFP in plasma or CSF is specific for non-seminomatous GCT (teratoma) while HCG may be elevated in teratoma or germinoma.

Management and prognosis

Raised serum and tumor markers obviate the need for a biopsy. Otherwise a biopsy is stereotactically guided or performed under direct or endoscopic vision. In the presence of hydrocephalus, patients may be considered for shunting. However, if germ cell tumor is suspected, shunting may increase the risk of systemic seeding, and should be delayed to enable spontaneous drainage which occurs following successful primary therapy.

Surgical excision is a potentially hazardous procedure with no obvious benefit in germinoma, pineoblastoma or glioma. However, the excision of a residual teratoma following chemotherapy and radiotherapy or the primary excision of localized pineocytoma may be curative.

Radiotherapy is the treatment of choice in localized pineal germinoma and is curative in most patients. This involves local radiotherapy to the pineal region and cranio-spinal irradiation which is given selectively depending on staging and the perceived risk of CNS seeding.[10] Spinal irradiation reduces the risk of spinal relapse, but this should be balanced against the potential toxicity of extended field irradiation, particularly in children with incomplete skeletal growth and in girls whose ovaries may be included in the radiation field. Localized germinoma is treated with cranio-spinal irradiation to 25–30 Gy except in pre-pubertal children and women where this should be given on an individual basis. This is followed by a boost to the primary site to a total dose of 40–45 Gy.

Like their systemic counterparts cranial GCTs are chemosensitive and potentially chemocurable. Platinum-based regimens are being exploited as part of primary treatment in disseminated or locally extensive germinoma and as the treatment of choice in verified teratomas. Disseminated germinoma is treated with a short course of cisplatin/carboplatin containing chemotherapy followed by craniospinal irradiation to a dose of 25–30 Gy and a local boost to 40–45 Gy. Teratomas are best treated with primary chemotherapy with platinum/carboplatin containing regimens used in systemic testicular tumors. This is followed by cranio-spinal axis irradiation and boost to primary site. Residual masses in the pineal region are best excised.

Patients with pineoblastoma are treated with cranio-spinal axis irradiation followed by a boost as other PNETs. The role of radiotherapy in the management of pineocytoma is not clear, and the appropriate therapy is surgical excision.

Primary cerebral lymphoma

Primary cerebral lymphoma (PCL) is a non Hodgkin's lymphoma (NHL) localized to the CNS and is usually a B cell diffuse large cell type. PCL is associated with immune deficiency (part of AIDS or following organ transplantation) or arises sporadically where the frequency increases with age.

The clinical presentation of PCL is indistinguishable from other brain tumors. On CT scanning there are single or multiple masses which are iso or hyperdense with frequent evidence of subependymal spread. An additional feature suggestive of lymphoma is an apparent CT response to corticosteroids. However, the imaging features are not sufficiently diagnostic and histological confirmation is therefore mandatory. Following the histological diagnosis of PCL further staging is restricted to CSF cytology and formal slit-lamp examination of the eyes. In the absence of a known preceding history of NHL there is no need for systemic staging.

Management and prognosis

Sporadic PCL

Surgery should be confined to a diagnostic biopsy and debulking surgical excision has no therapeutic role. Historically radiotherapy had been the mainstay of treatment and produces dramatic radiological and clinical response but the median survival is only 12 to 18 months with the majority of patients relapsing in the CNS and no long-term cures.[11,12]

Patients with PCL respond to chemotherapy which includes conventional NHL protocols (such as CHOP or MACOP-B) or regimens designed to cross the blood brain barrier such as high dose Methotrexate. They have been given in the adjuvant setting either before or after radiotherapy. While there are no randomized studies comparing these approaches, the excellent initial responses to chemotherapy and the effectiveness of chemotherapy in systematic NHL would therefore argue in favor of a combined modality approach in which chemotherapy is given first. The inclusion of intrathecal chemotherapy with methotrexate is recommended in patients with positive CSF cytology. In suitable patients this approach to treatment is associated with a long-term survival rate of 30–40%, which is comparable to that seen in advanced systemic high grade NHL. Patients unable to tolerate intensive treatment, either because of age or poor general condition, should receive radiotherapy alone.

AIDS-related PCL

The management of malignant disease in patients with AIDS depends on the severity of the AIDS complex. In patients with frequent opportunistic infections the presence of PCL has a further adverse effect on prognosis and treatment is aimed at palliation. The usual regimen is whole brain irradiation to a dose of 30 Gy in 10 fractions. More aggressive radiotherapy or combined treatment is reserved for patients with normal bone marrow reserve where PCL is the only presentation in an HIV positive patient.

Brain metastases

Tumors with particularly high risk of brain and meningeal metastases include small cell lung cancer, lymphoblastic and Burkitt's type lymphoma and acute lymphatic leukemia. Because of the high incidence of other solid tumors metastatic disease in the brain is seen most frequently in patients with breast and non-small lung cell cancer. Brain metastases present usually as multiple intracranial lesions or less frequently as solitary masses or as meningeal disease.

Clinical presentation is similar to a primary brain tumor with focal or global neurological impairment frequently with confusional state and multiple deficits. One or more enhancing masses seen on CT or MRI should be distinguished from other multiple lesions such as abscesses, rare opportunistic infections or primary cerebral lymphoma. In the absence of known systemic malignancy patients should undergo limited investigations to exclude tumors treatable systemically such as breast, prostate or small cell lung cancer and rarely lymphoma or thyroid cancer. In the presence of known systemic malignancy biopsy is only indicated if there are unusual features such as a solitary lesion in a patient otherwise free of disease. Patients presenting with lesions suggestive of metastases without a known primary site must undergo a careful systemic examination including rectal and pelvic examination and chest X-ray, prior to biopsy to exclude a more accessible site for obtaining tissue.

Management and prognosis

The treatment of brain metastases is aimed at palliation. Multiple metastases of chemosensitive tumors such as testicular teratoma, lymphoma or small cell lung cancer can be treated with chemotherapy pro-viding the disease is considered chemosensitive. The majority of patients with multiple metastases should receive a short palliative course of whole brain irradiation such as 20 Gy in five fractions which achieves neurological improvement in 60–70% of patients. Higher doses of conventional radiotherapy with more protracted treatment have no further palliative or survival benefit.[13] The prognosis of patients with multiple metastases is poor with a median survival of 3–4 months and which is determined mainly by age, performance status, and extent of control of primary and other metastatic disease. Solitary metastases may be best treated radically either by surgical excision[14] or by stereotactic radiotherapy/radiosurgery.[15]

SPINAL CORD TUMORS

The incidence of primary spinal cord tumors is low and the majority of tumors affecting the spinal cord are metastatic in nature.

Metastatic spinal cord tumors

Metastatic spinal cord tumors usually arise from bone or surrounding soft tissue masses and cause spinal cord compression. The aim of therapy is functional improvement and pain control. The most important determinant of functional outcome is pretreatment functional status. Early diagnosis of spinal cord compression before complete loss of neurological function may forestall paraplegia and allow for recovery of useful function.

Patients with suspected spinal cord compression are treated as a neurological emergency and should have initial plain spinal X-ray followed by spinal MR. In the absence of known primary disease, tissue should be obtained for histological examination. Initial treatment in patients with suspected spinal cord compression includes corticosteroids. Further treatment decision depends on the patient's general condition, functional status, tumor type and the extent of primary and metastatic disease.

Spinal cord compression by tumors of unknown histology progression of neurological deficit despite radiotherapy are indications for surgery. However, long-standing paraplegia rarely recovers and surgery may be withheld. Patients with tumors of known poor radio-responsiveness should also be considered for surgery first. Posterior cord compression is best relieved by posterior approach through a decompressive laminectomy. Disease arising from a vertebral body may be approached through a lateral or anterior approach. Removal of a vertebral body requires grafting and the spine may need subsequent stabilization. Such an intensive procedure is only suitable for patients with good long-term prognosis and limited metastatic disease. Patients with radioresponsive tumors and with common solid tumors such as breast, lung and prostatic carcinoma may be considered for initial radiotherapy. Chemotherapy can be used as initial treatment in tumors such as teratoma or lymphoma. The prognosis of patients with metastatic spinal cord compression is determined by the overall disease status and the degree of functional impairment.

Primary spinal cord tumors

Low grade cauda equina and conus medullaris ependymomas arise as intradural extramedullary tumors which can usually be completely excised with no need for further therapy. Complete resection of intramedullary tumors elsewhere is frequently difficult and may lead to severe neurological deficit. Following incomplete excision, local radiotherapy confined to the region of the tumor with a margin is recommended. The prognosis in patients with spinal ependymomas relates largely to the tumor grade and in low grade tumors to the extent of excision. Following partial excision and radiotherapy the 10-year progression-free survival is ~50%.[16]

Spinal astrocytomas are rare intramedullary tumors which histologically resemble cranial astrocytomas. The treatment includes surgery and radiotherapy although complete excision is usually not possible because of the infiltrative nature of the tumors. Patients with high grade tumors have a poor prognosis with frequent intracranial recurrence of disease.

Pituitary adenomas

Pituitary adenomas are slowly proliferating benign tumors arising from the cells of the anterior pituitary. Their management is described in Chapter 25.

References

1. Kleihues, P., Burger, P.C. and Scheithauer, B.W. (1993). The new WHO classification of brain tumours. *Brain Pathol.*, **3**(3), 255–268.

2. Bleehen, N.M. and Stenning, S.P., on behalf of the Medical Research Council Brain Tumour Working Party. (1991). A Medical Research Council trial of two radiotherapy doses in the treatment of grades 3 and 4 astrocytoma. The Medical Research Council Brain Tumour Working Party. *Br. J. Cancer*, **64**(4), 769–774.

3. Stenning, S., Freedman, I. and Bleehen, N. (1987). An overview of published results from randomized studies of nitrosoureas in primary high grade malignant glioma. *Br. J. Cancer*, **56**, 89.

4. Shapiro, W.R. (1986). Therapy of adult malignant brain tumours: What have the clinical trials taught us? *Semin Oncol.*, **13**, 38–45.

5. Shaw, E.C., Daumas-Duport, C., Scheithauer, B.W. *et al.* (1989). Radiation therapy in the management of low-grade supratentorial astrocytomas. *J. Neurosurg.*, **70**(6), 853–861.

6. Jenkin, D., Angyalfi, S., Becker *et al.* (1993). Optic glioma in children: Surveillance, resection, or irradiation? *Int. J. Radiat. Oncol. Biol. Phys.*, **25**, 215–225.

7. Horwich, A. and Bloom, H.J.G. (1985). Optic gliomas: Radiation therapy and prognosis. *Int. J. Radiat. Oncol. Biol. Phys.*, **11**, 1067–1079.

8. Rajan, B., Ashley, S., Gorman, C. *et al.* (1993). Craniopharyngioma — long term results following limited surgery and radiotherapy. *Radiotherapy and Oncology*, **26**(1), 1–10.

9. Glaholm, J., Bloom, H.J.G. and Crow, J.H. (1990). The role of radiotherapy in the management of intracranial meningiomas: The Royal Marsden Hospital experience with 186 patients. *Int. J. Radiat. Oncol. Biol. Phys.*, **18**, 755–761.

10. Brada, M. and Rajan, B. (1990). Spinal seeding in cranial germinoma. *Br. J. Cancer*, **61**, 339–340.

11. Nelson, D.F., Martz, K.L., Bonner, H. *et al.* (1992). Non-Hodgkin's lymphoma of the brain: Can high dose, large volume radiation therapy improve survival? Report on a prospective trial by the Radiation Therapy Oncolog Group (RTOG): RTOG 8315. *Int. J. Radiat. Oncol. Biol. Phys.*, **23**, 9–17.

12. Brada, N.J., Dearnaley, D., Horwich, A. and Bloom, H.J.C. (1990). Management of primary cerebral lymphoma with initial chemotherapy: preliminary results and comparison with patients treated with radiotherapy alone. *Int. J. Radiat. Oncol. Biol. Phys.*, **18**, 787–792.

13. Coia, L.R. (1992). The role of radiation therapy in the treatment of brain metastases. *Int. J. Radiat. Oncol. Biol. Phys.* **23**, 229–238.

14. Patchell, R., Tibbs, P. Walsh, J. *et al.* (1990). A randomised trial of surgery in the treatment of single metastases to the brain. *New Engl. J. Med.*, **322**(8), 494–500.

15. Laing, R.W., Warrington, A.P., Hines, F., Graham, J.D. and Brada, M. (1993). Fractionated stereotactic external beam radiotherapy in the management of brain metastases. *Eur. J. Cancer*, **29A**, 1387–1391.

16. Whitaker, S., Bessell, E., Ashley, S. *et al.* (1991). Postoperative radiotherapy in the management of spinal cord ependynoma. *J. Neurosurgery*, **74**, 720–728.

Cancer of Brain and Nervous System

Slightly more common in men and a common site for children

Lifetime risk
in USA white
   M   1 in 140
   F   1 in 170

Relative five-year survival in 1983–87
in USA whites:
   M   24.5%
   F   27.9%

Risk factors
Ionizing radiation

Geographical variation in 1983–87
Highest rate
M: 10.5 per 100,000 in Brazil, Port Alegre
F: 6.6 per 100,000 in Italy, Trieste
Lowest rate
M: 1.3 per 100,000 in Kyrgyzstan
F: 1.1 per 100,000 in Philippines, Rizal

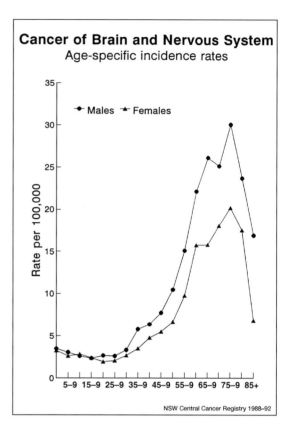

Cancer of Brain and Nervous System
Age-specific incidence rates

NSW Central Cancer Registry 1988–92

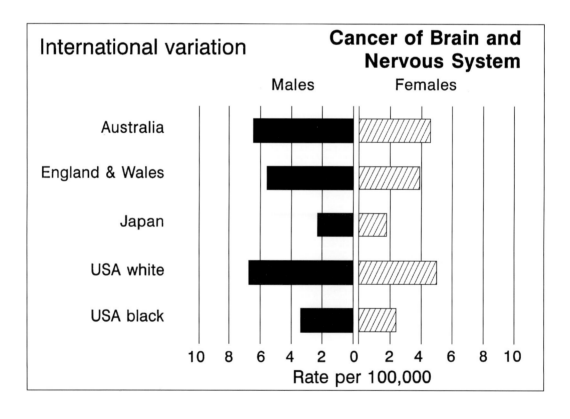

International variation

Cancer of Brain and Nervous System

Males   Females

Australia
England & Wales
Japan
USA white
USA black

Rate per 100,000

13. Cancer of the Head and Neck

JOHN E. de B. NORMAN

St. George Private Medical Centre, Kogarah, Australia

Primary malignant epithelial tumors of the head and neck may be of mucosal, cutaneous or glandular, including thyroid, salivary and lacrimal origin. The commonest form of oropharyngeal malignancy is the squamous carcinoma of the floor of mouth, tongue, and retromolar triangle. Mesenchymal malignancies and secondary carcinoma are uncommon, but the metastases of skin cancer (predominantly squamous carcinoma and malignant melanoma) constitute the commonest malignant tumor of the parotid gland. Malignant lymphoma may present in the head and neck, and non-Hodgkin's lymphoma is more common than Hodgkin's disease, while Burkitt's lymphoma tends to be localized to specific geographic areas such as Africa and Papua New Guinea. Accurate observation of the anatomical position of the cancer, its size, the involvement of the cervical lymph nodes and presence of distant metastasis allows comparison of treatment modalities between various centers, and one such classification is provided (Table 13.1).

ETIOLOGY

In the so-called developed countries, oropharyngeal cancer is linked to the use of alcohol, and smoking and chewing tobacco, and the combination of the two is synergistic. Reverse cigar, clay pipe and hookli smoking are also of etiological significance. In India and the south Pacific basin where the betel nut habit is endemic, oral cancer is common, and it is the slaked lime and tobacco (khaini) and other additives in the betel quid which are carcinogenic. The use of snuff is associated with carcinoma of the mucosal cheek, and the lesions may be fungating, ulcerative, rampant, diffuse or verrucous. Chronic irritation and oral sepsis are doubtful factors in carcinogenesis. Syphilitic interstitial glossitis and luetic leukoplakia are premalignant, as are chronic candidiasis and erosive lichen planus. The anemic woman with a negative iron balance over many years may develop oropharyngeal erythroplasia which may progress to *in situ* and later invasive squamous carcinoma, representing the oral equivalent of the Plummer–Vinson syndrome. Submucous fibrosis of the mouth, oropharynx and esophagus is common in Nepal and India, resulting from hypersensitivity to condiments and causing an epithelial atrophy which is more susceptible to carcinogens. The high incidence of nasopharyngeal carcinoma amongst the Chinese has long been recognized.

Oral *leukoplakia* is defined as a white patch on the mucosal surface which cannot be rubbed off, and is differentiated from frictional keratosis, pseudomembranous and hyperplastic candidiasis (thrush), congenital epithelial naevi, which appear white, spongy and sodden, and confluent papular or hypertrophic lichen planus. Leukoplakia is classified as plain (56%), speckled or erosive (17%) or verrucous (27%), the latter having the appearance of thick white paint, cracked and irregular. Hairy

Table 13.1. American Joint Committee on Cancer (AJCC) TNM classification and staging, with ICD numbers for some head and neck cancers.

Primary tumor (T of TNM classification)

TX	Primary tumor, not able to be assessed
T0	No evidence of primary tumor
Tis	Carcinoma in situ
T1	Tumor < 2 cm diameter
T2	Tumor > 2 cm, not > 4 cm
T3	Tumor > 4 cm
T4	Tumor invades adjacent structures, bone, muscle, skin

Regional lymph nodes (RLN)

NX	RLN cannot be assessed
N0	RLN metastasis
N1	Single ipsilateral RLN, < 3 cm
N2	Single ipsilateral RLN, > 3 cm, not > 6 cm
N2a	Metastasis, single ipsilateral RLN, > 3 cm, not > 6 cm
N2b	Metastasis, multiple ipsilateral RLN, none > 6 cm
N2c	Metastasis, bilateral or contralateral RLN, none > 6 cm
N3	Metastasis in RLN > 6 cm

Distant metastasis (M)

MX	Distant metastasis cannot be assessed
M0	No distant metastasis
M1	Distant metastasis

Staging

Stage I	T1 N0 M0
Stage II	T2 N0 M0
Stage III	T3 N0 M0; T1 N1 M0; T2 N1 M0; T3 N1 M0
Stage IV	T4 any N M0; any T, N2 or N3, M0; any T, any N, M1

ICD-O (AJCC, 1988)

140	Lip
141	Oral tongue (ventral tongue WHO 141.3)
142	Salivary gland
143	Alveolar ridge/gum
144	Floor of mouth
145	Hard palate (oral mesopharynx)

CLINICAL PRESENTATION

In the differential diagnosis of lesions and ulcers of the mouth, tongue and pharynx the most serious diagnosis should be first excluded,[1] and the diagnosis of mouth cancer is established by biopsy and not exfoliative cytology. A careful history should include the patient's use of tobacco, alcohol or betel. A middle-aged patient who is a heavy drinker and smoker and complains of a firm and persistent ulcer of the tongue associated with glossodynia and otalgia in the absence of aural disease has a tongue cancer until proved otherwise. A patient with carcinoma of the hypopharynx or upper esophagus may present with no more than deep-seated otalgia and dysphagia with solids. A patient with a similar history of hoarseness present for four weeks, has a carcinoma of the larynx until proved otherwise by direct laryngoscopy. Any cancer arising from the lining membranes of the upper aerodigestive tract may present in the first instance with a lump in the neck, and a small carcinoma of the mouth or pharynx may give rise to a large nodal mass in the ipsilateral neck. All too frequently this patient will be treated with repeated courses of antibiotics, and the diagnosis of the primary cancer will be delayed. A hard lump in the neck of an adult may be the first and outward sign of a carcinoma of the mouth or pharynx. The highest degree of suspicion must be maintained, and the patient investigated promptly or referred to the appropriate specialist. It should be emphasized that in 1997 biopsy of a cervical lymph node will be one of the last investigations carried out, if at all, and a fine needle aspiration (FNAC) by a competent cytopathologist readily establishes the diagnosis of malignancy.

PROGNOSTIC FACTORS

Stage I and II squamous carcinomas of the mouth have a high recurrence rate,[2,3] and the significant prognostic factors (1–3 below) include the following:

1. The status of the margin of the excised cancer: clear, close (2 mm) or positive, i.e. cancer to the margin of excision.
2. Tumor thickness. This is measured with an ocular micrometer in exactly the same fashion as for malignant melanoma. In the case of a mouth

leukoplakia is encountered in the latter stages of HIV–AIDS. Contrary to popular belief, leukoplakia is not necessarily premalignant, and only 10% proceed to carcinoma. It is the speckled and erosive forms about which there should be most concern.

The three areas of the mouth particularly predisposed to cancer are the oral tongue, the floor of mouth and retromolar trigone. Squamous carcinoma of the lip is more common on the lower lip, and related to sun exposure. The lip should be palpated and inspected with magnification and a bright light. The use of cutaneous surface microscopy (oil epiluminescence dermatoscopy) has refined the diagnosis of pigmented lesions of the skin.

cancer, tumor thickess > 5 mm implies a three-fold increase in the likelihood of recurrence.

3. The presence of cervical metastases. Metastatic cancer in the lymph nodes of the neck is the most important of the prognostic factors.

4. Perineural invasion. Squamous, mucoepidermoid and adenoid cystic carcinoma have a propensity for neural invasion, and this malignant neurotropism is also shared, to a lesser extent, by malignant melanoma and acinic cell cancers. The patient presents with sensory or motor neuropathy, and in particular, but not exclusively, with involvement of the trigeminal and facial nerves.

5. Sex and age of the patient.

6. Location and stage of the tumor.

7. Histopathological grading is on the Broder classification, and varies between well differentiated (G1), moderately well differentiated (G2), poorly differentiated (G3) and undifferentiated (G4).

8. Desmoplasia and lymphovascular invasion.

9. Inflammatory response.

(After Jones, *et al*, 1992[2]).

EXAMINATION

The examination of the head, neck and upper aerodigestive tract is carried out in a systematic fashion, with the neck fully exposed, and the patient comfortably seated or supine on the couch. A good light source is essential. Inspect the neck, comparing the right with the left side. Is there evidence of previous surgery, the scarring of cervical tuberculosis, loss of normal contour, muscle wasting, asymmetry or spasmodic torticollis? Identify the swelling, noting its anatomical position and general outline, and recording this, together with its size in centimeters, on a small drawing. Is the palpable surface of the lump smooth or bosselated? Is it deep to the sternomastoid, and is the overlying skin freely mobile, or adherent and associated with a discharging sinus? If there is a discharge it should be submitted for cytological examination and culture, remembering that "sulphur granules" are encountered not only in actinomycosis, but also in a necrotic carcinomatous lymph node. If there is a complaint of pain, ask the patient to indicate with one finger only the point at which the pain commences, and

where it radiates. If the patient is pyrexial, the swelling lies within the submandibular triangle, and the overlying skin is warm, red and tender, it may be no more than an abscess secondary to an infected tooth or submandibular salivary gland. It may be that the neck lump is a metastasis from a squamous carcinoma or malignant melanoma excised or "burned off" 12 months earlier. The skin of the neck, face and scalp is examined, and if there is a suspicion that the lump is a nodal metastasis from a primary cutaneous malignancy the nurse gently combs through the scalp using a hairdryer and illumination.

It is the author's preference to palpate the patient's neck from behind, commencing with the submental triangle and moving posteriorly to the submandibular triangle and its nodes, never neglecting the pre- and post-vascular facial lymph nodes which may lie on the lateral aspect, inferior or infero-medial border of the mandible. Attention is directed to the jugulo-digastric or tonsillar nodes, and on to the face, gently palpating those nodes contained in and around the parotid gland and immediately adjacent to the preauricular skin crease. Do not neglect the ear, since infection of a pierced ear may give rise to preauricular lymphadenitis. Palpate the sulcus between the parotideal margin of the mandible and the mastoid process, identifying the transverse process of the axis, and move on to the suboccipital triangle. While suboccipital lymphadenopathy may be the result of cutaneous malignancies of the scalp, it is also encountered in glandular fever, lymphoma, rubella and infestation with head lice. The fingers are now moved down and beneath the anterior border of trapezius, flexing the patient's head in order to feel beneath the edge of that muscle and identify any nodes lying on the muscular floor of the posterior triangle. Make a mental note of Erb's point, rolling the greater auricular nerve trunk beneath the fingers. Surgeons practicing in the tropics include this assessment in the examination of the patient with leprosy. Erb's point is also a reasonable surface guide to the accessory nerve as it emerges through the posterior border of the sternomastoid and proceeds superficially across the posterior triangle in company with five or six lymph nodes, slipping beneath trapezius at the junction of its lower third and upper two-thirds. Examine the base of the posterior triangle before palpating the jugular (Concatenate) chain of lymph nodes beneath the sternomastoid. Move now to the suprasternal notch, confirming that the trachea is central, before identifying the sternoclavicular joints and palpating the supraclavicular nodes from medial to lateral. Palpate the thyroid gland carefully, and ascend the neck in the midline, assessing the cricoid cartilage, larynx and hyoid, and completing your examination at the submental triangle. If you are unable to satisfy yourself in regard to the lump of which the patient has complained, repeat the examination with the patient supine.

There are aids to diagnosis. These include transillumination of a mass in a dark room, in the presence of a chaperone — the cystic hygroma transilluminates brilliantly. A swelling lying against the carotid artery will transmit arterial pulsation. It is generally believed that while a thyroid mass moves on swallowing, a thyroglossal cyst gives a characteristic tug when the tongue is protruded. A matted submental nodal mass or a dumb-bell shaped dermoid cyst perforating the mylohyoid diaphragm also gives rise to this physical sign, while a submental lipoma does not. Normal structures which are sometimes mistaken for pathology, particularly following cervical lymphadenectomy, include the transverse process of the second cervical vertebra, the greater horn of the hyoid, the carotid bulb, and an enlarged, partially subluxated sternoclavicular joint. The large bulge overlying the median third of the clavicle encountered following a neck dissection and myocutaneous flap repair is likely to be muscle and not recurrent disease. This regional examination of the head and neck is carried out in concert with a full physical examination.

First inspect the face for any sign of asymmetry or obvious cranial nerve lesion. Whereas facial or hypoglossal palsy may be immediately obvious, careful examination of the cranial nerves should be carried out in any head and neck case. Attention is now directed to the lining membranes of the upper aerodigestive tract. Inspection of the nasal airway is accomplished by rhinoscopy, utilizing a Thadacum nasal speculum and light source. The presence of an offensive or bloodstained unilateral discharge in an adult may be the signpost to sino-antral or nasopharyngeal carcinoma. In a child or baby it is usually indicative of a foreign body. Further examination of the postnasal space and nasopharynx requires fibreoptic nasopharyngoscopy. The ears are inspected, and the helix examined for any telltale scar. The pinna has two surfaces, and the ear should be turned forward and the junctional skin inspected

before the ear canal and tympanic membrane are scrutinized with the auriscope. The examination of the mouth requires a good light and two dental mirrors or retractors. A systematic inspection of the mucosal surfaces of the lower lip, cheek and adjacent gum is followed by examination of the hard and soft palate, and then the anterior or oral two-thirds and posterior or pharyngeal third of the tongue, its lateral margins and ventral surface and the adjacent mouth floor. Attention is directed to the posterior lingual gutter, and if the patient gags, spray the area with a topical anaesthetic to reduce this reflex. The gloved finger is inserted into the mouth floor, and when the finger tips the hilum of the submandibular gland it is 7 cm from the mandibular incisor teeth. Bimanual examination of the submandibular triangle and its contents and the sublingual gland is carried out, and the tongue is firmly but gently re-palpated from back to front. The almost symmetrical bony lump lying slightly medial to the maxillary tuberosity of the junctional hard and soft palate is the pterygoid hamulus, and not a tumor.

The parotid gland on each side is gently palpated from the glenoid lobe overlying the jaw joint through the body and accessory lobes to the tail of the gland, and the deep lobe may be palpated bimanually by a gentle clinician without unduly discomfiting the anxious patient.

TUMORS OF THE NECK

Cervical tumors of neurogenous origin

The Schwannoma is usually a slowly growing, solitary tumor, and the neurofibroma is associated with von Recklinghausen's disease. The former is encapsulated, sometimes painful and rarely malignant, and the latter is asymptomatic, albeit unsightly, and approximately 10% undergo malignant change. If the sympathetic chain is involved the patient may present with a Horner's syndrome.

Carotid body tumor (chemodectoma)

A slowly developing tumor, with a strong family history, presenting with a painless lump in the neck, the oft-quoted axiom that the lump does not move up and down, but does move from side to side, is of little value, since it can be applied to many neck lumps. There may be involvement of the lower four cranial nerves, in addition to a Horner's syndrome. The diagnosis is made on angiography, and a small number of tumors undergo malignant transformation and metastasis.

Cervical metastasis

The presence or absence of a cervical metastasis is known to be the most important prognostic factor in squamous carcinoma of the mouth and pharynx. It is the cervical lymph nodes which form a temporary barrier to the progress of the cancer, spreading initially by local invasion and infiltration and later by permeation of the peritumoral lymphovascular spaces. In the early stages the tumor cells grow through the lymphatics and colonize the next lymph node in the chain, and tumor emboli hasten the process. Tumors occurring in the three prevalent sites of mouth cancer commonly metastasize to lymph node levels I, II and III. The occult involvement of the cervical lymph nodes is present in approximately 30% of patients with T1 and T2 disease, and prognostic factors are discussed above.

The clinical recognition of cervical metastases by palpation has been shown to be unreliable, and other methods of assessment have been sought, including ultrasound, computed tomography, magnetic resonance imaging, PET and fine needle aspiration.

Fine needle aspiration cytopathology (FNAC or FNAB)

Fine needle aspiration of body organs as a means of diagnosis was first described in 1847, and by 1933 Martin, Ellis and Stewart had reported on 2500 tumors examined by this method. Parotid tumors were particularly suited to aspiration, but as a general technique it found little favor with pathologists. Other forms of exfoliative cytology were more widely used. There are limitations as to what can be deduced from smears prepared from an aspirate of a lymph node or tumor, and FNAC is an aid to diagnosis, and is considered along with the history, clinical findings and other special investigations, including forms of imaging. For deepseated tumors, the needle is guided by means of ultrasound or CT.[4] The technique of biopsy using a Trucut needle is favored by some, but not the writer.

SURGICAL MANAGEMENT

Cancers of the mouth and pharynx are in the main managed by either surgery or a combination of surgery and radiotherapy. The constraints of space preclude other than a broad discussion of the fundamentals, and the case of a T2 carcinoma of the tongue is illustrative. First, it is important to establish the diagnosis.

Case study

A 52-year-old man who smokes 25 cigarettes per day and is a heavy drinker presents to his family doctor with an indurated and painful ulcer of the lateral tongue and adjacent mouth floor. He complains of pain in the tongue and otalgia, in addition to a hard 2.5 cm mass in the right jugulo-digastric region. A full physical examination is carried out, in addition to the regional assessment and digital rectal examination. He undergoes a hematological and biochemical survey in addition to a chest radiograph and ECG. He is admitted into the ward on a day care basis for an examination under anesthesia (EUA) and triple endoscopy. The patient with a carcinoma of the tongue may have a second primary cancer elsewhere in the aerodigestive tract. Frozen section examination of the excised biopsy specimen confirms the diagnosis of well-differentiated squamous carcinoma, and FNAC of the cervical lymph node confirms metastatic squamous carcinoma.

A joint consultation with surgeon and radiotherapist is held in the combined clinic. The treatment strategy is determined, and surgery is advised, followed by irradiation therapy.[5] Supplementary consultations are arranged with the clinic dental officer, social worker, speech therapist and dietitian. The operation is discussed with the patient and family, and informed consent obtained for hemiglossectomy in continuity with a right modified radical neck dissection. Complications of this operation are discussed in a compassionate fashion, avoiding the use of jargon and without unduly alarming the patient. As this patient is a manual worker, the importance of the spinal accessory nerve is emphasized, and it is explained that while every attempt will be made to preserve the nerve, a functional deficit may result, and whilst it may only be partial and temporary, no surgeon could guarantee that it will not be permanent. The complications of surgery in general are also discussed and documented, and it is the author's practice to have this record of interview signed by the patient and witnessed.

RADIOTHERAPEUTIC MANAGEMENT

Radiotherapy plays an important role in the curative treatment of head and neck cancer patients, either by itself, or more commonly as an adjunctive treatment to sterilize microscopic residual cancer following surgery. Indications for post-operative radiotherapy include a large primary SCC, incomplete surgical resection (i.e. positive margins), cervical lymph node metastases and/or aggressive histopathologic features such as significant lymphovascular invasion, perineural infiltration or high grade.

In some anatomic sites such as the posterior one-third of the tongue, vallecula, epiglottis, nasopharynx or vocal cords, radiotherapy alone is the sole treatment of choice and results in rates of cure between 50–80%. In frail patients with accessible tumors (< 3 cm in size), a radioactive implant (brachytherapy) over a 3–5 day period may be curative.

Radiotherapeutic planning in the head and neck region requires impeccable attention to detail in order to adequately treat the cancer, yet minimize damage to critical normal tissues such as the ocular lens, brain, spinal cord, auditory apparatus, salivary glands and mandible. Treatment plans must be designed on an individual basis and the patient advised to maintain strict oral hygiene. During a course of high dose radiotherapy to the head and neck region, troublesome side effects frequently include loss of taste (ageusia), dry mouth (xerostomia), thick saliva, mucosal inflammation and ulceration, candidal overgrowth and skin erythema. In many patients, dry mouth and a tendency to candidal overgrowth become permanent.

All patients require a meticulous dental assessment prior to commencing radiotherapy in order to maximize oral hygiene; dental extractions may occasionally be required prior to commencing radiotherapy, but should rarely (as a general rule) be considered following treatment lest mandibular osteo-radionecrosis occur.

CHEMOTHERAPY

Cytotoxic chemotherapy has had a disappointing

impact on head and neck cancer cure rates. Although cytotoxic combination of drugs such as cisplatin, methotrexate, 5-fluorouracil and bleomycin can significantly reduce the size of primary head and neck cancers in up to 80% of cases, an overall improvement in survival has not been demonstrated in numerous published studies. Cytotoxics administered concomitantly with radiotherapy may result in a survival advantage, but at a far higher rate of significant toxicity. In patients with laryngeal cancer, a combination of cytotoxic followed by radiotherapy may reduce the need for radical surgery (i.e. laryngectomy).

THE NECK

The surgical management of the neck in patients with mucosal, cutaneous and salivary cancers is based on the various risk factors. It is the cornerstone of treatment, and the names associated with the operation include George Crile[6] and Hayes Martin.[7] These surgeons described the operation of radical neck dissection (RND), which involves the *en bloc* removal of all cervical lymphatics from the lower border of the mandible to the clavicle, and from the anterior border of the trapezius to the midline of the neck and contralateral submental triangle. The non-lymphatic structures which are removed include the submandibular salivary gland, the tail of the parotid gland, the internal jugular vein (IJV), the sternomastoid (SCM) and omohyoid (OH) muscles, and the spinal accessory nerve (SAN). It has been appreciated that some structures, particularly the spinal accessory nerve, can be safely preserved. If this nerve is sacrificed, some patients may develop severe disability, including pain and weakness of the ipsilateral shoulder. In the light of important clinical research at the Memorial Sloan-Kettering Cancer Center[8,9] and the MD Anderson Hospital, amongst others, modifications of the neck dissection have been developed.[10] It is no longer appropriate to carry out radical neck dissection as a routine in the management of cervical metastases, although it is the procedure with which other forms of lymphadenectomy are compared. Neck dissection is now classified as comprehensive (radical or modified radical) or selective, and in the latter case it is customary to specify the nodal levels dissected (I–V) and the anatomical structures preserved.[11,12] Three types of MRND, in

Table 13.2. Modified and selective cervical lymphadenectomy.

MRND 1	Preserves SAN
MRND 2	Preserves SAN + IJV
MRND 3	Preserves SAN + IJV + SCM
SND	Preserves SAN + IJV + SCM – levels II-IV (LND)
SND	Preserves SAN + IJV + SCM – levels II-V (LND)

each of which nodal levels I-V are dissected, are described (Table 13.2) and the techniques continue to evolve.[13]

SALIVARY GLANDS

Salivary gland neoplasms are more common in the parotid, and while 80% are benign, 20% are malignant.[14] Tumors of the parotid gland are more common in the body and tail of the gland, and only rarely present in the oropharynx, arising in the deep lobe. Cancers of the parotid may present as an isolated lump, readily mistaken for a benign pleomorphic adenoma, or as a diffuse swelling. The latter may be the presenting sign of an aggressive squamous or adeno-carcinoma or malignant lymphoma. If, in addition to the mass, there is a lower motor neurone facial paralysis, the lesion is almost certainly malignant. Parotid malignancies may be primary or secondary, and the latter are more common and arise from adjacent squamous carcinoma or malignant melanoma of the scalp, face or ear. Some parotid cancers present with a rock-hard swelling, surface ulceration, facial palsy and cervical nodal involvement. Submandibular malignancies are less common. The primary carcinomas of salivary gland origin include mucoepidermoid and adenoid cystic carcinoma, acinic cell adenocarcinoma, squamous carcinoma and adenocarcinoma ex pleomorphic adenoma, or malignant mixed tumor. A brief summary of management of these glandular malignancies[16] is given in Table 13.3. An unusual form of malignant lymphoma of MALT type occurs in patients with Sjögren's syndrome.

Malignant tumors of the minor salivary glands are minor in name only, and in the main arise from the salivary gland cushion of the hard and soft palate. They may, however, occur anywhere in the upper aerodigestive tract, and from the ear to the larynx.[17]

Table 13.3. Management of salivary gland malignancy. TNM classification applies only to major salivary glands.[15] (Reproduced by courtesy of *Modern Medicine*[16]).

Staging
CT scan clavicle to skull base
CT scan thorax
Nuclear scintigraphy, technetium/gallium
Other investigations on an individual basis

Parotid gland

Low grade	Parotidectomy + facial nerve preservation
Intermediate	Parotidectomy + facial nerve preservation + MRND[a]
High grade	Parotidectomy + facial nerve preservation + MRND + RTX[b] If perineural infiltration VII obvious, and prognosis otherwise good, facial neurectomy + nerve grafting is considered. If skin is involved, it is excised widely in continuity, and the defect resurfaced with either a local or distant flap, or a vascularized free flap.

Submandibular gland

Low grade	Submandibular sialadenectomy ± MRND
Intermediate	Submandibular sialadenectomy + MRND
High grade	Submandibular sialadenectomy + MRND + RTX

[a]MRND = modified radical neck dissection
[b]RTX = external beam radiotherapy

CARCINOMAS OF OTHER SITES IN THE HEAD AND NECK

Carcinoma of the maxilla may arise *de novo* from the overlying mucoperiosteum, and this is almost invariably squamous carcinoma. Sino-antral malignancies and those arising primarily in the maxillary sinus may invade the alveolus, causing dental pain, the loosening of teeth, an extraction socket which fails to heal, or displacement of a denture in the edentulous patient. If the cancer grows medially, it will give rise to nasal obstruction and a foul, blood-stained nasal discharge. A cancer of the antrum invading the orbit will give rise to non-axial proptosis, epiphora and pain and later anesthesia in the infra-orbital dermatome. As a general rule, carcinoma of the maxilla is treated by maxillectomy and radiation therapy. With modern techniques of reconstruction, it is possible to close the surgical defect with a transfer or free flap, which may incorporate bone. The development of osseous integrated implants has allowed the surgeon and the dentist ultimately to restore a portion of the patient's dentition in a selected group of these patients.

The methods of reconstruction now available are many and varied, and the use of a variety of tissue transfer techniques employing vascularized flaps and, more recently, free flaps of bone and soft tissue has revolutionized the immediate reconstruction and rehabilitation of the patient who has undergone a complex resection of mouth, pharynx, jaw and neck. The description of these operations is beyond the scope of this chapter.

CONCLUSION

Although the majority of head and neck cancers occur in a readily accessible area, late diagnosis is unfortunately by no means uncommon. The clinician should maintain a high index of suspicion when examining an indolent ulcer of skin or mucosa, or a lump in the neck. Pain radiating to the ear in the middle-aged or elderly is a common symptom of oropharyngeal cancer, and dysphagia or difficulty in swallowing solids is very suspicious of cancer of the hypopharynx or esophagus. Hoarseness persisting for more than 4 weeks should raise the suspicion of laryngeal cancer, and warrants immediate specialist referral. Proptosis associated with cheek swelling and anaesthesia in the infra-orbital dermatome is indicative of malignant antrum, as is a unilateral bloodstained nasal discharge in an adult. An ocular paresis and lump in the neck in a Chinese patient should immediately raise the possibility of nasopharyngeal carcinoma. Prompt examination and specialist referral will in many cases increase the strength of possibility of cure.

References

 1. Butlin, H.T. (1885). Clinical manuals for practitioners and students of medicine. Diseases of the tongue, pp. 258–302. London: Cassell and Company.
 2. Jones, K.R., Lodge-Rigal, R.D., Reddick, R.L., Tudor, G.E. and Shockley, W.W. (1992). Prognostic factors in the recurrence of stage I and II squamous cell cancer of the oral cavity. *Archives of Otolaryngology and Head and Neck Surgery*, **118**, 483–485.
 3. Beahrs, O.H., Henson, D.E., Hutter, R.V.P. and Myers, M.H. (1988). Manual for Staging of Cancer. American Joint Committee on Cancer, 3rd edn. Philadelphia: JB Lippincott Company.
 4. Young, J.A. (1993). Technique. In Fine needle aspiration cytopathology, edited by J.A. Young, pp. 48–67. Oxford: Blackwell.
 5. Goffinet, D.R., Fee, W.E. and Goode, R.L. (1984). Combined surgery and postoperative irradiation in the treatment of cervical lymph nodes. *Archives of Otolaryngology*, **110**, 736–738.
 6. Crile, G. (1906). Excision of cancer of the head and neck with special reference to the plan of dissection based on one hundred and thirty-two operations. *Journal of the American Medical Association*, **47**, 1780–1788.
 7. Martin, H.E., Del Valle, B., Ehrlich, H. and Cahan, W.G. (1951). Neck dissection. *Cancer*, **4**, 441–499.
 8. Andersen, P.E., Shah, J.P., Cambronero, E. and Spiro, R.H. (1994). The role of comprehensive neck dissection with preservation of the spinal accessory nerve in the clinically positive neck. *American Journal of Surgery*, **168**, 499–502.
 9. Strong, E.W. (1969). Preoperative radiation and radical neck dissection. *Surgical Clinics of North America*, **49**, 271–276.
10. Spiro, R.H., Gallo, O. and Shah, J.P. (1993). Selective jugular node dissection in patients with squamous carcinoma of the laryunx or pharynx. *American Journal of Surgery*, **166**, 399–402.
11. Robbins, K.T., Medina, J.E., Wolfe, G.T., Levine, P.A., Sessions, R.B. and Pruet, C.W. (1991). Standardizing neck dissection terminology. *Archives of Otolaryngology and Head and Neck Surgery*, **117**, 601–605.
12. Shah, J.P. and Andersen, P.E. (1995). Evolving role of modifications in mech dissection for oral squamous carcinoma. *British Journal of Oral and Maxillofacial Surgery*, **33**, 3–8.
13. Diaz, E.M., Austin, J.R., Burke, L.I. and Goepfert, H. (1996). The posterolateral neck dissection: technique and results. *Archives of Otolaryngology and Head and Neck Surgery*, **122**, 477–480.
14. Norman, J.E. de B. and McGurk, M. (1995). Color Atlas and Text of the Salivary Glands: Diseases, Disorders and Surgery, pp. 139–172. London: Mosby-Wolfe.
15. Hermanek, P. and Sobin, L.H. (1987). Classification of Malignant Tumors, 4th edn. Berlin: Springer.
16. Norman, J.E. de B. (1996). Tumors and allied swellings of the parotid and other salivary glands. *Modern Medicine*, **39**, 48–64.
17. Norman, J.E. de B. and Badcock, C.-A. (1995). Tumors of the minor salivary glands. In Color Atlas and Text of the Salivary Glands: Diseases, Disorders and Surgery, edited by J.E. de B. Norman and M. McGurk, pp. 197–228. London: Mosby-Wolfe.

Cancers of Head and Neck

Distinctly more common in men

Worldwide: 4th most common in men
             8th most common in women

Lifetime risk
in USA whites: for oral and pharyngeal cancers
  M   1 in 70
  F   1 in 140

Relative five-year survival in 1983–87
in USA whites:
  M   53.3%
  F   58.5%

Risk factors
Tobacco: lip, mouth, pharynx, larynx
Alcohol: mouth, pharynx, larynx
         together account for ≈ 90% of
         oropharyngeal cancers
Nutritional deficiencies: mouth, pharynx
Betel nut chewing: mouth, pharynx
Epstein Barr virus: nasopharynx
Salted fish: nasopharynx
Sunlight: lip

Geographical variation in 1983–87
Highest rate — all except nasopharynx
M: 68.3 per 100,000 in France, Bas Rhin

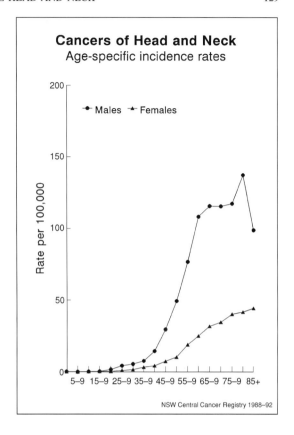

F: 14.3 per 100,000 in India, Madras
Highest rate — nasopharynx
M: 28.5 per 100,000 in Hong Kong
F: 11.2 per 100,000 in Hong Kong

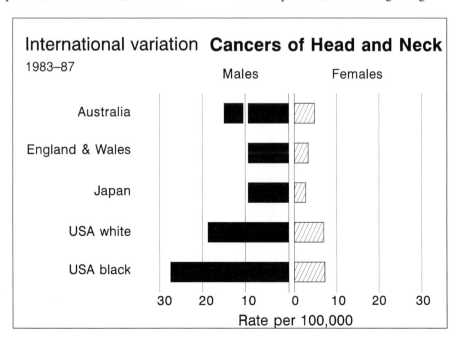

14. Breast Cancer

JO MARSDEN[1] and MICHAEL BAUM[2]

[1] *Institute of Cancer Research, The Royal Marsden Hospital, NHS Trust, London, UK*
[2] *University College Hospital, London, UK*

EPIDEMIOLOGY

Breast cancer is the commonest malignancy affecting women with more than half a million new cases every year. It accounts for 4% of all female deaths and is the commonest cause of mortality in women aged between 30 and 60 years.

PREDISPOSING AND RISK FACTORS

Epidemiological studies have identified many potential risk factors for breast cancer but these only account for approximately 10–20% of disease occurrence. As second-generation Japanese women living in the USA have assumed the incidence rates of their adopted country, environmental factors appear to be more important than racial characteristics in the development of the disease.

Familial breast cancer

A woman's risk of breast cancer is doubled if a first-degree relative (i.e. mother, sister or daughter) develops the disease before the age of 50 years; this is increased by four to six times if the disease is bilateral or if two first-degree relatives are affected.

Approximately 90% of all breast cancers that occur are sporadic, that is, there is no significant family history of the disease. Of the 10% of breast cancers that have a familial association approximately half are due to an inherited gene mutation. Such familial cancers are characterized by an early age at presentation (i.e. < 50 years), the occurrence of bilateral disease, involvement of several relatives and a history of related epithelial cancers (e.g. colon, ovary, endometrium). The inheritance is complex being autosomal dominant with a limited penetrance. This means that mutated genes can be transmitted by either sex but carriers of the gene do not necessarily develop breast cancer themselves. Two genes, BRCA-1 and BRCA-2, probably account for two-thirds of these breast cancers and currently genetic testing will only be offered to families where there is a strong possibility that a gene mutation has caused the familial incidence (e.g. where more than four cases of breast cancer have been identified, or where ovarian cancer exists in addition to three or more cases of breast cancer). Presently, the only preventative measure that can be offered to women with an undoubted genetic predisposition is bilateral prophylactic mastectomy with or without breast reconstruction. Obviously, the implications for patients demonstrated to be at high risk emphasizes the importance of counseling before testing.

Family history clinics can be used to identify women who are at high risk of developing breast cancer. These women are usually seen annually and undergo breast examination although this is of unproven value. Debate also exists as to whether mammographic screening of high risk women from the age of 35 years onwards will be of benefit in reducing mortality.

Hormonal risk factors

Epidemiological studies implicate exposure to endogenous estrogen as one of the main factors for the development of breast cancer. The female preponderance of breast cancer, early menarche, late menopause, nulliparity, obesity and an older age at first full-term pregnancy have all been shown to be associated with an increased risk, whereas there is a 40% reduction in incidence in women undergoing surgical oophorectomy before the age of 35 years. Despite these observations, no clinical studies in humans have definitively demonstrated that the administration of exogenous estrogens promotes the growth or spread of breast cancer cells.

The oral contraceptive pill

It has been reported that there is a small increase in the risk of developing breast cancer during current use of the combined oral contraceptive pill and for 10 years after stopping it. This amounts to an excess risk of 0.5 cancers per 10,000 women for use at age 16–19 yrs and increases with age. The cancers detected are less advanced in pill users than in non-users.

Hormone replacement therapy

The most recent and comprehensive review of studies investigating HRT and breast cancer risk suggest that there may be a slightly increased risk of breast cancer with a long duration of HRT use (i.e. > 10 years), however, this small risk rapidly declines after HRT is stopped. In advising a woman about the benefits of HRT (in alleviating menopausal symptoms and a reduction in morbidity and mortality from osteoporosis and cardiovascular disease by 50%) it is important to explain there may be a relation with breast cancer but any definitive evidence is lacking.

Dietary factors

Countries with a diet high in fats have a high incidence of breast cancer. It is not clear from epidemiological studies whether dietary restriction of fats (saturated or unsaturated) has any impact on the incidence of breast cancer. The relation between alcohol intake and breast cancer risk is inconclusive.

Radiation

Exposure to ionizing radiation is associated with increased risk of breast cancer, the sensitivity appears to be greatest in childhood when exposure can occur during periods of rapid breast formation and differentiation.

Benign breast disease

Benign breast disease describes a variety of non-neoplastic conditions with differing etiologies and only some are associated with an increase in risk of subsequent breast cancer. Women with atypical ductal or lobular hyperplasia have a four to five times increase in the risk of developing breast cancer. There is a very slight risk associated with proliferative breast changes without atypia (e.g. multiple cysts, duct papillomas and sclerosing adenosis) and no relation between non-proliferative benign breast disease (e.g. solitary cysts, ectasia or adenosis) and breast cancer has been observed.

Pathology

Breast cancer arises from the epithelium of breast ducts and lobules and may be classified as either *in situ* (non-invasive) or invasive. *In situ* disease is confined to the breast ducts and/or lobules without breaching the basement membrane, whereas invasive carcinoma involves growth into the surrounding breast tissue.

In situ carcinoma

There are two types of *in situ* breast disease, ductal carcinoma *in situ*, (DCIS), and lobular carcinoma *in situ* (LCIS). Lobular *in situ* disease can be considered to arise from the epithelium of breast lobules, whereas ductal *in situ* disease arises from the epithelium of terminal ductules.

Lobular carcinoma *in situ*

This is usually diagnosed as an incidental finding in a breast biopsy performed for some other reason. Approximately 30% of women with this finding will develop an invasive ductal or lobular cancer (which can occur in either breast) with long-term follow-up. At present there is no method for determining which patients are likely to progress to invasive disease and as a result there is debate as to whether patients should be managed by observation alone or prophylactic bilateral mastectomy, although most authorities favor a policy of close observation.

Ductal carcinoma *in situ*

DCIS may present as a nipple discharge, a palpable breast lump, an incidental finding at biopsy or as a screening abnormality on mammography. The association of DCIS with infiltrating carcinoma is stronger than that of LCIS. DCIS has been subdivided into two broad categories: (a) large cell, comedo and (b) small cell, or papillary, cribriform type. Although the former has a greater potential to progress to invasive disease it has been postulated that the malignant potential of DCIS may in fact be related to nuclear grade. The optimal treatment of DCIS has not been established and currently a national UK trial is under way to evaluate the use of post-biopsy radiotherapy and tamoxifen treatment for DCIS detected during mammographic screening.

Invasive breast carcinoma

Some invasive cancers have distinctive features, are termed as special type and they generally have a better prognosis (e.g. papillary, tubular and mucinous cancers). The majority of the remaining carcinomas are either lobular (constituting 5% of invasive cancers) or ductal (70–80% are of this type).

Ductal carcinoma

These cancers can be classified into three grades according to the degree of glandular differentiation and nuclear pleomorphism. The histological grading (after Bloom and Richardson) is related to prognosis, well-differentiated, grade I, tumors being associated with a better survival than poorly differentiated, grade III, cancers.

Lobular carcinoma

The microscopic appearance is characterized by a fibrous matrix through which run loose strands of small tumor cells in a linear arrangement known as Indian filing. Synchronous or metachronous bilateral carcinomas are not uncommon. The prognosis is similar to invasive ductal carcinoma.

The spread of breast cancer

(1) *Local spread.* As a tumor increases in size it can involve greater proportions of the breast, overlying skin, underlying pectoral muscles and the chest wall.

(2) *Lymphatic spread.* This occurs either by direct invasion of lymphatic vessels by carcinoma cells or by tumor emboli entering draining lymphatics. The ipsilateral axillary lymph nodes and internal mammary chain are usually involved at an early stage.

(3) *Blood spread.* The common sites involved include the skeleton (ribs, lumbar and thoracic vertebrae, femur and skull), liver, lungs and brain.

Lobular carcinoma can exhibit an unusual spread of metastases, for example, meningeal infiltration in the central nervous system and diffuse retroperitoneal/serosal spread in the abdomen.

SCREENING

Reduction in mortality from breast cancer could be achieved by preventing the disease from occurring (i.e. primary prevention), detecting the disease at an early stage (i.e. secondary prevention) and provision of the best treatment once diagnosed (i.e. tertiary prevention).

Primary prevention is not yet possible for breast cancer as no clear causative factors have been identified. However, as breast cancer patients treated with tamoxifen have a lower incidence of contralateral breast primaries, tamoxifen is currently being evaluated as a preventative agent in women at high risk of developing breast cancer in studies in the UK, USA, Europe and Australia.

Mammographic screening

The aim of mammographic screening is to detect and treat breast cancer at an early, asymptomatic stage before it has had a chance to spread. It is an example of secondary prevention. National screening programs have been instituted following randomized controlled trials which overall have shown a 28% reduction in mortality from breast cancer in women screened over the age of 50 years (but not younger than this).

Initial population screening is termed the prevalent (or basic) round, subsequent screening rounds are called incident screens. Interval cancers are those cancers arising between screening rounds. They are usually faster growing and more aggressive than screen-detected cancers which are usually smaller, well differentiated and more likely to be non-invasive (20% are DCIS). Decreasing the screening interval (currently three years in the UK) may not necessarily reduce their incidence and has yet to be evaluated. Furthermore as the optimum treatment for DCIS is not known it may be that many women attending for screening are being overtreated.

Successful implementation of mammographic screening will require a high participation of the eligible population; however, it is not without its adverse effects. Unnecessary recall for further investigations or biopsy generated by false positive results may contribute towards patient anxiety. Detecting cancers at an earlier asymptomatic stage can result in a patient having to live with her diagnosis for a longer period without any survival benefit thus affecting her quality of life. The increased risk of breast cancer caused by radiation of the breast during mammography has been estimated to be less than 0.05 of the natural incidence in this age group and is therefore negligible.

If an impalpable abnormality is detected on mammography (up to 70% are) further assessment is necessary. Aspiration cytology can be performed under ultrasound or X-ray (stereotaxic) guidance.

An impalpable lesion requiring excision may be localized before surgery by placing a percutaneous hooked wire adjacent to the lesion under mammographic guidance. The surgeon can then carry out a limited excision based on palpation of the needle tip. Excision can be confirmed by an X-ray of the excised specimen at the time of surgery.

Self-examination for breast cancer

As most breast cancers are found by women themselves there is a need to optomize the chances of a woman finding a cancer. Routine breast self-examination (which was promoted to encourage women to detect breast lumps) has not been shown to be an effective method of screening for breast cancer. It has a high false positive rate and some women are unhappy about it and have difficulty in performing it. Furthermore, breast self-examination increases biopsy rates with no detectable effect on mortality. There is a case, however, for encouraging women to become breast aware and report any changes (not just lumps) in their breasts promptly to their doctor for assessment especially as mammographic screening is not an absolute test for breast cancer and carcinomas can develop between screening rounds.

CLINICAL PRESENTATION

Primary disease

The commonest presentation of breast cancer is that of a painless lump, the majority occurring in the upper outer quadrant and axillary tail of the breast. The stroma surrounding a cancer can become fibrosed, shorten Coopers's Ligaments and cause dimpling of the overlying skin or nipple inversion. Edema (Peau d'orange) occurs when dermal lymphatics are infiltrated by tumor.

Less than 2% of carcinomas are associated with a nipple discharge. Single duct discharge indicates a local cause such as intraduct papilloma or carcinoma and a blood-stained discharge should always be investigated. Multiple duct or bilateral discharge is usually benign.

Inflammatory carcinoma clinically resembles acute inflammation with erythema, swelling, skin edema and tenderness. It accounts for up to 4% of all cancers and is often rapidly progressive.

Clinical examination to detect involvement of ipsilateral axillary lymph nodes is often inaccurate and up to 40% of breast cancer patients with clinically normal nodes have metastatic axillary disease. Rarely axillary lymphadenopathy may be the only sign of an impalpable, occult breast carcinoma.

Paget's Disease is usually associated with an underlying intraduct or infiltrating ductal carcinoma. The characteristic changes of nipple discharge, inflammation and ulceration clinically mimic eczema (although the former is usually unilateral) and often it is only diagnosed by performing an incision biopsy of the nipple.

Secondary disease

Breast cancer can be locally advanced with fixation to the underlying muscles and chest wall or to the skin with ulceration. Alternatively the patient may

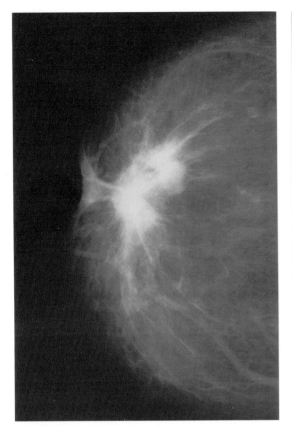

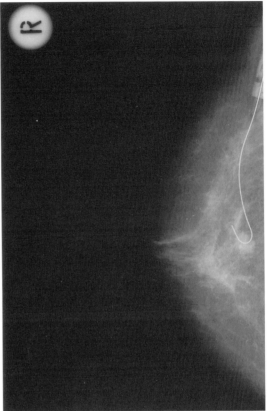

Figure 14.1a. Mammogram demonstrating large, irregular density with architectural distortion — a carcinoma. Reproduced with kind permission of Dr. E. Moskovic.

Figure 14.1b. Localization of an impalpable, mammographically suspicious lesion with a percutaneous hook wire. (Lesion lies alongside the curve of the wire). Reproduced with kind permission of Dr. D. Blunt.

present due to symptoms from widespread metastases in the liver, skeleton or brain.

INVESTIGATION

The aim of investigations is to determine the nature of the abnormality. If a cancer is diagnosed a patient should be fully counseled before definitive treatment. Clinical examination, mammography, aspiration cytology and ultrasound scanning combined have a very high positive predictive value with a low false positive rate.

If a breast cancer is clinically confined to the breast and/or regional lymph nodes (i.e. it is localized or operable), extensive investigations (e.g. bone or liver scans) are not necessary to assess the presence of subclinical, micrometastatic disease as in the absence of signs and symptoms these have a very low positive yield.

Mammography

Cancers can present as: (see Figure 14.1)

1. densities (which may be irregular or spiculated),
2. architectural distortions,
3. edema,
4. calcifications within the breast. Malignant calcifications vary in size, density and alignment and may be clustered, linear or branching. They usually indicate DCIS and to a lesser extent invasive ductal carcinoma. Benign calcifications in contrast are commonly uniform in size and density.

Ultrasound scan

This can be used as an adjunct to mammography especially in differentiating between solid and cystic masses. Malignancies are usually irregular, of mixed echogenicity and vascular on color doppler scanning.

Fine needle aspiration cytology

Aspiration cytology can be used to determine whether palpable lumps are solid or cystic or in the evaluation of impalpable mammographic lesions where a sample of cells can be aspirated under mammographic or ultrasound guidance. It is a safe and reliable out-patient procedure. The commonest complication is hematoma formation. Infection and pneumothorax have been documented, but are extremely rare.

Trucut biopsy

This can be performed under a local anesthetic in the out-patient clinic and used to confirm the nature of a suspicious lump.

Excision biopsy

There are a small proportion of breast lumps whose nature cannot be determined with these investigations and excision biopsy is required. If this is necessary, the breast incision should always be placed in a position that is (1) cosmetic and (2) could be incorporated in a further resection specimen if it proved to be a carcinoma.

Staging

Staging groups of patients according to the extent of their disease has been promoted as being useful in choosing treatment for individual patients, estimating prognosis and comparing the results of different treatment programs. The TNM and UICC systems have been developed for use in breast cancer patients. These are shown with five-year survival date in Table 14.1.

As staging is dependent on clinical examination (which is observer biased), the surgery performed and the use and availability of imaging techniques, accurate comparisons between patients worldwide are not possible. Furthermore if a patient has operable disease treatment decisions are based on the histological features of the primary tumor and the ipsilateral axillary lymph nodes and not on the clinical TNM staging.

Table 14.1.   The TNM staging of breast cancer.

T-stage reflects the size of the tumor

Tis	Carcinoma *in situ*
T1	< 2 cm diameter without skin fixation
T2	2–5 cm diameter without skin or pectoral fixation
T3	5–10 cm diameter, skin ulcerated over the lump, pectoral fixation
T4	Any size but direct extension to the overlying skin of chest wall

N-stage reflects the presence or absence of regional lymph node involvement

N0	No regional nodes
N1	Palpable mobile ipsilateral axillary lymph nodes
N3	Palpable immobile ipsilateral axillary lymph nodes
N4	Ipsilateral infra-clavicular or supraclavicular lymph nodes

M-stage indicates the presence or absence of metastatic tumor

M0	No evidence of distant metastases
M1	Distant metastases present

Correlation of UICC (International Union of Cancer) and TNM staging with breast cancer survival

UICC stage	TNM stage	Five-year survival
I	T1, N0, M0	84%
II	T1, N1, M0	71%
	T2, N0–1, M0	
III	any T, N2, N3, M0	48%
	T3, any N, M0	
	T4, any N, M0	
IV	any T, any N, M1	18%.

TREATMENT

A breast cancer patient is best cared for by a multidisciplinary approach between the surgeon, medical oncologist, radiotherapist and specially trained nurse counselor who can provide invaluable psychological support. Breast cancer is regarded as being a systemic disease from the outset where long-term survival is determined by the control of occult micrometastases. Treatment of operable breast cancer therefore requires local control (with surgery) combined with adjuvant therapies to treat systemic disease. Advanced disease is more appropriately treated primarily with endocrine therapy, chemotherapy or radiotherapy.

Surgery

Patients with operable disease may be offered breast conserving surgery or mastectomy. Breast conservation (i.e. excision of the tumor with a surrounding margin of normal tissue) with radiotherapy provides similar disease control and equivalent survival to mastectomy with a superior cosmetic result. However, it would be inappropriate for a large tumor in a small breast, if the cancer was multifocal, if the risk of recurrence in the breast is high (e.g. tumor extending to excision margins), or if a patient herself wishes to have a mastectomy.

Mastectomy involves excision of all the breast tissue with some of the overlying skin and all patients should be offered either immediate or delayed breast reconstruction. There is no evidence that immediate reconstructive surgery prevents the detection of local recurrence or affects survival. The aim of reconstruction is to provide symmetry with the opposite breast. There are many techniques including insertion of subpectoral silicone implants or tissue expanders and myocutaneous latissimus dorsi or rectus abdominous flaps.

The psychological outcome in patients undergoing conservative or more radical surgery has not been shown to differ indicating that it is the diagnosis itself which affects mental well-being.

Treatment of the axilla

Axillary lymph nodes are the principal site of regional metastases from breast cancer. They are the most important prognostic indicator as their involvement indicates that a patient has a high risk of relapse from metastatic disease. The greater the number of involved nodes the worse a patient's survival. Axillary surgery provides nodal tissue for histological examination and by removing axillary tissue prevents regional recurrence. Formal axillary dissection is better than either node biopsy or sampling which can provide prognostic information but at the expense of inadequate local control. Treating the axilla does not have any effect on survival.

Radical axillary radiotherapy achieves equivalent local control rates to axillary dissection, but prognositc information is unavailable.

RISKS OF TREATMENT

Complications after breast surgery include hematoma (which require evacuation) and seroma formation (these can be aspirated), infection and flap necrosis with mastectomy which rarely necessitates debridement and grafting. Radiotherapy can induce skin reactions such as erythema and telangiectasia. Radiation pneumonitis affects less than 2% of patients. Axillary surgery can cause damage to the intercostobrachial nerve with subsequent parasthesia or numbness, restricted shoulder movement and lymphoedema. Physiotherapy, arm massage and compression bandaging can relieve these latter complications. Supraclavicular radiotherapy is associated with a small risk of damage to the brachial plexus which can lead to intractable pain and loss of arm function. Avoidance of combined axillary surgery and radiotherapy has dramatically reduced the incidence of severe lymphoedema.

Risk evaluation and prognosis

In routine management of patients axillary node status is used to determine which patients should receive adjuvant chemotherapy; however, there are a proportion of patients without involved nodes who will have a poor prognosis and might benefit from adjuvant treatment. Unfortunately at present there is no accurate method of predicting who these patients are. Tumor size, histological grade and the presence of vascular or lymphatic invasion can be of use in these circumstances. Many other factors have been identified as correlating with prognosis, e.g. measures of tumor proliferation (S-phase fraction, thymidine-labelling index), C-erb2 oncogene but they do not appear to have practical significance and do not contribute towards patient management.

ADJUVANT SYSTEMIC TREATMENT

In an overview of 133 randomized trials of adjuvant therapies in the treatment of early breast cancer the benefits of different adjuvant treatments in pre- and post-menopausal women were defined. Systemic adjuvant therapy decreases the risk of relapse or death by up to 30% at 10 years, although the absolute overall benefits are much more modest (4–12%).

In women less than 50 years of age, a significant reduction in the annual rates of recurrence and death can be achieved by the use of polychemotherapy and ovarian ablation. Common side effects of chemotherapy include lethargy, nausea and vomiting, alapecia (temporary), risk of infection, mucositis and diarrhea. Ovarian ablation induces a premature menopause.

The effects of pre-operative (i.e. neoadjuvant) chemotherapy on the survival of patients is currently being investigated including the possibility that tumors can be downstaged so enabling conservative surgery to take place (thus avoiding mastectomy).

Tamoxifen prescribed to post-menopausal women reduces the annual rate of death by 17%, recurrence by 25% and the incidence of contralateral breast cancer by 39%. Trials are underway to evaluate whether two or five years is the optimum duration of treatment. Long-term use has been associated with thickening of the endometrium and possibly endometrial hyperplasia or carcinoma; this, however, has still to be fully evaluated. Investigation of patients is presently recommended only if they are symptomatic (e.g. abnormal or post-menopausal bleeding). Over the last 10 yrs, mortality from early stage breast cancer has fallen by 10% in England and Wales. This has been attributed to more widespread use of adjuvant tamoxifen and chemotherapy.

Table 14.2. Treatment of the complications of advanced breast cancer.

Complication	Treatment
Hypercalcemia	Rehydration, Calcium-lowering drugs, e.g. bisphosphonates
Pathological fracture	Internal fixation and radiotherapy
Cord compression (emergency as risk of paraplegia)	Radiotherapy (before paraplegia) Surgical decompression +/- stabilization spine and radiotherapy (if signs of paraplegia)
Cerebral metastases	Dexamethasone and radiotherapy
Pain control	Analgesia (use in a graduated fashion) Pain clinics (if appropriate and available) Nerve block, cordotomy

TREATMENT OF METASTATIC DISEASE

Metastatic disease is incurable and once detected the average duration of survival is two years. Disease palliation while maintaining a good quality of life is the management goal.

Endocrine treatment is usually the first-line therapy. Tamoxifen is the drug of choice in post-menopausal women while zoladex (a gonadotrophin releasing hormone analogue) or ovarian ablation can be used in pre-menopausal patients. The response is usually of the order of 25–30% but may be as much as 60% in estrogen receptor positive tumors. If there is no response or relapse at multiple sites second line hormonal therapy (e.g. progestogens or aromatase inhibitors) can be used but the clinical response rates are usually not as marked. Chemotherapy is indicated in endocrine resistant disease, rapidly progressive or life-threatening disease and younger patients. Approximately 60% of patients will have a response of an average duration of six months. Further treatment with second- and third-line chemotherapy regimes can be used but the response rates are less.

Secondaries can arise at any site and should be treated appropriately (see Table 14.2). Close liaison between hospital staff, the palliative care team and the family practitioner is essential in the manage-

ment and emotional support of terminally ill patients and their relatives.

FOLLOW-UP

Patient follow-up involves the diagnosis and treatment of recurrent disease, evaluation of the effectiveness of therapies (including patients treated within clinical trials), monitoring for long-term complications of treatment and patient rehabilitation and psychological support. Routine re-staging investigations to detect recurrence do not appear to yield any more information than that obtained from a history, examination, mammography and additional tests as dictated by patient symptoms and have no effect on patient survival. Mammography can be used to detect local relapse after breast conserving surgery and to screen the opposite breast for metastatic disease or a new primary. Psychological problems are common (30% of patients have significant depression and anxiety one year post diagnosis) and efforts need to be made to improve identification of patients at such risk.

References

Barr, L.C. and Baum, M. (1992). Time to abandon TMN staging of breast cancer? *Lancet*, **339**, 915–917.

Bostwick, J. III. (1990). *Plastic and Reconstructive Breast Surgery*. St Louis, Missouri: Quality Medical Publishing Inc.

Ciatto, S., Pacini, P., Azzini, V., *et al.* (1988). Preoperative breast cancer investigations: a multicentre study. *Cancer*, **61**, 1038–40.

Collaborative Group on Hormonal Factors in Breast Cancer (1997). Breast cancer and hormone replacement therapy: collaborative reanalysis of data from 51 epidemiological studies of 52,705 women with breast cancer and 108,411 women without breast cancer. *Lancet*, **350**, 1047–1059.

Collaborative Group on Hormonal Factors in Breast Cancer (19967). Breast cancer and hormonal contraceptives: collaborative reanalysis of individual data on 53,297 women with breast cancer and 100,239 women without breast cancer from 54 epidemiological studies. *Lancet*, **347**, 1713–1727.

Early Breast Cancer Trialist's Collaborative Group. (1992). Systemic treatment of early breast cancer by hormonal, cytotoxic of immune therapy. *Lancet*, **339**, 1–15, 71–85.

Easton, D.F., Narod, S., Ford, D. and Steel, M. on behalf of the Breast Cancer Linkage Consortium. (1994). The genetic epidemiology of BRCA1. *Lancet*, **344**, 761.

Fallowfield, L.J., Baum, M. and Maguire, G.P. (1986). Effects of breast conservation on psychological morbidity associated with diagnosis and treatment of primary breast cancer. *British Medical Journal*, **293**, 1331–34.

Fisher, B., Redmond, C., Poisson, R., *et al.* (1989). Eight year results of a randomized trial comparing total mastectomy and lumpectomy with or without radiotherapy in the treatment of breast cancer. *New England Journal of Medicine*, **320**, 822–828.

Tomiak, E. and Piccart, M. (1993). Routine follow-up of patients after primary therapy for early breast cancer: Changing concepts and challenges for the future. *Annals of Oncology*, **4**, 144–204.

140

Breast Cancer

200 times more common in women

Worldwide: most frequent in women
  3rd most common in world

Lifetime risk
in USA whites:
  M 1 in 1000
  F 1 in 8

Relative five-year survival in 1983–87
in USA whites:
  F 80.1%

Risk factors
Family history of breast cancer
Reproductive factors: late age at first birth,
nulliparity, early menarche, late menopause
Obesity in post-menopausal women
Ionizing radiation
Breast feeding possibly confers protection
Dietary fat suspected but not established
Alcohol may increase risk
Environmental factors appear to be more important
than racial characteristics in the development of the
disease (e.g., 2nd generation Japanese women liv-
ing in the USA)

Geographical variation in 1983–87
Highest rate

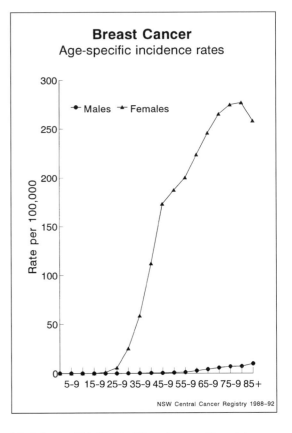

M: 2.2 per 100,000 in Kuwait, non-Kuwaitis
F: 104.2 per 100,000 in USA, Bay Area, whites
Lowest rate
M: 0.2 per 100,000 in Japan, Osaka
F: 9.5 per 100,000 in China, Qidong

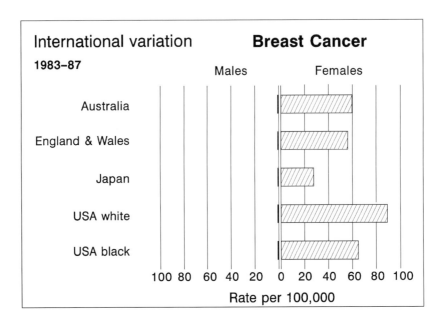

15. Lung Cancer

CHRIS WILLIAMS

Institute of Health Science, Oxford, UK

INTRODUCTION AND ETIOLOGY

Lung cancer is easily the commonest malignancy in the western world — a fact made more poignant since it is one of the most recent and preventable of all cancers. The rise in incidence of the tumor this century is really remarkable. In a major monograph on thoracic pathology in 1912, Adler says, "On one point, however, there is nearly complete consensus of opinion, and that is that primary malignant neoplasms of the lungs are amongst the rarest forms of disease." Contrast this with the current incidence rates in western countries (about 110 per 100,000 for men and 30 per 100,000 for women) and the extent of the epidemic becomes clear.

Any discussion of the etiology of lung cancer must take into account this dramatic change in its incidence. While there are probably a number of factors that play a part in the cause of the tumor, one, cigarette smoking, is by far the most important. Although tobacco has been used in western countries for 400 years, it was the development of the cigarette at the end of the last century, with cured tobacco that could be inhaled deeply into the lungs, that led to the epidemic of this disease. As with many other cancers caused by chemical carcinogens, there is a long "lag period" between the start of exposure to cigarette smoke and the development of lung cancer. This is usually in the region of 20–40 years, a finding which fits well with the sudden increase in lung cancer in men which began in the 1930s. This being some 20 years after the

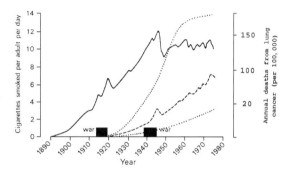

Figure 15.1. Cigarette consumption (mean number smoked per adult per day) and lung cancer mortality from 1890 to 1980.

First World War — the first time that cigarette smoking really became common. It was General Pershing, in 1917, who said that cigarettes are "as indispensable as the daily ration." The incidence in women didn't start to rise till the late 1940s, women having started to smoke some 10–20 years after men. Figure 15.1 shows the annual per capita consumption of cigarettes, by sex, from the beginning of this century and the rising death rate from lung cancers that starts some two decades later. The death rates are similar to the incidence rate since the long-term survival rates of this disease are so poor (approaching 5% at 10 years).

There are many other strands of evidence linking cigarette smoking to lung cancer. Amongst these are:

1. The incidence of lung cancer rises with increasing consumption of cigarettes.

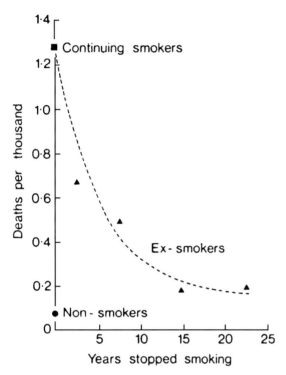

Figure 15.2. Mortality rate (per thousand) from lung cancer in the years from stopping smoking.

western countries is resulting in a fall in lung cancer deaths.

Other factors implicated in the development of lung cancer, apart from smoking, include:

1. Genetic predisposition. Although lung cancer is not an inherited disease, there is strong evidence that first-degree relatives have an increased risk of cancer, including lung cancer. One possible explanation for this may be inherited difference in enzymes involved in the metabolism of carcinogens in cigarette smoke. Tentative evidence does indeed link lung cancer to several such enzymes. Another alternative explanation is that, since two hits are necessary to inactivate a recessive oncogene, one of these mutations could be inherited in the germ line from the parents. For instance, patients successfully treated for inherited retinoblastoma subsequently have a greatly increased risk (more than 15-fold) of developing small cell lung cancer. Similarly some families with the inherited condition Li-Fraumeni syndrome (mutation of the p53 gene) have a propensity to develop lung cancer.

2. Diet low in vegetables and fruit. A number of studies have shown that there is an inverse relationship between serum levels of vitamin A and lung cancer. However, recent randomized controlled trials of vitamin supplementation, using carotenes, has failed to show any reduction in the incidence of lung cancer — though in one study low pre-treatment serum levels of carotene were correlated with a higher risk of developing lung cancer.

3. Pollution. Although lung cancer has a higher incidence in urban areas, the influence of air pollution on the causation of lung cancer is thought to be relatively small compared to cigarette smoking. However, a small number of individuals exposed to carcinogens (asbestos, chromates, nickel, arsenic, radioactive materials, mustard gas and the products of coal distillation) at work do have a definite increase in risk of lung cancer. Of these asbestos is the most important factor — there is likely to be an epidemic of both lung cancer and mesothelioma in the next several decades related to asbestos exposure. The risk of these diseases is increased in a synergistic fashion if the exposed individual is also a smoker (the risk of devel-

2. Even more persuasive is the fall in incidence of lung cancer that occurs when a group of smokers give up the habit. Figure 15.2 shows that there is a gradual fall in risk of lung cancer after stopping smoking, till it is only marginally higher than that of a life-time non-smoker. A similar pattern is found for cardiovascular disease.

3. Risks vary according to smoking habit — for example, the length of butt left, the tar content, the use of filters and age at starting — those at greatest risk are smokers who keep the cigarette in their mouth between puffs and who relight half-smoked cigarettes.

These sorts of findings have been duplicated in multiple retrospective and prospective studies in over 20 countries. Even in countries with lower incidence rates than Western countries, the findings are remarkably homogenous. Unfortunately, the habit of cigarette smoking has recently been exported to many other countries and the incidence of lung cancer is increasing in the rest of the world — just at a time when the reduction in smoking in

Table 15.1. Histological classification of lung cancer.

Squamous carcinoma
Small cell carcinoma
Adenocarcinoma
   Bronchogenic
   Acinar
   Bronchioalveolar
Large cell carcinoma
   With or without mucin
   Giant cell
   Clear cell
Mixed tumors
Other tumors
   Carcinoid
   Cylindroma
   Sarcoma

oping lung cancer for someone exposed to asbestos who is also a smoker is 45-fold greater than the normal population).

PATHOLOGY

Lung cancer is primarily a disease of the large and medium-sized bronchi — it rarely arises in the true lung parenchyma. Although there is much variation in histological appearance and there are often admixtures of different histological types, it is customary to divide it into four major histological groups (Table 15.1). Current evidence suggests that these different types of lung cancer develop from a common precursor cell that has the capacity to differentiate into a variety of histological types. The stem cells in the large bronchi may , however, differ from those in smaller bronchi.

Squamous cell lung cancer

This is the commonest histological type of lung cancer. It is characterized by the presence of keratinization and/or intercellular bridging. It is often subdivided on the basis of cellular differentiation. They generally develop in large airways and are usually central tumors, though they can be seen in the peripheral lung. Since there is no squamous epithelium in the bronchi it seems likely that malignant change is preceded by squamous metaplasia.

Adenocarcinoma

These tumors show the typical appearance of tumors derived from glandular epithelium with formation of acini, papillae and mucus. Adenocarcinomas may sometimes arise in scar tissue and fibrotic lung disease. They are more often peripheral in site than the other types of lung cancer and are less clearly related to cigarette smoking. They appear to be somewhat commoner in women. Interestingly, there appears to be an increase in incidence of this histological type of lung cancer in western countries. Bronchiolo-alveolar cell carcinoma is an uncommon variant that presents with multifocal tumors spread widely in the lung.

Large cell undifferentiated

This histological group of tumors, which is fairly uncommon, has a variable appearance. The cells are large with a featureless cytoplasm and they have little tendency to keratinization or acinar formation. Some may, however, produce mucin and have ultrastructural features that are typical of adenocarcinoma. The tumor often arises in the more distal bronchi.

Small cell carcinoma

This tumor is characterized by the presence of a diffuse growth of small cells with finely granular nuclei, inconspicuous nucleioli and scanty cytoplasm. The cells are often tightly packed and molded. They are often very fragile, with smearing of DNA and a high proportion of pyknotic cells. Neurosecretory granules are often seen on electron microscopy. They usually arise in the larger bronchi and are nearly always central tumors. They have a high tendency to both local invasion and lymphatic and blood-borne spread so that surgery is rarely helpful. These tumors are thought to derive from APUD (amine precursor uptake and decarboxylase) cells which contain neurosecretory granules. In keeping with this is the observation that small cell lung cancer is the malignant tumor most often implicated in the ectopic production of hormones (ADH, ACTH and calcitonin most commonly).

Making the diagnosis

Although lung cancer cells can be found in the sputum of 80% of patients with the disease, examination of isolated sputum specimens is not a reliable method of diagnosis, with a pick-up rate of only 50%. This rises to nearly 80% when four sequential specimens are examined; however, time

Table 15.2. Signs and symptoms of lung cancer. Those that are common are shown in a **bold** type face.

General effects
  Weakness
  Cachexia
Ectopic endocrine effects
  SIADH
  Hypercalcemia
  Cushing's syndrome
  Carcinoid syndrome
  Paraneoplastic syndromes
    Acanthosis nigricans
    Autonomic overactivity
    Hypertrophic pulmonary osteoarthropathy (**clubbing alone is common**)
    Disseminated intravascular coagulation
    Tylosis
    Non-bacterial thrombotic endocarditis
    Migratory venous thrombosis
    Neurological syndromes: Encephalopathy
                    Cortical cerebellar degeneration
                    Peripheral neuropathies
                    Myasthenia-like (Eaton-Lambert)
Local effects
  Cough
  Dyspnoea
  Chest pain
  Hemoptysis
  Wheeze or stridor
  Pneumonic (fever, productive cough)
Regional effects
  Recurrent laryngeal nerve palsy (hoarseness)
  Phrenic nerve palsy (elevation of hemidiaphragm)
  Superior vena caval obstruction
  Pleural effusion
  Pericardial tamponade
  Cardiac arrhythmia
  Esophageal compression causing dysphagia
  Bronchesophageal fistula
Metastatic
  Liver
  Contra-lateral lung
  Brain
  Spinal cord
  Bone (including marrow)
  Adrenal

should not be wasted waiting for the results of such tests before organizing other more definitive tests. At bronchoscopy, biopsy, brush and lavage specimens will usually make the diagnosis cytologically or histologically and will be a more accurate guide to histological subtype. Where there are palpable enlarged lymph nodes, likely to be involved by tumor, fine needle aspiration is very useful.

CLINICAL FEATURES

The median age of onset is about 70 years and the sex ratio is 2.5:1 males to females. Most patients with lung cancer present with symptoms caused by the presence of the tumor in their chest. Since they usually have a history of chronic obstructive airways disease, being smokers, their symptoms (Table 15.2) are often similar to those they chronically or intermittently suffer from. It is, therefore, not surprising that the diagnosis is often delayed until the patient has failed to respond to several courses of antibiotics given for a "chest infection."

Intrathoracic

Cough is extremely common and is often paroxysmal in character gradually becoming more frequent and troublesome. Hemoptysis is less commonly seen but should always be taken seriously; 50% of men in developed countries over 40 years of age who have hemoptysis turn out to have lung cancer. Pain in the chest, when it is not due to pleuritic involvement, is often non-specific and may even be on the opposite side to the tumor. The symptoms of the cancer are often sufficiently different in quality from those that the patient normally experiences for them to respond by giving up smoking. Over half the patients seen with lung cancer give a history of having "given up" smoking in the preceding few months.

Peripheral tumors often present late with involvement of the structures of the chest wall. This frequently causes pain due to extension of tumor into ribs and the pleura. Tumors at the apex of the lung may cause a characteristic syndrome (Superior sulcus or Pancoast's) due to invasion of the brachial plexus. This leads to pain in the chest, shoulder and arm and to weakness of the small muscles of the hand which is caused by C8/T1 motor loss. Rib destruction is very common and sometimes there is involvement of vertebra.

Central tumors are more common and lead to a number of specific symptoms in addition to those seen in chronic lung disease. These may be broken down by whether they are secondary to endobronchial growth or pressure. These include dyspnoea due to obstruction of a central airway with consequent collapse of the segment of the lung supplied by that airway and wheeze and stridor caused by severe narrowing of a major airway. Other symptoms of central disease already mentioned include cough, hemoptysis and infection. Central tumors also cause symptoms by pressure and invasion of other structures in the mediastinum. These include obstruction of the superior vena cava. The superior vena cava formed by the junction of the innominate veins runs downward to the heart along the right sternal border and is thus more likely to be obstructed by right sided tumors. Just before entering the peri-cardial sac the superior vena cava is joined by the azygous vein, and the clinical picture seen in superior vena caval obstruction depends on whether the obstruction is proximal or distal to this venous junction. When the obstruction is above the junction with the azygous vein there is distention of the arm and neck veins, suffusion or oedema of the face, neck and arms, and the presence of dilated, tortuous collateral vessels on the upper chest and back. Obstruction of the vena cava proximal to the junction of the azygous vein causes a more severe picture, with more extensive collateral circulation along the anterior and posterior abdominal walls in order to reach the systemic circulation via collaterals to the inferior vena cava. Small cell lung cancer is the commonest cause of this syndrome.

Involvement of the pericardium may lead to an effusion and occasionally tamponade. Arrhythmias are sometimes seen as a consequence of pericardial tumor extension. Involvement of the pleura commonly results in a pleural effusion. Other structures commonly involved by these tumors include the left recurrent laryngeal nerve and the phrenic nerve on either side. The course of the left recurrent laryngeal nerve around the arch of the aorta makes it especially vulnerable to damage by central tumors on the left. This causes a weak hoarse voice with a characteristic bovine cough. Once established this seldom returns to normal, despite treatment of the underlying cancer. Phrenic nerve damage causes paralysis of the diaphragm on the involved side.

Involvement of the esophagus by lung cancer is relatively uncommon. Patients may develop symptoms due to external pressure on the esophagus or there may be direct invasion of the esophagus which may go on to form a broncho-esophageal fistulae.

Extrathoracic

Lung cancer commonly metastasizes so that presentation with clinically obvious metastatic disease at one or more sites is common. The organs most commonly involved are:

- bones
- liver
- draining lymph nodes
- brain
- skin
- adrenals
- contralateral lung

Other syndromes

Lung cancers are one of the commonest causes of a variety of paraneoplastic syndromes. These are listed in Table 15.2. Of these, the syndrome of inappropriate secretion of antidiuretic hormone (SIADH) is the commonest, being found in up to one-half of patients with small cell lung cancer. Occasionally it may be severe, resulting in a very low serum sodium and fits.

Hypercalcemia is relatively uncommon, being seen most often in association with squamous carcinoma of the lung. The symptoms associated with a raised calcium include obtundation occasionally leading to frank coma, nausea and vomiting, constipation and polyuria.

Clubbing is common in lung cancer though rarely symptomatic, but the painful condition hypertrophic pulmonary osteoarthropathy is rare. In addition to clubbing of the fingers and toes there is pain and tenderness over the distal ends of the tibia, fibula, radius and ulna, caused by periostitis. It is most commonly seen in adenocarcinoma of the lung (12% of cases).

Neurological syndromes, such as Eaton Lambert, are rare and may start several years before the cancer is diagnosed. They rarely respond to treatment of the underlying cancer.

MANAGEMENT

The management of lung cancer is classically lumped together and separated into two main groups — small cell lung cancer and the other histological subtypes amalgamated together and called collectively non-small cell lung cancer. This is done because of differences in the underlying biology of the two groups which results in different clinical behavior and response to treatment. The key difference, clinically, is the different outcomes seen with surgery and chemotherapy between the two groups.

The first step in management is making the diagnosis. The differing emphasis in management for the two main clinical subtypes means that it is very important to differentiate small cell tumors from the other sorts of lung cancer. This can often be done cytologically. Brochoscopy and other invasive methods of making the diagnosis should not be delayed.

Small cell lung cancer

These tumors are aggressive, invading and spreading locally, by lymphatics and through the bloodstream, Obvious metastases are found in a half of patients at presentation and nearly all the rest prove to have microscopic metastases which become evident later. Most of these tumors are central and not technically amenable to surgery. Thus, surgery plays little part in the care of these patients. Historic series showed very few survivors (1%) in the minority of patients who had tumors that could be operated on. The only exception to this is the very rare patient who presents with a small peripheral lung mass. In this situation up to a third of patients may survive 5 or more years. Since surgery is rarely indicated for patients with small cell lung cancer, there is no need for detailed staging of the extent of the cancer and the staging system used simply divides patients into two groups — limited (disease confined to one hemi-thorax with or without involved lymph nodes in the low neck) and extensive (any disease more extensive than limited).

Trials of radiotherapy as primary management carried out in the 1960s and 70s showed that it was as ineffective as surgery, a result which was not surprising since the main problem with this disease is the propensity to early metastatic spread.

Chemotherapy

During the early 1970s a number of chemotherapy agents were found to be active in this disease and by the middle of that decade trials of combinations of cytotoxic drugs were starting to appear. Combinations of three or four individually active cytotoxic drugs will regularly produce high response rates (Table 15.3). The great disappointment for workers in this field is that there has not been a concomitant progressive increase in long-term survival. While

Table 15.3. Chemotherapeutic agents in small cell lung cancer.

Cytotoxic drugs with a 20% or higher response rate:

Tenoposide	65%
Carboplatin	50%
Etoposide	45%
Cyclophosphamide	40%
Vincristine	35%
Doxorubicin	30%
Methyl CCNU	25

Activity of 2 to 4 drug combinations:

Limited disease
  Overall response rate — 70–80%
  Complete remission rate — 40–50%
  Partial remission rate — 30–40%
Extensive disease
  Overall response rate — 40–50%
  Complete Remission rate — 10%
  Partial remission rate — 30–40%

some tumors, like testicular cancer for instance, were in the same position as small cell lung cancer (SCBC) in the 1970s and have gone on to have higher and higher cure rates, this has not happened in SCBC. This has been despite the use of increased doses and intensity of therapy and the introduction of new classes of active agents.

Although chemotherapy has yet to produce the improved long-term survival rates that were hoped for, it has become the primary therapy of this disease. Because of the high risk of metastases systemic therapy is required. The optimal chemotherapy regimen is unclear; recognized combinations of drugs using two to four of the following drugs should be considered: carboplatin, etoposide, cyclophosphamide, vincristine, doxorubicin.

High dose chemotherapy, with hemopoetic growth factor support or peripheral stem cell support (autologous bone marrow support in the past), remains experimental, there being no evidence that it results in increased survival.

Treatment with chemotherapy will increase median survival by 6–12 months, but rarely produces long-term disease control. Thus, the median survival for patients with localized disease is about 15–18 months while that for patients with extensive disease is 10–12 months. These results (Figure 15.3) are derived from clinical trials, which may exclude some of the sicker patients, so that the true figures in routine practice are probably somewhat lower. However, despite the side effects of chemotherapy, many patients have a good temporary response and feel better and return to a more normal life style for

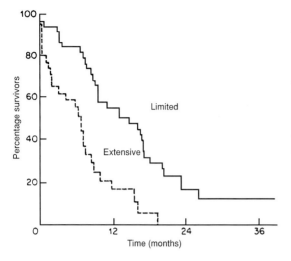

Figure 15.3. Survival curves for patients with limited and extensive small cell lung cancer treated with combination chemotherapy. Median survival for extensive disease is less than a year and for limited disease is about 15–18 months. Untreated, the median survival figures are 9 and 11 weeks respectively.

a period of time. Because of this many clinicians and patients feel that the treatment is worthwhile, even though it is not curative.

Radiotherapy

Although it is not used as a primary treatment for SCBC anymore, radiotherapy still plays an important role in the management of this disease. Where patients have localized disease, apparently limited to the mediastinum, radiotherapy may be combined with chemotherapy in order to get the best possible control of the primary tumor. The best way to combine these therapies is unclear. Concomitant use increases toxicity but might improve local disease control; use of radiotherapy after chemotherapy is the usual alternative which is adopted. A series of randomized trials comparing chemotherapy alone with chemotherapy and radiotherapy have shown that local control rates and survival rates were a little better (about 5%) when both treatments were used.

Radiotherapy also has a role as a palliative treatment for patients with progressive or relapsing disease. It should be remembered that such treatment will not affect survival, its intended effect being symptom control only. Because of this prolonged fractionation schedules and toxic treatments should be avoided. Radiotherapy also has a role in the prevention of brain metastases in patients responding well to primary therapy. During the course of the disease up to a half of patients will develop clinically significant brain metastases (30–40%) or will be found to have unrecognized brain metastases at autopsy (10%). Randomized trials comparing a policy of prophylactic whole brain radiotherapy after primary treatment with no initial whole brain radiotherapy, have shown that the incidence of clinically evident brain metastases is reduced from 25 to less than 10%. There is, however, little or no effect on overall survival — patients developing brain metastases usually relapse at other sites at around the same time. At present many centers who offer such treatment confine it to those with less extensive disease who respond well to initial chemotherapy.

Surgery

As noted above the routine role of surgery in SCBC is limited to the occasional patient who presents with a small isolated peripheral lung lesion. Clinical trials in the past few years have been asking whether surgery after, or during, chemotherapy may be beneficial in patients who have localized disease and who respond well to initial chemotherapy. Current trials are inconclusive and such therapy, often combined with radiotherapy to the mediastinum, remains experimental in nature.

Small cell lung cancer is a highly aggressive tumor that despite good initial responses to chemo — and other therapies nearly always relapses. Five-year survival rates for unselected patients are around 5%. However, good temporary symptom control is gained with treatment and therapy is normally worth considering in all but the sickest patient. Response to therapy should always be monitored closely. Failure to respond or progression after an initial response should always result in the treatment being reappraised — where the intent of therapy is primarily palliative, unnecessary treatment should always be avoided.

Non-small cell lung cancer

The main reason that these tumors are lumped together and separated from SCBC is that the mainstay of their treatment for potential cure is surgery. Every effort should be made to identify those patients whose tumor may be amenable to

Table 15.4. Investigation used to stage non-small cell lung cancer prior to surgery.

History and physical examination
Chest X-ray
Bronchoscopy
Hematology and biochemistry
If there is then no contra-indication to surgery, proceed to selected tests from these options:
    CT scan of thorax
    MRI of the thorax
    Mediastinotomy/oscopy
    Ultra sound/CT scan/MRI of the abdomen

surgical intervention. Unfortunately the proportion who fall into this group is relatively small.

When the diagnosis has been confirmed, patients should be assessed for surgery. Some patients will have obvious metastatic disease on routine examination or will be too unwell and will be ruled out straight away — half of all patients fall into this category. The remaining half will need further investigations to be carried out. These are outlined in Table 15.4. Bronchoscopy should always be carried out and CT scan is often useful. Mediastinoscopy or mediastinotomy is frequently needed to look for the presence of involved lymph nodes in the center of the chest — CT can be misleading whether or not enlarged glands are seen. Routine biochemistry and hematology should be carried out with special attention to the possibility of hypercalcaemia (most commonly in squamous carcinoma) and changes consistent with involvement of the bone marrow with cancer. The finding of a low sodium, suggesting SIADH, should always suggest the possibility that the tumor is an SCBC.

There is no consensus on whether special tests to look for metastatic disease should be done routinely. Some centers will only carry out such studies when there is a symptom, physical finding or blood test result that suggests that there may be organ involvement. Others routinely carry out more extensive investigation of the likely sites of metastatic involvement. Some assessment of respiratory function is also needed to see if the patient will have sufficient respiratory capacity after excision of part or all of the affected lung.

At the end of this process only about 25% of presenting patients will be suitable for a surgery. One measurement of excellence in a thoracic surgery center is the rate of unnecessary thoracotomies. This should be about 5–10% — high rates mean

that there is an unacceptable number of patients who are going through the morbidity of surgery for no benefit at all. The art of selecting patients is to pick out all of those who might benefit, while avoiding those who will prove to have disease found to be too extensive to resect at thoracotomy.

The surgical procedure used will be tailored to the situation found at operation and may vary from a tissue conserving operation such as a segmentectomy to complete removal of the affected lung. Mortality of the operation will be governed by the extent of the operation and the fitness of the patient prior to surgery. Age in itself is not a bar to surgery, it is fitness that is crucial. Since nearly all the patients have been long-term smokers they will frequently have other severe illnesses. Mortality will vary from 2–6% in most centers. Morbidity is quite severe. In addition to the usual post-operative complications of surgery, pain in the chest can be a long-term problem for some patients.

Not surprisingly, the long-term outcome following surgery is closely connected to the stage of the disease at the time of surgery. The full staging

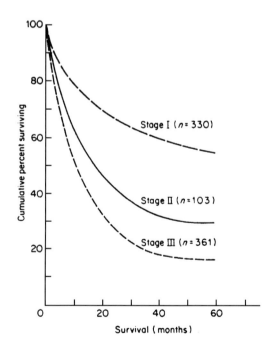

Figure 15.4. Survival, by stage, for patients with non-small cell lung cancer treated by surgical resection. Although, in this series, a substantial number of patients operated on had stage 1 disease, this figure is inflated by selection — there are many more patients with stage 3 disease who are either inoperable or on the borderline of operability.

system is very complicated, with multiple clinical and pathological stages, and beyond the scope of this book. The staging system is simplified by condensing the multiple groups into four stages, stages 1–3 being increasing disease within the chest and stage 4 being metastatic disease. Figure 15.4 shows the survival of patients with resectable disease. Unfortunately most patients with surgically resectable disease present with relatively advanced cancer (stage 3), so that the optimistic results for stage 1 and 2 disease are confined to a very small proportion of all patients presenting with lung cancer.

Adjuvant therapy

Over the past couple of decades attempts have been made to improve the outcome of patients with early stage lung cancer by adding chemotherapy or radiotherapy to surgery. The usefulness of this approach has not been clearly shown in these trials and there is no consensus on when or how to use this approach. A recent systematic review of the literature found that the addition of modern (cisplatin containing) chemotherapy modestly improved the long-term outlook for patients treated with primary surgery and/or radiotherapy. Because the data was based on many small trials and the results were not clear cut, the use of adjuvant chemotherapy after primary therapy is currently being tested in large-scale trials. One finding that was clear from this systematic review was that patients who were treated in the past with alkylating agent monochemotherapy fared worse, with significantly shorter survival times. Chemotherapy is also being tested to see if its use prior to considering surgery can increase the number of patients who are able to undergo a resection of their tumor. The group targeted in these trials is those patients with quite extensive intrathoracic disease who are on the borderline of resectability.

Radiotherapy

The main role of radiation in non-small cell lung cancer is palliative. It is sometimes used as part of the primary therapy in relatively early stage lung cancer, often these days in conjunction with chemotherapy. Radical radiotherapy may also be used in patients who have a surgically resectable cancer but who cannot undergo surgery for other reasons, such as poor respiratory reserve.

For the great majority of patients the disease is too advanced to consider curative therapy and the intent of radiation treatment is symptom control. In this situation the disease that is causing problems may be in the chest (cough, hemoptysis, collapse of lung, superior vena caval obstruction) or it may be metastatic (bone pain/fracture, brain metastases, spinal cord compression, lymph node masses). When radiotherapy is used for intrathoracic disease, the treatment should be made as simple as possible so that unnecessary discomfort is avoided. A British Medical Research Council trial has recently shown that a short course of radiotherapy (two fractions) is just as effective as a longer course (10 fractions). Similar studies of the management of bone metastases have shown that short courses of therapy are as effective as longer courses and are much easier for patients. It should always be borne in mind that the median survival from presentation for unresectable non-small cell lung cancer is only about 4–6 months.

A further dilemma facing radiotherapists is when to use therapy in patients who are not currently particularly symptomatic. One school of thought says that the majority of patients will develop symptoms from the tumor in their chest before they die and that this should be irradiated straight away. Others argue that since treatment is palliative it should only be used when the patient has significant symptoms that could be palliated by radiotherapy. There is no clear evidence as to which is the best approach from the patient's point of view and such randomized trials are currently being carried out. Even short courses of radiotherapy cause moderate side effects, their intensity being amplified by the poor general condition of this group of sick patients. The main side effects are temporary increase in cough, soreness on swallowing and malaise. In general radiotherapy is fairly effective in palliating some of the symptoms of advanced lung cancer (Table 15.5).

Table 15.5. Symptomatic response to radiotherapy in lung cancer.

Symptom	Response rate (%)
SVCO	95%
Hemoptysis	80%
Pain	75%
Dyspnoea	70%
Brain metastases	65%
Atelectasis	55%
Vocal cord paralysis	5%

Chemotherapy

Has been little used in this disease till the past few years. This was because of poor response rates to therapy, the fact that there was no effect on survival and there was quite marked toxicity. The introduction of drug combinations including cisplatin has resulted in improved response rate (50% or more shrinkage of tumor) to therapy (increased to 40–50%), though at the expense of moderate to severe toxicity. A recent meta-analysis of chemotherapy showed that there was a statistically significant improvement in survival in trials comparing a policy of chemotherapy and best supportive care with best supportive care alone. However, the advantage was small — patients only surviving some extra six weeks or so. There is debate as to whether such a small gain is worthwhile and a new generation of large trials has begun to try to answer the question more clearly. One of the major deficits in all previous lung cancer trials has been a failure to measure the quality of life of those individuals in the trials. Since most of the treatment is palliative and the therapeutic gains have been modest at best, it is essential that we now try to measure what subjective benefit or deficit patients experience when treated for this disease.

Conclusions

Lung cancer, whatever the histologically subtype, is a devastating disease with a very high death rate. The five-year survival rate for non-small cell lung cancer is not much more than 5% for non-small cell lung cancer (usually in surgically resectable patients), a figure that is similar to that seen in patients with small cell lung cancer when it is treated with chemotherapy. The principal guiding light in therapeutic decisions should be finding ways to best palliate while causing the minimum of side effects and discomfort. Patients should be included in the decision-making process so that their concerns are properly addressed. Current studies are concentrating on the use of combined modalities of therapy to see if modest improvements in survival and quality of life will result. There continues to be a desperate need for new, more effective and innovative therapies. Patients who wish it may be suitable for inclusion in trials testing such treatments.

It is salutary to remember, in the light of these depressing facts, that lung cancer is the most easily avoided of all cancers.

MESOTHELIOMA

This is still a relatively uncommon cancer, though its incidence is rapidly increasing in most developed countries. There is evidence, gathered over the past several decades, that this malignant tumor is closely related to exposure to asbestos. Because exposure has often been industrial (ship yards, docks, lagging, railway manufacture, etc.) mesothelioma is often concentrated in those localities where these industries were common (Figure 15.5). Although it most commonly affects the pleura, it may also arise in the peritoneum and other sites. The median age of onset is about 55 years with a 2:1 male to female sex ratio.

The period between exposure to asbestos and development of the tumor (the latent interval) may be very long (40 or more years) and the exposure need not be heavy or prolonged. Those heavily exposed are, however, at highest risk. The risk is multiplied in smokers since there seems to be a synergistic interaction between cigarette smoking and asbestos exposure — this results in an increase in the numbers of both mesotheliomas and lung cancer. The families of those exposed industrially are also at increased risk, presumably because of exposure to asbestos carried home in work clothes. Those living in the vicinity of asbestos factories are also at an increased risk compared with the general population. Clear evidence of asbestos exposure is present in 80% of cases of mesothelioma and it is suspected that nearly all the rest have been unknowingly exposed to asbestos at some time.

The risk depends on the type of asbestos — there are two main type of asbestos fibre:

- chrysotile, which is silky and serpentine, and
- amphiboles, which are straight and rod-like.

Mesothelioma risk is mainly related to the amphiboles. They in turn are divided into several subtypes. Of these crocidolite is said to carry the greatest risk though none is safe. Autopsy studies in asbestos miners show that there is preferential clearing of the chrysotile fibres compared to the amphibole fibres

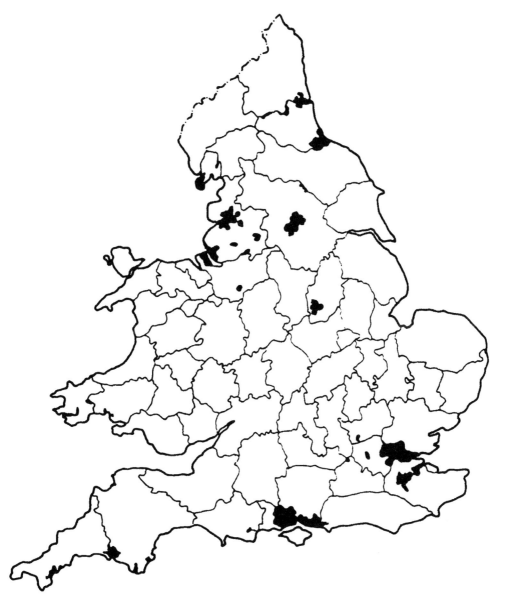

Figure 15.5. Distribution of mesothelioma in England and Wales. Areas of high incidence (black areas) are all in parts of the country where ship building, ports, railway manufacture, asbestos manufacture and other industries using asbestos are located.

— possibly as a consequence of the fibre size. The mechanism whereby the fibres induce malignant change in the pleura or peritoneum has yet to be fully elucidated.

Pathology and natural history

The primary sites for this tumor are pleura (by far the commonest), peritoneum (more common in asbestos miners), pericardium, tunica vaginalis, ovary, fallopian tube and uterus. It spreads by direct invasion with distant metastases being less common than in lung cancer. Pleural mesotheliomas often invade the chest wall and ribs.

Histologically they appear sarcomatous, though epithelial, fibrous and biphasic forms are described. Electron microscopy and immunohistochemistry may help distinguish between mesothelioma and poorly differentiated carcinoma — a not uncommon clinical problem.

The presenting features of mesothelioma will depend on the site of primary involvement. Thus:

- tumors of the pleura cause: chest pain
                                dyspnoea
                                weight loss
                                fever
- tumors of the
  peritoneum cause: abdominal swelling from
                      ascites
                      weight loss
                      abdominal pain

These symptoms are generally relentlessly progressive and are little changed by specific anticancer therapies.

Management

A good biopsy is essential as there may be doubt over the type of tumor since carcinomas may mimic mesothelioma. This information is important in planning therapy and in some countries in claims for compensation arising from exposure to asbestos. Extensive staging and investigation is rarely indicated since therapy is essentially palliative in nature. Where assessment of response to therapy is important, in a trial for instance, CT scans give a much better indication of what is happening than chest X-rays.

Treatment is in nearly all cases simple palliation. Surgery is used in some situations though its effectiveness has not been demonstrated in clinical trials. Occasional localized mesotheliomas can be removed macroscopically though most of these patients will go on to relapse and die of their disease. Excision of the pleura, where possible, is said to help control recurrent pleural effusions in some cases, though there are no controlled clinical trials to back this up. Radiotherapy is generally ineffective providing temporary pain relief in a minority of patients. Intracavitary radiocolloids have been of little value. Chemotherapy is also ineffective. Though there are a number of drugs and combinations of drugs that will cause some shrinkage of these tumors in up to 20–30% of patients, there is no evidence from randomized clinical trials that they cause patients to live longer or feel better

The disease is usually remorselessly progressive with most patients living 6–18 months. Less than 10% of patients survive three or more years. Good supportive care is essential; the main problems encountered by patients are pain, dyspnoea or bowel obstruction depending on the primary site, fevers, gross malaise and anorexia and weight loss.

References

Peto, R., Lopez, A.D., Boreham, J., Thun, M. and Heath, C. Jr. (1994). *Mortality from Smoking in Developed Countries, 1950–2000.* Oxford: Oxford University Press.

Non-small Cell Lung Cancer Collaborative Group. (1995). Chemotherapy in Non-small Cell Lung Cancer: a Meta-analysis Using Updated Data on Individual Patients from 52 Randomised Clinical Trials. *Brit. Med. J.*, **311**, 899–910.

Johnson, B.E. and Johnson, D.H. (1995). *Lung Cancer.* New York, USA: Wiley-Liss Inc.

Medical Research Council Lung Cancer Working Party. (1991). Inoperable Non-small Cell Lung Cancer (NSCLC): A Medical Research Council Randomised Trial of Palliative Radiotherapy with Two Fractions or Ten Fractions. *Brit. J. Cancer*, **63**, 265–270.

Girling, D.J. (1994). Recent Clinical Trials in Advanced Lung Cancer. In *New Perspectives in Lung Cancer*, edited by N. Thatcher and S. Spiro, pp. 105–119. British Medical Journal Publishing Group.

Lung Cancer

More common in men

Worldwide: Most common in world
Decreasing in developed countries;
increasing in developing countries

Lifetime risk
in USA whites:
 M 1 in 12
 F 1 in 20

Relative five-year survival in 1983–87
in USA whites:
 M 3.7%
 F 6.2%

Risk factors
Tobacco
 Accounts for 80–85% of lung cancers
Asbestos
Radon
Arsenic
Ionizing radiation

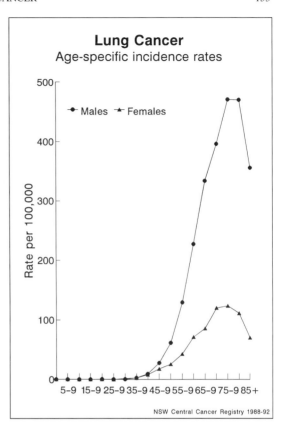

Geographical variation in 1983–87
Highest rate
M: 119.1 per 100,000 in New Zealand, Maoris
F: 62.2 per 100,000 in New Zealand, Maoris

Lowest rate
M: 4.8 per 100,000 in Mali, Bamako
F: 1.4 per 100,000 in India, Madras

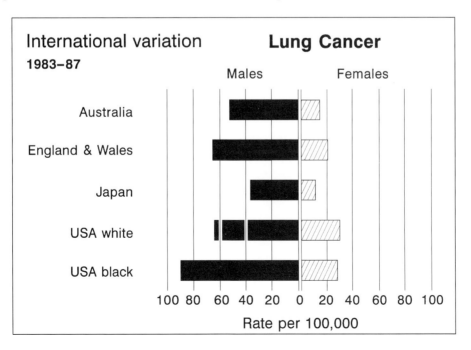

Mesothelioma

Rare but more common in men
Occurs in pleura, peritoneum or pericardium
Increasing in men in USA and Australia

Lifetime risk
in New South Wales:
   M   1 in 325
   F   1 in 2300

Relative five-year survival in 1977–90
in South Australia:
   M   9.4%
   F   7.4%

Risk factors
Asbestos
   Accounts for 80% of mesothelioma in industrial
   countries

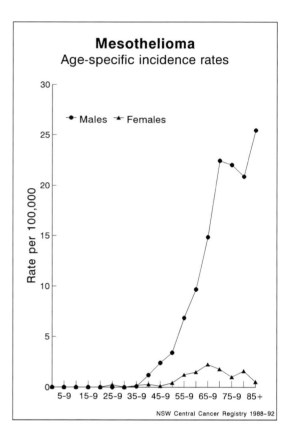

16. Cancer of the Esophagus

SIMON LAW and JOHN WONG

Department of Surgery, University of Hong Kong Medical Centre, Queen Mary Hospital, Hong Kong

EPIDEMIOLOGY

Esophageal cancer is the sixth most common cancer worldwide. Squamous cell carcinoma and adenocarcinoma are the two major pathologic types and they vary widely in incidence in different populations.

Squamous cell cancer has a very high incidence in the coastal areas of the Caspian Sea, in northern Iran, in the Transkei province of South Africa, in the former Soviet republics of Turkmenistan, Kazakhstan and northern Siberia, in Afghanistan, as well as the Henan province in northern China, and along the coast of southern China. Over 200 cases per 100,000 populations has been reported. By contrast, this cancer is relatively uncommon in the United States, Canada, Australia and most areas of Europe with the notable exceptions in certain parts of France and Italy. In low incidence areas, only 3–10 cases per 100,000 population are affected. Such variations, even within close geographic regions, suggest environmental factors as the main etiologic agents.

In the French provinces of Normandy and Brittany, in Italy and the United States, smoking and alcohol consumption play a major pathogenic role.

Table 16.1. Etiologic agents in the pathogenesis of esophageal cancer.

Environmental factors	Other associated conditions
Smoking	Lye corrosive stricture
Alcohol	Long-standing achalasia[†]
Hot beverages and maté drinking[§]	Tylosis
Nitrosamines	Plummer–Vinson syndrome[‡]
Opium	Chronic mid-third esophagitis with dysplasia[*]
Poor nutrition	Other aerodigestive malignancy[*]
Betel nut chewing	Barrett's esophagus[#]
Food contamination with fungi like *Geotrichum candidum* and *Fusarium species*	
Deficiency of vitamin A and C, molybdenum, copper, zinc	

[*] Predisposed to squamous cell carcinoma
[#] Predisposed to adenocarcinoma
[†] Typically squamous cell carcinoma of the middle third
[‡] Also known as Peaterson–Kelly syndrome or sideropenic dysphagia
[§] Tea made from the herb *Llex paraguensis* which is drunk at very hot tempeature in Uruguay

In Asia, other dietary patterns are implicated (Table 16.1). In high risk areas of China, of particular interest is the finding of chronic esophagitis together with severe dysplasia in the middle third of

Correspondence: Professor John Wong, Department of Surgery, University of Hong Kong Medical Centre, Queen Mary Hospital, Hong Kong. Tel: (852) 28554610, Fax: (852) 28551897

the esophagus not associated with gastroesophageal reflux disease; this has been identified to predispose to squamous cell carcinoma. Patients with other aerodigestive malignancies have a 5–8% risk of developing synchronous or metachronous esophageal squamous cancer, probably because of exposure to the same environmental carcinogens.

Esophageal cancer typically affects patients in the sixth and seven decades of life, with a male to female ratio ranging from 1:5 to 8:1, the former in high incidence areas. This predilection for men, is reversed in those regions with a high incidence of Plummer–Vinson syndrome. This syndrome typically affects women and consists of iron deficiency anemia, glossitis, cheilosis, koilonychia, brittle fingernails, and dysphagia due to a post-cricoid web formed by hyperkeratotic and desquamated mucosal membrane. It predisposes to post cricoid cancer.

In Asian countries, more than 80% of esophageal cancers are of squamous cell origin. In western countries, there has been an unexplained increase in adenocarcinoma of the lower esophagus and gastric cardia in the past two decades and in the United States it is the fastest growing tumor. This is not paralleled by similar increases in squamous cell tumors of the esophagus and cancers of the rest of the stomach. In some series, nearly 50% of primary esophageal cancers are adenocarcinomas. The prevalence of gastroesophageal reflux disease and the associated development of Barrett's esophagus is likely to be the contributing factor.

PATHOLOGY

The thoracic esophagus is divided into the upper third, from the superior portion of the aortic arch upwards; the middle third, from the inferior pulmonary vein up to the superior portion of the aortic arch; and the distal third, from the inferior pulmonary vein to the gastroesophageal junction. The most common site of squamous cancer is the middle third of the esophagus (60%), followed by the lower third (25%). Squamous cancers of the upper third and abdominal esophagus are uncommon. Because of the high frequency of middle third esophageal involvement, the tumor can infiltrate the tracheo-bronchial tree, left recurrent laryngeal nerve, pericardium, adjacent lungs and aorta. Liver secondaries from a squamous cancer is rare compared with an adenocarcinoma of the cardia. Symp-

toms therefore correspond to the site of the primary tumor and the extent of invasion. Most esophageal cancers are advanced on presentation, except where screening programs are carried out as in Japan.

Early lesions are uncommon. Intraepithelial cancer or mucosal cancer may appear as flat lesions like leukoplakia. More advanced tumors can be ulcerative or protuberant, the latter is being far more common. Microscopically, most squamous tumors contain islands of atypical squamous cells that infiltrate the underlying adjacent normal tissues and contain keratin pearl formation and intercellular bridges between tumor cells.

Barrett's esophagus is a premalignant condition characterized by metaplastic replacement of the esophagus with columnar epithelium as a result of chronic gastroesophageal reflux. By convention, it is diagnosed when columnar epithelium extends for more than 3 cm above into the tubular esophagus. Specialized columnar mucosa defined by biopsy and which extends for less than 3 cm up the tubular esophagus is now termed short segment Barrett's esophagus. Its malignant potential is at present unclear. Men are seven times more commonly affected than women. A prospective study of patients with Barrett's epithelium shows rates of one case of cancer per 52 to 152 patient-years, equivalent to a 30–40 fold risk for cancer compared to the general population.

Dysplasia in Barrett's epithelium shows an increased nuclear/cytoplasmic ratio, loss of basilar orientation of the epithelial cells along the basement membrane, irregular chromatin clumping, hyperchromatic nuclei, and prominence of nucleoi. Approximately 40% of patients with high grade dysplasia at the time of biopsies have adenocarcinoma found in the resected specimen and therefore is an indication for surgery, although this policy remains controversial.

Other cancers, all of which are uncommon, include mucoepidermoid carcinoma, small cell carcinoma, adenoid cystic carcinoma, sarcoma, lymphoma and melanoma.

Spread of tumor is by direct infiltration, subepithelial extension, lymphatic and hematogenous metastases. Subepithelial extension is longitudinal and can be continuous or skip lesions. An *in vivo* proximal esophageal margin of 10 cm should be the aim at resection to avoid this spread. Once the submucosal layer is breached, lymph node metastases are present in at least 30% of patients.

SCREENING

Cytologic screening of high risk asymptomatic populations has been carried out in China with swallowed balloon catheter. Similarly, an encapsulated brush has also been developed in Japan. The capsule, which is attached to a string, is swallowed. As the capsule dissolves, a contained polyurethane sponge ball expands and is withdrawn through the esophagus and cytologic examination can be carried out from cells obtained on its surface. In most countries with a lower incidence, the method is not cost-effective.

In the premalignant condition of Barrett's esophagus, patients should be enrolled into a regular endoscopic surveillance program, especially in those with dysplasia. There is no convincing evidence that Barrett's epithelium will regress even after successful treatment of reflux, although the progression to dysplasia may be halted or slowed down. The value, optimal interval of endoscopy, and cost effectiveness of surveillance programs however remains undefined. Treatment of Barrett's esophagus with ablative therapy (e.g. photodynamic therapy) followed by intensive acid suppression (medical or surgical) is also investigated.

CLINICAL PRESENTATION

Progressive dysphagia is the presenting symptom in over 90% of patients and it may not be apparent until two-thirds of the lumen has been obliterated. This is particularly true for squamous cancers. Patients also tend to modify their diets until severe dysphagia and weight loss has occurred before presentation. Regurgitation (as distinct from vomiting of gastric content), and pain on swallowing (odynophagia) are common. Hoarseness may signify recurrent laryngeal nerve involvement. There may be signs of pneumonia from aspiration or the development of an esophageal–respiratory fistula. Metastases may be palpable in supraclavicular or cervical lymph nodes. Hypercalcaemia in the absence of bony metastases is not uncommon. Hypertrophic osteoarthropathy and dermatomyositis have been described in association with squamous cell tumors.

For adenocarcinomas of the cardia, patients may also present with gastrointestinal bleeding. For both squamous and adenocarcinomas, physical examination usually yields no positive signs except for weight loss. Only in very advanced diseases can signs of dissemination be detected.

Table 16.2. TNM staging of esophageal cancer.

Primary tumor (T)

Tx	Primary tumor cannot be assessed
T0	No evidence of tumor
Tis	Carcinoma *in situ*
T1	Tumor invades lamina propria or submucosa
T2	Tumor invades muscularis propria
T3	Tumor invades adventitia
T4	Tumor invades adjacent structures

Regional lymph nodes (N)

Nx	Regional lymph nodes cannot be assessed
N0	No regional lymph node
N1	Regional lymph node metastases

Metastasis (M)

Mx	Distant metastases cannot be assessed
M0	No distant metastases
M1	Distant metastases

Stage groupings

Stage	T	N	M
Stage 0	Tis	N0	M0
Stage I	T1	N0	M0
Stage IIa	T2	N0	M0
	T3	N0	M0
Stage IIb	T1	N1	M0
	T2	N1	M0
Stage III	T3	N1	M0
	T4	any N	M0
Stage IV	any T	any N	M1

From Beahrs, O.H., Henson, D.E., Hutter, R.V.P., Myers, M.H. (eds) (1988). *Manual for staging of cancer*, 3rd ed. American Joint Committee on Cancer. Philadelphia: JB Lippincott.

INVESTIGATIONS AND STAGING (Table 16.2)

A chest radiograph may show a hilar mass, tracheal compression and deviation, aspiration pneumonia or metastases. The presence of tuberculosis and emphysema may influence the choice of therapy. A barium swallow identifies the location and length of narrowing, mucosal irregularity, and "shouldering" made by the upper border of the tumor (Figure 16.1). Tortuosity, angulation, axis deviation from the midline, sinus formation and frank fistulation into bronchial tree suggest advanced disease. It also

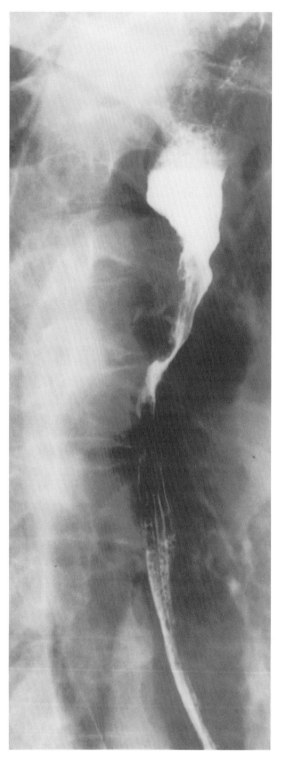

Figure 16.1. Barium swallow showing narrowing of the esophagus by tumor, and hold up of contrast material proximally.

provides the exact relationship of the tumor to other thoracic structures, information not provided by endoscopy. Flexible endoscopy allows biopsy of the tumor, together with brush cytology if necessary; a histologic diagnosis can be made in over 95% of patients. In early cancer or dysplastic lesions, Lugol's iodine or toluidine blue solution aids in their detection. The former stains normal mucosa brown and leaves dysplastic areas unstained. The latter stains abnormal mucosa blue. Suspicious areas can be identified for further biopsy. Bronchoscopic examination documents tracheobronchial involvement. Signs include external compression, widened carina from subcarinal lymph node, tumor infiltration or fistulation. The last two features preclude surgical resection.

Computed tomography (CT) scans and Magnetic Resonance Imaging (MRI) both lack sensitivity and specificity when used to assess the depth of esophageal wall infiltration and regional lymph node metastases except in overtly advanced cases, with large lymph nodes and liver metastasis. Endoscopic ultrasonography is currently the most accurate method in assessing T and N staging and is around 90% accurate. The probe cannot be passed through the tumor stenosis in about 30% of tumors, limiting its use. However, most tumors with that degree of stenosis will be T3 or T4 lesions. Small mini-probes which can be passed through the working channel of an endoscope are now used, making high grade stenosis lesions less problematic. As CT scans allow better detection of distant lymph nodes and organ metastases such as in the abdominal lymph nodes and liver, the two techniques are complementary.

Early experience on the use of laparoscopy and thoracoscopy in staging has been reported, but they have the disadvantage of necessitating general anesthesia.

PROGNOSTIC FACTORS

The two pathologic features that have overriding prognostic power are the depth of invasion of the tumor into the esophageal wall and beyond (T stage), and the lymph node status (N stage). Very detailed lymph node examination may place the disease at a more advanced stage than when such thorough examinations are not done ("stage migration"). This

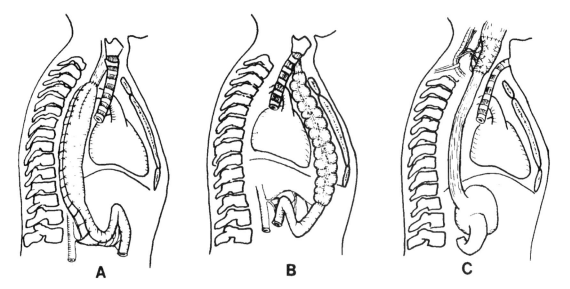

Figure 16.2.   Reconstruction after (a) Lewis–Tanner operation, (b) colonic interposition brought up to the neck via the retrosternal route, and (c) jejunal interposition after resection of a postcricoid tumor.

phenomenon must be kept in mind when comparing treatment results from different centers and especially from different parts of the world.

Immunologic markers and DNA ploidy analysis are the additional factors studied besides histologic features to assess the prognosis of esophageal cancer. Of the immunologic markers, squamous cell carcinoma-related antigen (SCC-RA) is the most sensitive. It is positive in about 50% of patients and this rate increases with progressive histologic invasion, nodal metastases, clinical stage and tumor volume. It is usually negative in benign esophageal disease. It is rarely positive in early cancer and in poorly differentiated cancers regardless of stage. Epidermal growth factor receptor (EGF-R) expression also correlates with the propensity of lymph node metastases, differentiation and mitotic index. Both markers have been linked to poorer prognosis.

DNA aneuploidy has also been linked to greater incidence of lymph node metastases, higher recurrence rate and poorer survival. Advances in molecular biology have identified various gene/gene products in association with esophageal cancer, e.g. *ras, p53, myc,* and *c-erbB-1*. The value of such markers and DNA ploidy remains controversial. None has been shown superior to histologic features and staging in assessing prognosis. These markers may have potential clinical application in the early diagnosis of cancer in high risk patients in the future, for example in Barrett's esophagus.

TREATMENT

Most patients present with clinically advanced disease, with the exception of certain centers in China and Japan. The main treatment objective therefore is to provide effective and expedient palliation. In general, for patients who are suitable for major surgery and in the absence of distant visceral organ metastases, the primary tumor should be resected because successful surgery offers the best quality of palliation and a reasonable chance of cure. In those with advanced disease who have risk factors which would make surgery hazardous, alternative treatments should be considered to restore some swallowing ability.

Operative treatment (Figure 16.2)

Direct infiltration or fistulation into the tracheobronchial tree, and distant organ metastases contraindicate resection. Aortic infiltration also precludes resection although the later diagnosis may not be ascertained by pre-operative imaging studies alone.

Potential surgical candidates should stop smoking. Intensive chest physiotherapy and practice on incentive spirometry are instituted. Malnutrition requires pre-operative enteral (by nasogastric feeding) or parenteral nutrition.

The surgical approach depends on the level of cancer, and whether a thoracotomy is deemed necessary in tumor extirpation. or tolerable by patient status.

For tumors of the middle and lower third of the esophagus, the most often performed operation is the Lewis–Tanner operation. The stomach is first mobilized via a laparotomy, the vascular supply of which is based on the right gastric and gastroepipleoic vessels. A pyloroplasty is performed for effective gastric drainage. The esophagus is then resected through a right thoracotomy. The stomach is delivered into the thorax through the esophageal hiatus to anastomose with the proximal divided esophagus. In cancer of the gastroesophageal junction, resection can also be carried out via a left thoracotomy or a left thoracoabdominal approach; however, the exposure and the length of esophagus that can be removed are limited.

In upper third cancers, esophagectomy can be carried out through a thoracotomy. By simultaneous left cervical and abdominal incisions, the stomach is then prepared and delivered up to the neck for anastomosis. The stomach can be placed in the original esophageal bed (orthotopic), or behind the sternum (retrosternal). The upper half of the sternum can also be split to gain access to the part of the esophagus behind the sternum and so avoid a thoracotomy.

Cervical and post-cricoid cancers mandate the resection of the larynx and pharynx, with the construction of a terminal tracheostomy. The stomach is used to restore continuity (pharyngo-laryngoesophagectomy). Radiotherapy is an alternative primary treatment to preserve the larynx. However, there is a high incidence of recurrence in advanced stages.

In patients with poor pulmonary reserve, esophagectomy can be performed without a thoracotomy. Simultaneous cervical and abdominal incisions are made and the esophagus is bluntly shelled out by the surgeon's hand introduced into the posterior mediastinum via the diaphragmatic hiatus (transhiatal esophagectomy). This partly "blind" procedure increases the risk of bleeding, injury to the membranous trachea and the left recurrent laryngeal nerve. The risk is higher for tumors of the middle third since mobilization of this part of the esophagus cannot be done under direct vision. It has also been criticized that this operation is an inadequate cancer operation, although reported survival rates in uncontrolled studies are apparently similar to more extensive resections.

Recent advances in video-assisted thoracoscopy allows esophagectomy under vision without a thoracotomy. While adequate lymphadenectomy can be performed, operating time and duration of one-lung anesthesia are lengthened. The procedure remains experimental.

The extent of optimal lymphadenectomy remains controversial. Most surgeons perform lymphadenectomy of the upper abdomen and mediastinum (two-field dissection). Some advocate the addition of bilateral neck dissection (three-field dissection). Only a controlled trial can determine if either method is superior.

The stomach is most commonly used for esophageal substitution because of its good blood supply, ease of preparation, and the need for only one anastomosis. Potential late problems include gastric stasis, dumping, ulceration, duodenogastric reflux and reflux esophagitis. For those with previous gastric surgery or for other indications, the right, or left colon, or the jejunum can be used. The colon is durable, relatively easy to prepare, and offers good conduit function. In post-cricoid tumors, resection may not need to involve the thoracic esophagus and a free jejunal graft or the pectoralis major myocutaneous flap can be placed in the neck to restore continuity.

The esophageal substitute, when brought to the neck for anastomosis, can traverse the posterior mediastinum (orthothopic), retrosternal space, or subcutaneous space. The orthothopic route should be avoided when adjuvant radiotherapy to the posterior mediastinum is planned so as to avoid radiation injury. The subcutaneous route is unsightly and a longer length of substitute is required; it is now rarely employed except where there is an extensive superior mediastinal tumor mass or lymph nodes.

In patients whose general condition is fit for surgery but with locally unresectable tumor, a bypass procedure offers good palliation. Most commonly the stomach conduit is brought up to the neck behind the sternum and anastomosed to the cervical esophagus; the distal esophagus is drained via a Roux-en-Y loop (Kirschner bypass) (Figure 16.3).

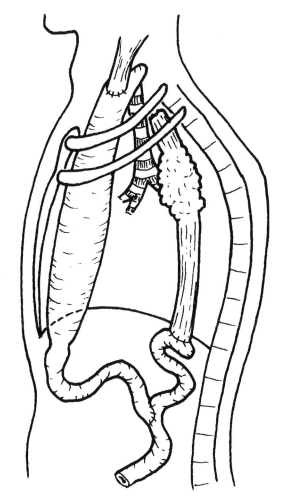

Figure 16.3. Reconstruction after a Kirschner bypass procedure for an unresectable middle-third esophageal tumor.

Careful selection is mandatory in this group of patients with locally advanced cancers; and if poor medical risk is found, non-operative alternatives should be employed.

Complications of surgery

Cardiopulmonary problems are the most common complications encountered and the major causes of death. Bronchoscopic sputum suction, early or prophylactic tracheostomy in patients with poor cough effort, especially in those with vocal cord paralysis, is invaluable. Careful attention should be paid to fluid balance to avoid overloading especially in hypoalbuminemic patients.

Anastomotic leakage which was once a common event (25%) should now be rare in experienced centers (<5%). Other specific surgical complications include post-operative bleeding, tracheobronchial injury, chylothorax from damage to the thoracic duct, and recurrent laryngeal nerve injury, the latter predisposes to aspiration. Most surgical complications should be uncommon and in specialized centers, and the 30-day mortality after esophagectomy is under 5%.

Non-operative treatments

Chemotherapy and radiotherapy

External-beam radiation or brachytherapy is offered as the main alternative to surgery. There are no random control trials comparing survival after surgery or radiotherapy for squamous cell carcinoma. Radiotherapy is often employed in those with advanced tumor or those unfit for surgery. In terms of palliation, relief of dysphagia is slower and less complete than surgery. Stricture from radiation and recurrent disease can develop in over 50% of patients.

As neoadjuvant or adjuvant therapy with surgery, neither radiotherapy nor chemotherapy has demonstrated overall survival benefit compared to surgery alone. Pre-operative (neoadjuvant) chemotherapy produces reduction in tumor bulk in 50% of patients and in some patients no residual evidence of tumor is found; it is still not clear that this will improve long-term survival. Radiotherapy when given preoperatively with chemotherapy (chemoradiation) aims at enhancing local tumor control and effecting eradication of systemic micrometastases. Chemotherapeutic agents like cisplatin and mitomycin-C are also radiosensitizers. This therapy produces complete histologic remission in 20–35% of patients who undergo subsequent resection. Tumor may still recur despite apparently complete response. Responders to pre-operative treatment tend to have better survival. In patients with palliative resections, post-operative radiotherapy reduces the incidence of local recurrence, such as to the tracheobronchial tree. All adjuvant treatments have potential disadvantages such as prolonging treatment time, toxicities and increasing perioperative morbidity. The ultimate impact of these protocols await further studies.

Other treatment options

For early mucosal lesions, "mucosectomy" can be performed via the endoscope. The mucosal cancer is "raised" by injecting saline in the submucosal plane, and then snared by an electrocautery loop as in polypectomy. The number of patients suitable for this treatment is minimal.

Placement of a prosthetic tube across the tumor stenosis may be indicated in patients not suitable for surgery. The tube can be inserted by laparotomy (e.g. Celestin tube, Mousseau–Barbin tube) or esophagoscopy under sedation or anesthesia (e.g. Atkinson tube, Souttar tube). The tumor stenosis is first dilated by a bougie or balloon dilator and the prosthesis pushed down across the tumor. A variety of expensive self-expanding membrane-coated metallic prostheses are also available. Expansion is gradual over 24 hours and placement is less traumatic. Problems of intubation are esophageal perforation, compression of adjacent airway, tube migration and repeated blockage. Patients with cervical cancer tolerate a prosthesis poorly because of foreign body sensation in the upper esophagus and sometimes pain. Laser therapy (Neodymium: yttrium-aluminium-garnet Nd:YAG laser) vaporizes the tumor to restore luminal patency. The risk of perforation is less than intubation, but repeated treatment sessions are required as the effect is temporary.

Other less commonly employed non-surgical options include photodynamic therapy, intralesional ethanol injection, bicap probe electrocoagulation, hyperthermia and immunotherapy. The choice of therapy depends on availability, expertise, cost, and consideration of efficacy. In selected patients, single modality or combinations are effective in restoring esophageal luminal patency. Apart from surgery, most treatment options cannot restore complete swallowing ability. The type of food that can be consumed remains only soft puree to liquid diets for most patients given non-operative treatment.

RESULTS OF TREATMENT

Except in early cancers, the prognosis of esophageal cancer with whatever treatment modality is unsatisfactory although surgery still offers the best results. Depth of tumor penetration through the esophageal wall, the presence and number of involved lymph nodes remain the main determinants of prognosis.

With mucosal cancer, five-year survival rates of over 80% are reported. For tumors involving the submucosa, the five-year survival rate is about 55%. Even after apparently curative resection where all gross tumors have been removed, the median survival is around two years and the five-year survival about 35%. The respective figures for palliative resection are eight months and 5%. The five-year survival rates for stage I, IIa, IIb, III and IV diseases are 57%, 31%, 42%, 14% and 2% respectively. The majority of patients with recurrence will present within two years after initial treatment, mostly within the first.

References

1. Fok, M., Wong, J. (1995). Squamous cell carcinoma. In *Esophageal surgery*, edited by F.G. Pearson, J. Deslauriers, R.J. Ginsberg, C.A. Hiebert, M.F. McKneally and H.C. Urschel Jr, pp. 571–586. New York, Churchill Livingstone.
2. Orringer, M.B. (1993). Tumors, injuries, and miscellaneous conditions of the esophagus. In *Surgery, scientific principles and practice*, edited by C.J. Greenfield, M.W. Malholland, R.T. Oldham and G.B. Zelenock. Philadelphia: JB Lippincott.
3. Review in depth: Esophageal Cancer, edited by Watson, A. (1994). *European Journal of Gastroenterology and Hepatology*, **6**, 645–648.
4. Esophageal cancer, edited by Tytgat, G.N.J. (1994). *Current opinion in gastroenterology*, **10**, 455–464.
5. World progress in surgery: Squamous esophageal cancer, edited by Wong, J. (1994). *World Journal of Surgery*, **18**, 307–405.
6. Roth, J.A., Lichter, A.S., Putnam, J.B. and Forastiere, A.A. (1993). Cancer of the esophagus. In *Cancer: Principles and practice of oncology*, edited by T. Vincent, R. De Vita, Jr., S. Hellman and S.A. Rosenberg. Philadelphia: JB Lippincott.

Cancer of Esophagus

Distinctly more common in men

Worldwide: 6th most common cancer
            4th in developing countries

Lifetime risk
in USA whites:
    M   1 in 150
    F   1 in 400

Relative five-year survival in 1983–87
in USA whites:
    M   8.8%
    F   10.7%

Risk factors
Tobacco
Alcohol
    Together account for 80–90% of esophageal
    cancer in North and South America, Europe and
    Japan
Fresh fruit and vegetables confer protection

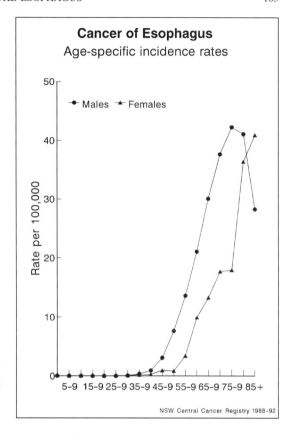

Cancer of Esophagus
Age-specific incidence rates

NSW Central Cancer Registry 1988–92

Geographical variation in 1983–87
Highest rate
M: 26.5 per 100,000 in France, Calvados
F: 8.8 per 100,000 in India, Bangalore

Lowest rate
M: 1.3 per 100,000 in Israel, Jews born in Africa
   or Asia
F: 0.5 per 100,000 in Eastern Europe

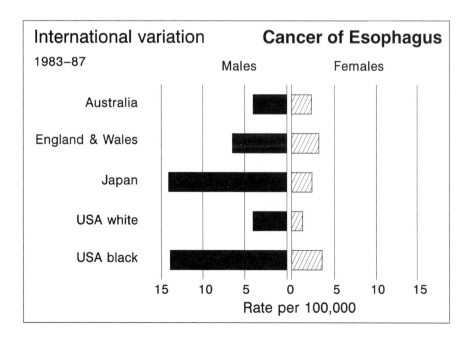

International variation — Cancer of Esophagus
1983–87

17. Gastric Cancer

FRANK J. BRANICKI and DAVID G. GOTLEY

Department of Surgery, University of Queensland, Australia

EPIDEMIOLOGY

Despite a remarkable decline in incidence of gastric cancer in the past 50 years, the disease remains the second leading cause of cancer deaths worldwide with over 650,000 cases reported annually. High incidence rates are evident in the Far East (Japan and Korea), parts of Europe (Germany, Poland) and South America (Chile); these vary from 8.2 (USA), 30 (Chile, China, Iceland, Poland, Korea) and 70 (Japan) per 100,000 population. The disease is most common in the fifth to seventh decades of life, with a male to female ratio of 1.6, two-thirds of patients being more than 65 years of age. In the United States, less than 10% of patients are less than 50 years of age. While the overall prognosis with gastric cancer remains poor with less than 15% of patients surviving five years there is recent evidence for an improved outlook for those undergoing surgery with curative intent. Contributing factors might include a decrease in surgical mortality rates, better preoperative selection and earlier diagnosis, improved perioperative care, and perhaps more radical surgery.

PREDISPOSING AND RISK FACTORS

Although familial gastric cancer is known to occur, genes related to inherited susceptibility have not as yet been cloned. Environmental influences are believed to be important in the multifactorial pathogenesis of the disease. A high salt intake, preserved, smoked or pickled foodstuffs, a high animal fat and carbohydrate intake with low fruit and vegetable ingestion and a lack of trace elements are regarded as etiological considerations. The initial stages of gastritis and atrophy are linked not only to excessive salt intake but to Helicobacter pylori (H. pylori) infection. It is speculated that the introduction of dietary change and domestic refrigeration, with reduction perhaps of H. pylori infection, has been accompanied by a spectacular decline in disease incidence. Sequentially, chronic gastritis, gastric atrophy, intestinal metaplasia and dysplasia may progress to gastric cancer. Pre-malignant conditions include gastric polyps, Menetrier's disease, gastric ulcer, pernicious anemia and previous gastric operation designed to reduce acid output.

Achlorhydria in pernicious anemia is believed to predispose to malignancy by enabling the overgrowth of bacteria with degradation of nitrates to form carcinogenic nitrosamines. In this disorder, there is a three to six-fold increase in the relative risk of gastric cancer. Whether the post-surgical stomach (vagotomized or partially resected) is more likely to undergo malignant change is unsettled, as

Correspondence: F.J. Branicki, Department of Surgery, Queen Mary Hospital, The University of Hong Kong, Pokfulam Road, Hong Kong

there is some evidence to suggest that this may occur a decade or more after operation. The question as to whether long-term peptic ulcer maintenance drug therapy is also likely to lead to an increased risk of gastric cancer is as yet unproven.

Recent attention has focused on H. pylori which is now widely regarded as having an etiological role in the "intestinal" type of gastric cancer which occurs particularly in countries with a high incidence of the disease. Serum tests for antibodies to H. pylori have indicated a 40% correlation between antibody prevalence and gastric mortality in geographical areas with a high incidence of stomach cancer such as China. It is, however, unlikely that H. pylori alone is causative.

Borrman's classification for gastric cancer describes four types:

I.   solitary polyploid lesions
II.   sharply defined ulcer
III. less well defined ulcers with infiltrative margins
IV.   diffuse cancer (linitis plastica).

Tumors may be well or poorly differentiated and papillary, tubular, mucinous and signet ring cell types are described. Lauren's histological classification of "intestinal", "diffuse" and "indeterminate" types of gastric cancer has been found to be useful in clinical practice. Ming described "expanding" and "infiltrative" types corresponding to the "intestinal" and "diffuse" lesions of Lauren. The presence of involved lymph nodes more than halves the expected survival rate in gastric cancer from 40–50% to less than 20%. Prognosis is also related both to the distance from the tumor of lymph node involvement and the number of lymph nodes involved. Predictably, the extent and distribution of lymph node involvement is dependent on the location of the primary tumor and has an important bearing on operative strategy.

EARLY GASTRIC CANCER

Patients with early gastric cancer subjected to surgical treatment have an excellent prognosis comparable to an age and sex matched control population. Early gastric cancer is gastric adenocarcinoma confined to the mucosa or submucosa irrespective of whether lymph nodes are involved. The mean prevalence of early gastric cancer in published series from North America is 4%, whereas between 30 and 40% of gastric malignancies in Japan are detected at an early stage. Macroscopic subtypes include:

I.   protruded
IIa. superficial elevated
IIb. flat
IIc. superficial depressed
III. excavated lesions

Combined types, e.g. IIc + IIa, are also recognized. Lymph node metastasis occurs in approximately 5% of patients with intramucosal cancer and 15% of patients with a lesion invading the submucosa.

PROGNOSTIC FACTORS

Gastric cancer displays multiple genetic disturbances involving oncogenes, growth factors or cytokines, cell cycle regulators, tumor suppressor genes and cell adhesion molecules. The two main types of gastric cancer described by Lauren display different genetic alterations on different chromosomes in gastric tumor cell lines and tissues. Alterations in the ras family, c.erb.B-2, c-met and K-sam genes are relatively frequent in gastric cancer; point mutations may, however, have an important role in development and progression. Loss of heterozygoity (LOH) is believed to play an important role in the inactivation of tumor suppressor genes, APC, p53 and DCC. Abnormalities of several growth factor receptor systems have been found in gastric cancer. Genetic alterations are also involved in tumor invasion and metastasis to nodes and liver. Increased coexpression of ras and transforming growth factor $\propto$ (TGF$\propto$) correlates with stage, grade, depth of invasion, metastasis and poor prognosis. CD44 expression has been reported to be correlated with distant metastases at presentation and with recurrence following RO-UICC resection. E Cadherin (a cellular adhesion molecule) mutations are believed to contribute to the development of metastasis. Urokinase plasminogen activator (uPA) and plasminogen activator inhibitor type I (PAI-I) have been shown to have potential as independent negative prognostic factors for gastric cancer because of a role in metastasis. High levels of proliferating cell nuclear antigen (PCNA), a measure of cellular growth rate or index, also have prognostic significance. To date, however, prognostic factors have not modified therapeutic approaches to gastric cancer.

SCREENING

Endoscopic and double contrast radiographic screening in asymptomatic patients over the age of 40 years have been in widespread use in Japan and has produced high proportions of early cancers together with a reduction in population mortality in areas where screening has been used. Routine screening has not proved to be cost-effective in low incidence areas but some surgeons advocate endoscopic surveillance for patients at high risk, e.g. in pernicious anemia or a decade following gastric resection for peptic ulcer.

CLINICAL PRESENTATION

In 75% of patients symptoms have been present for less than six months. Unfortunately, epigastric pain, obstructive symptoms, gastrointestinal bleeding and perforation are generally manifestations of advanced disease. The earliest symptom is often nausea and weight loss may be a prominent feature in advanced cancer. Back pain is suggestive of contiguous or direct pancreatic involvement. Gastrointestinal bleeding may be chronic and occult in nature giving rise to iron deficiency anemia or profuse and life threatening.

INVESTIGATIONS AND STAGING

Investigations

Accurate and standardized staging is essential for any meaningful comparison of results. Traditionally, pathological staging for carcinoma of the stomach has been different in Japan compared to the Western world, and this may be one reason for discrepancies observed in the outcomes of treatment. In the west, variations of the TNM classification have been traditionally used to stage carcinoma of the stomach. The Japanese Research Society for Gastric Cancer (JRSGCS) categorizes four tiers of lymph node involvement (N_{1-4}) for each of three areas of the stomach designated cardiac (C), middle (M) and antral (A) tumors. Staging is based on presence of peritoneal, hepatic, and lymph node metastases and serosal infiltration; in Stage 1 tumors none are involved, in Stage IV disease each of these features is positive.

An iron deficiency anemia and/or deranged liver function tests may be noted, metastatic disease often giving rise to an elevated alkaline phosphatase. CEA or Ca 19.9 levels may be raised. Upper endoscopy is essential for diagnostic purposes and enables biopsy confirmation of malignant disease. Upper endoscopy also provides invaluable information concerning the proximal and distal extent of disease and this is essential for the decision-making process as regards operative approach and the extent of resection. There is little place for contrast radiology for gastric pathology as endoscopy will be necessary even in the absence of radiological abnormalities. Endoscopic ultrasound with a radial sector probe is now regarded as more sensitive than computed tomography (CT) in the evaluation for T and N status for staging purposes. CT may understage or overstage extent and is unlikely to identify peritoneal carcinomatosis. In contrast, laparoscopic assessment enables peritoneal seedings to be visualized and laparoscopic ultrasound may be useful in the assessment of liver and pancreatic status. The detection of cytokeratin positive cells in bone marrow enables the detction of microbone metastasis using a monoclonal antibody to cytokeratin.

TREATMENT

Surgery

Pre-operative preparation may include blood transfusion, rehydration, gastric washouts and in the case of advanced lesions, a bowel preparation as for colonoscopy because tumor involvement of the transverse mesocolon and/or colon itself may occasionally necessitate resection. A single injection of a cephalosporin is recommended one hour before surgery for prophylaxis against infection following resection. Operative staging of lymph node involvement is unreliable. Radical gastrectomy includes removal of the primary lesion with *en bloc* removal of any organ directly invaded by tumor, resection of one or more tiers of lymph nodes and removal of the greater omentum and superior leaf of the transverse mesocolon. Splenectomy is believed to be detrimental to post-operative recovery and is now usually reserved for the treatment of bulky tumors involving the greater curvature or gastric fundus when splenic hilar gland metastasis is considered probable. Radical gastrectomy with nodal dissection has been shown to yield > 90% five-year survival figures in patients with early gastric cancer. Retropancreatic gland dissection is not considered necessary for early gastric cancer, a 2 cm gastric resection margin now being regarded as sufficient. If more than 7–8 lymph nodes are involved by tumor, prognosis is dismal.

Whenever possible a distal subtotal gastric resection is preferred to total gastrectomy provided that an adequate proximal gastric resection margin can be obtained because of better functional results. Following resection for early gastric cancer a Billroth I type (gastro-duodenal) anastomosis may be preferred and is regarded as more physiological for digestive purposes; there is, however, a greater risk of local recurrence with obstruction of the conduit if continuity is restored in this way following excision of advanced gastric cancer. This is best avoided by fashioning a gastro-jejunal anastomosis, either directly to a loop of jejunum (Billroth II or Polya) or to a Roux-en-Y jejunal limb which will prevent bile reflux. Subtotal proximal gastrectomy with anastomosis of the distal gastric remnant to the esophagus often leads to gastric or esophageal bile reflux and is not usually recommended.

In the majority of patients gastric resection is only palliative but does provide relief of symptoms from the primary lesion, and is recommended in the absence of gross ascites, peritoneal carcinomatosis or widespread liver disease in the patient otherwise deemed fit for surgery. Even in the presence of bilobar liver metastases good palliation may be achieved for 6–12 months by gastric resection without lymphadenectomy. Excisional surgery is not advised when there are features of advanced disseminated disease with abdominal distention from ascites, jaundice from metastatic liver disease or nodal obstruction of the porta hepatis or marked cachexia. Paracentesis, repeated if need be, and blood transfusion may provide symptomatic benefit.

Physical signs are often lacking in early gastric malignancy. Advanced malignant disease may be evident as left supraclavicular lymphadenopathy, i.e. Troiser's sign in Virchow's node. Jaundice, abdominal distension with ascites, a palpable epigastric or pelvic mass are signs of advanced disease, although the primary tumor alone may be palpable, gross hepatomegaly is usually secondary to liver involvement. On rectal examination, metastatic tumor due to transcaelomic spread to ovaries (i.e. Krukenberg tumors), or extensive spread to the pelvic side walls, Blumer's shelf are occasionally encountered.

In Japanese series the mortality rate for gastric resection is usually 1–3% compared with around 5% in Western series. Anastomotic leakage from a gastro-jejunal suture or staple line is uncommon but leakage is more frequent following esophago-jejunostomy after total gastrectomy; the latter is also usually managed conservatively. Long-term post-operative sequelae specific to gastric resection include diarrhea and dumping, iron, vitamin B_{12}/folate deficiency, bile reflux and the possibility of cancer developing in the gastric remnant.

Minimal access surgery

Laser therapy for early gastric cancer in elderly high risk patients has gained popularity in the past decade with long-term results comparable to surgical outcomes. Endoscopic mucosal resection or "strip biopsy" has been more widely practiced and is indicated in the absence of nodal disease on endoscopic ultrasound for well-differentiated, non-depressed early gastric cancer. More recently, laparoscopic wedge resection of the stomach has been introduced as well as totally laparoscopic or laparoscopic-assisted partial or total gastrectomy for more advanced lesions. Laparoscopic intragastric surgery has also been described with direct laparoscopic removal of early lesions from within the lumen of the stomach.

ADJUVANT THERAPY

To date little benefit has been shown for chemotherapy alone or in combination with radiation therapy, partial response rates even for combination therapy are low and a complete response very unlikely. Preoperative chemotherapy has so far failed to show a clear increase in the rate of complete tumor removal in patients with resectable disease. Effective drug combinations are lacking and either novel drug therapies or entirely new approaches to treatment need to be developed. The outcome of external beam radiation therapy in the post-operative period has not been shown to be of benefit. Cimetidine, the ulcer healing H_2 antagonist, has been shown to significantly but modestly improve survival in gastric cancer; the mechanism may relate to its immunological effects or to growth factor antagonism. There is still much skepticism in western practice regarding immunochemosurgery as practiced in Korea and which utilizes Corynebacterium parvum for immunomodulation although some early data have been reported.

References

1. Longmire, W.P., Jnr M.D. (1993). A Current View of Gastric Cancer in the US. *Annals of Surgery*, **218** (5), 579–582.
2. Deakin, M. and Elder, J.B. (1994). Gastric Cancer. *Medicine International*, 236–240.
3. Kim, J., Kim, Y., Yang, H. and Noh, D. (1994). Significant Prognostic Factors by Multivariate Analysis of 3926 Gastric Cancer Patients. *World J Surg*, **18**, 872–878.
4. Sawyers, J.L. (1995). *Gastric Cancer Current Problems in Surgery*, **XXXII** (2), 101–188.
5. Hermanek, P. and Wittekind, C. (1995). News of TNM and Its Use for Classification of Gastric Cancer. *World J Surg*, **19**, 491–495.
6. Tahara, E. (1995). Molecular Biology of Gastric Cancer. *World J Surg*, **19**, 484–490.
7. Siewert, J.R., Sendler, A., Dittler, H.J., Fink, U. and Höfler, H. (1995). Staging Gastrointesstinal Cancer as a Precondition for Multimodal Treatment. *World J Surg*, **19**, 168–177.
8. Bonenkamp, J.J. and van de Velde, C.J.H. (1995). Lymph Node Dissection in Gastric Cancer. *British Journal of Surgery*, **82**, 867–869.
9. Harrison J.D. and Fielding, J.W.L. (1995). Prognostic Factors for Gastric Cancer Influencing Clinical Practice. *World J Surg*, **19**, 496–500.
10. Macdonald, J.S. and Schnall, S.F. (1995). Adjuvant Treatment of Gastric Cancer. *World J Surg*, **19**, 221–225.

Stomach Cancer

About twice as common in men

Worldwide: 2nd most frequent cancer
but decreasing

Lifetime risk
in USA whites:
    M   1 in 80
    F   1 in 130

Relative five-year survival in 1983–87
in USA whites
    M   14.9%
    F   19.7%

Risk factors
Fresh fruit and vegetables confer protection. Introduction of refrigeration and consequent decline in
food preservation by salting, pickling and smoking
are thought to be linked to decreasing rates.

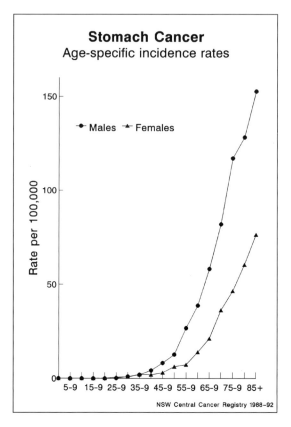

Geographical variation in 1983–87

Highest rate
M: 93.3 per 100,000 in Japan, Yamagata
F: 42.9 per 100,000 in Japan, Yamagata

Lowest rate
M: 2.1 per 100,000 in India, Ahmedabad
F: 1.5 per 100,000 in India, Ahmedabad

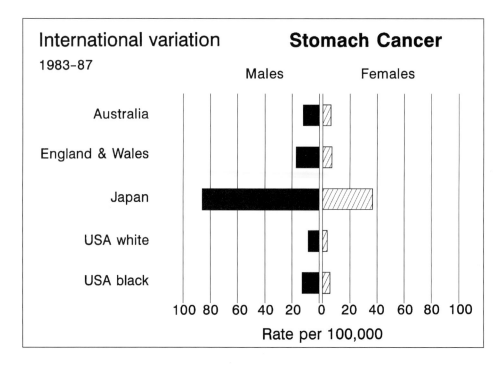

18. Lower GI Cancer

DENIS W. KING

The St. George Hospital, Kogarah, Australia

INCIDENCE

In countries such as the USA, UK and Australia, at least one person in 25 will develop colorectal cancer.

It is estimated that in the USA in 1993 there were 152,000 new cases of colorectal cancer comprising 13% of new cancers, with 57,000 deaths accounting for 11% of all cancer deaths. Colorectal cancer is now the commonest internal malignancy affecting Australians, and the second most common cause of cancer death after lung overall, and breast in women.

There appears to be a strong environmental or lifestyle association with colorectal cancer. Japanese families migrating to Hawaii at the end of World War II reached the North American incidence by the second generation. Migrants to Australia from the Middle East, where colorectal cancer incidence is one-tenth that of Australasia, have rates that tend to converge upon local rates, with the change first becoming apparent after about 10 years.

Incidence is generally greater in industrialized countries, but the degree of industrialization in itself would not appear to be a factor, as one of the lowest incidences is found in Japan.

There is a strong age association, with the incidence increasing rapidly after the age of 40 years, doubling each five years to 60 years, and then increasing more slowly to peak at over 80 years.

The total risk rises from 50 to 80 years by a factor of 2–3, with less than 10% of colorectal cancers occurring under the age of 55.

SEX/SITE

At least 50% of colon cancers occur distal to the splenic flexure. There appears to be an excess of right side tumors in females, and of rectal tumors in males.

The sex ratios change with age, with carcinoma of the rectum of approximately equal incidence to the age of 45 in both sexes in Australia, with men at proportionately greater risk with advancing age.

PREDISPOSING AND RISK FACTORS

Adenomatous, polyps and the polyp/cancer sequence

Adenomas are classified on morphological growth as tubular, tubulovillus and villus. At the time of surgery, approximately 30% of people with colorectal cancer are found to have adenomatous polyps in the colon, with a greater likelihood with right side cancers.

Supporting the proposition that many bowel cancers start as polyps are the observations that a small proportion of adenomas are found to have severe dysplasia or carcinoma *in situ*, that the likelihood of a villus component and malignant change within a polyp increases with the size of the polyp and that there is a correlation between prevalence of adenomas and deaths from colorectal cancer. Subsite distributions, which vary at different ages, are similar for both polyps and cancers, and residual adenoma is sometimes found in early cancer, with some adenomas undoubtedly progressing to carcinoma.

A population kept free of adenomas is less likely to develop carcinoma. In a study in Minnesota where 18,000 patients were followed for up to 25 years, periodic sigmoidoscopic screening and removal of polyps appeared to result in a reduction in rectal cancer incidence by up to 85%. Subsequent studies have confirmed that colonoscopic polypectomy reduces mortality from colorectal cancer.

Polyps are, however, very common; up to 70% of males in their sixties will have adenomatous polyps. The incidence of adenomas tends to reach a plateau at 70 years, whereas that of carcinoma continues to increase. Only a minority of polyps appear to proceed to cancer.

Hyperplastic polyps are not thought to have malignant potential, but do appear to be a marker of proximal adenomatous polyps: the presence of distal hyperplastic polyps is considered an indication for total colonoscopy.

Progressive gene mutations and deletions appear to explain the "polyp–cancer sequence" hypothesis. The process may take up to 30 years.

Family history

First-degree relatives of bowel cancer patients have a two to three-fold overall increase in likelihood of developing bowel cancer, the risk being greater if the index case develops the cancer before 55 years of age, presumably due to genetic associations.

APC gene mutations, of which over 120 have been identified, are among the first changes that appear in patients without Familial Polyposis Coli (FPC) who develop adenomatous polyps. The progression to invasive carcinoma appears to be associated with further mutations involving activation of genes such as the K-*ras* oncogene, and inactivation of genes such as p53. The specific gene mutations may have a bearing on the morphology of the preceding polyp, the biological behavior of the resultant carcinoma, and the prospects of survival of the patient.

Familial Polyposis Coli and HNPCC

FPC accounts for approximately 1% of colorectal cancers, and hereditary non-polyposis colorectal can-

cer (HNPCC), the Lynch Syndromes, for 5–10%. Studies of patients with FPC have shown genetic defects in the region of chromosome 5q, leading to the identification of the adenomatous polyposis coli (APC) gene, mutations of which cause FPC and Gardner's Syndrome.

A family suffering from the Cancer Family Syndrome, or hereditary nonpolyposis colorectal cancer (HNPCC) was first described in 1895. These families show an autosomal dominant pattern of inheritance with 80% penetrance. In one variant of HNPCC there is a higher incidence of urinary, upper GI, gynecological and other cancers. The colorectal cancers tend to occur at an earlier age and be more proximal than the sporadic type and there is a tendency to multiple cancers.

Association with previous cancer

Up to 5% of people with colorectal cancer develop a further colorectal cancer within 10–15 years, an incidence that is higher than that of the general population.

Inflammatory bowel disease

Ulcerative colitis and perhaps Crohn's Disease predispose to the development of carcinoma of the colon and rectum. With ulcerative colitis, the risk of developing colorectal cancer is largely confined to those with total colitis and appears related to the length of history of the disease and age of onset. Goligher suggested that any patient with total involvement of the colon and rectum for 20 years has a risk of developing carcinoma of at least 5% for each subsequent year but other studies have suggested a much lower rate.

The general distribution of carcinomas is the same as that in patients without colitis but there is a greater tendency to multiple carcinomas. Histologically, the cancers are more likely to be poorly differentiated and to be associated with surrounding premalignant mucosal changes. Survival following treatment is determined by the same criteria that apply to non-colitis cancers.

Ionizing irradiation

Pelvic irradiation appears to increase the risk of developing rectal cancer.

Dietary

In 1969, Aries *et al.* postulated that colorectal cancer is caused by metabolites produced by bacterial flora. Fermentable vegetable fiber may limit the exposure of the colonic mucosa to mutagens by increasing the colonic bacterial content, and increasing the rate of transit.

High dietary intake of saturated fat and meat appear to increase the risk of development of colorectal cancer, whereas crude fiber, particularly vegetables of the brassica family such as cabbage and spinach, and dairy products appear protective, the latter possibly because of high calcium levels, which have been shown to affect the rate of cell turnover in the rectum.

There is good epidemiological data linking red meat intake to the development of colorectal cancer within high risk societies, and the incidence of colorectal cancer in Japan is rising as meat intake increases.

Epidemiological studies suggest a clear relationship between low stool weight, correlating with low starch and dietary fiber intake, and a higher incidence of colon cancers.

Bile acids

The evidence that bile acids may act as tumor promoters is largely derived from animal studies. A relationship between bile acid concentration and colorectal adenomas and cancer has been demonstrated in a number of studies, and cholecystectomy has been found to be associated with an increased risk of right side tumors.

Hormonal

Increasing parity, early age of first pregnancy and use of oral contraceptives may protect against colorectal cancer, possibly because of the effect of estrogen on hepatic function and the composition of bile. This would explain the observation that there may be an increased risk of a second breast cancer and of prostate cancer following colorectal cancer, and that women with breast cancer have a higher incidence of colorectal cancer. It would also be consistent with the observation that smoking, which has an anti-estrogenic effect, may offer protection against colorectal cancer.

Gastrin appears to be a growth factor for colorectal cancer. High gastrin levels promote colorectal cancer in experimental animals and some colorectal cancer cells have functional gastrin receptors. Gastrin antagonists have been shown to slow the growth of colorectal cancer in animal models.

PATHOLOGY

Macroscopically, colorectal carcinoma starts as a firm area within a pre-existing adenoma or within normal mucosa. Most cancers then form either polypoid or ulcerating lesions.

The polypoid carcinoma is a fungating mass of tumor projecting into the lumen. The surface is firm and nodular initially, eventually becoming necrotic and ulcerated. Initially, there is little associated infiltration of the intestinal wall. Up to 10% of colorectal cancers are colloid and these are usually polypoid in nature.

The ulcerating carcinoma develops as a malignant ulcer with everted edges and a central area containing necrotic tissue. This type of cancer tends to infiltrate the bowel wall early, and is more likely to produce an anular and stenosing carcinoma and to be associated with external deformity and narrowing of the lumen.

Some bowel cancers diffusely infiltrate the bowel wall, in a manner similar to linitis plastica of the stomach, although there is usually mucosal ulceration at some point.

Although any type of tumor can occur in any part of the colon, polypoid tumors are more likely to occur on the right side and stenosing on the left. Proximal colon cancers are more likely than distal to be late-stage at the time of diagnosis.

As many as 30% of patients with carcinomas have associated adenomatous polyps and 3% have two or more carcinomas at the time of presentation.

The histological appearance can vary between well differentiated and anaplastic but most cancers are moderately well differentiated, with polypoid tumors better differentiated than ulcerating, and colon cancers better differentiated than rectal.

MODES OF SPREAD

The methods of spread of the primary tumor are by the lymphatics and bloodstream, by direct spread through the bowel wall to contiguous tissue, and by shedding of cells from the serosal surface into the peritoneal cavity.

Direct spread

Direct spread occurs in all directions within the bowel wall but appears to be more rapid circumferentially than in the long axis. Microscopic spread in lymphatics takes place in advance of macroscopic involvement but only for a few millimeters, unless there is extensive extramural lymphatic infiltration or the cancer is poorly differentiated. Distal mesorectal spread in rectal cancer may extend further than intramural spread, with significant implications for the surgical treatment of rectal tumors.

In the intraperitoneal rectum or colon, a breach of the peritoneal surface allows either transperitoneal spread or direct involvement of adjacent organs. Adherence to or invasion of other viscera is often seen, but adhesions may be inflammatory.

Transperitoneal spread carries a poor prognosis. Although macroscopic involvement of peritoneal surfaces may only be apparent adjacent to the tumor, the possibility of wider spread in such circumstances is high.

Implantation of exfoliated cancer cells may occur at the time of surgery. Apart from recurrence at the anastomosis, which in some instances appears to be related to the seeding of cells shed into the lumen, there are documented instances of cancer seeding in hemorrhoidectomy wounds and of isolated drain- and wound-site recurrences. This may be a more common problem following laparoscopic colectomy, with port site recurrence rates of up to 6% reported.

Lymphatic spread

Following involvement of the submucosal lymphatics, the first extramural lymphatic involvement usually occurs in the paracolic glands closest to the primary tumor, followed by progressive involvement of glands related to the blood supply. Although this spread is usually sequential, the tumor may bypass local groups of nodes.

The frequency of nodal metastases reported varies with the diligence with which metastases are sought by the pathologist, with up to 60% nodal involvement in some series. Involvement of regional lymph nodes is unusual, but not unknown in tumors that have not reached the serosa or pericolic tissues, and this becomes significant in the management of cancer apparently confined to polyps that have been removed colonoscopically.

In the rectum, the usual mode of spread to glands immediately adjacent to the tumor posterior to the rectum is followed by involvement of glands related to superior hemorrhoidal and inferior mesenteric vessels. There is also lymphatic spread within the lateral ligaments to the internal iliac glands and, if the cancer involves perianal skin and ischiorectal fat, to the inguinal lymphatics.

Blood-borne spread

The commonest site of blood-born metastasis is the liver. Fifty percent of people dying of bowel cancer have liver metastases. There is some evidence that direct invasion of thick-walled extramural veins is associated with a higher incidence of liver involvement.

Approximately one-fifth of patients dying of bowel cancer have lung metastases. Isolated lung metastases occur in approximately 2% of patients and are occasionally amenable to surgical treatment.

Blood-born metastases may also involve bones, brain, kidney and adrenals. The presence of malignant cells in the circulation at the time of surgery does not appear to influence prognosis.

PROTECTIVE FACTORS

With no major advance in the cure rate for established disease in recent decades, the best prospect of decreasing morbidity and mortality may lie in preventing the development of cancer, treatment of the precursors, and early diagnosis.

Non-steroidal anti-inflammatory drugs (NSAID) have been observed to inhibit the development of polyps and cancers. Sulindac was noted in 1983 to cause regression of rectal polyps in Familial Polyposis Coli (FPC) following colectomy and ileorectal anastomosis, and subsequently of diffuse polyposis, usually caused by FPC or a variant.

Aspirin in a dose recommended for thromboembolic prevention, 150 mg per day or less, may achieve a 30–50% reduction in incidence of colorectal polyps and carcinoma with prolonged use, although not all studies show such results. A prospective randomized trial established to resolve this issue was terminated early because of the significant lessening of cardiac problems in the treated group.

It has been suggested that vitamins C and E and beta Carotene may inhibit the development of colonic polyps, but a prolonged controlled trial recently reported has not demonstrated this effect.

CASE FINDING AND SCREENING

There are two types of fecal occult blood testing (FOBT) commonly available, guaiac tests (e.g. Hemoccult, Hemoccult SENSA), based on the pseudoperoxidase activity of hem, and immunochemical (HemeSelect, Hemolex) which utilize an antibody to human hemoglobin.

Prospective studies of FOBT in screening for colorectal cancer have demonstrated the relatively low specificity and sensitivity of currently available tests. Although the test itself is inexpensive, the cost of investigating the 1–3% who test positive is relatively high. Cancers are detected in 2–10% of those with a positive result, with the test failing to diagnose at least 30–60% of carcinomas depending on the technique used and the degree of adherence to recommended dietary restrictions.

Several studies have shown, however, that carcinomas detected by screening are at a significantly earlier pathological stage. A Minnesota study has shown a 33% decline in cumulative mortality over 13 years in those screened yearly as compared to control subjects, although the number that had colonoscopy during the study may have influenced the result. A Danish trial using non-rehydrated FOBT showed an 18% reduction in colorectal cancer mortality.

Screening for fecal occult blood reduces mortality from colorectal cancer but because of doubts about the cost-effectiveness of such programs, their place remains undetermined.

The American Cancer Society recommends yearly digital rectal examination from the age of 40 years, and FOBT from the age of 50 years, and encourages widespread availability of sigmoidoscopy, preferably flexible, performed by primary care physicians, every three to five years for people aged over 50.

Flexible sigmoidoscopy will not routinely detect polyps proximal to the splenic flexure but most polyps and cancers occur distal to that point and about one-third of people with proximal cancers will have an adenoma within reach of a flexible sigmoidoscope. Two recent case control studies have shown a reduction in colon cancer mortality in patients screened with sigmoidoscopy.

It may be that most of the benefits of annual FOBT and regular sigmoidoscopy from the age of 50 years could be obtained with colonoscopic surveillance of the 3–5% of patients found to have large (> 1 cm) or villus adenomas and who appear to have at least a fourfold increase in long-term likelihood of developing colorectal cancer.

Air contrast barium enema (ACBE) is not currently recommended for screening.

Surveillance of risk groups

Routine surveillance is recommended for those with colorectal cancer in one or more first degree relatives, chronic inflammatory bowel disease or a history of large or multiple colorectal adenomas or colorectal cancer. The recommended surveillance is colonoscopy, or ACBE with flexible sigmoidoscopy, every five years from the age of 35 to 50 years, depending on the age and number of the affected relatives. Members of HNPCC families require earlier and more intensive screening.

If an adenomatous polyp is found, colonoscopy should be performed to clear the colon of polyps, with follow-up colonoscopies each three to five years if several adenomas > 1 cm or adenomas with villus change are found.

CLINICAL PRESENTATION

Primary

The most common presenting symptom of large bowel cancer is rectal bleeding. Other symptoms include altered bowel habit, with constipation or diarrhea, iron- deficiency anemia, abdominal pain and weight loss, usually due to metastases.

Bright rectal bleeding which drips at the end of defecation, is on the paper, or sprays onto the bowl can be assumed to be arising from the anus or rectum and flexible sigmoidoscopy is sufficient investigation.

Complete investigation of the colon and rectum by colonoscopy, or a combination of flexible sigmoidoscopy and high quality air ACBE, is indicated when the blood is dark or mixed with the feces, if the patient is unsure of the nature of the bleeding, if bleeding persists despite treatment of the apparent local cause, or if there are associated bowel or abdominal symptoms. Colonoscopy is the preferred method, as it is generally more accurate and may be required in any case should a lesion be apparent on sigmoidoscopy or ACBE.

Carcinomas of the right side of the colon in particular may present with iron deficiency anemia, as well as a relatively minor change in bowel habit, a right iliac fossa mass or weight loss.

Carcinomas of the transverse and left colon are more likely to present with a change in bowel habit, usually increasing constipation. Blood and mucus may be seen with more distal tumors.

Carcinomas of the rectum or rectosigmoid region typically present with rectal bleeding, sometimes mixed with the stool and sometimes passed without feces.

In rectal cancer, the usual change in bowel habit may be described by the patient as diarrhea, but is more often a sense of incomplete evacuation. The patient experiences a call to stool, and may pass only a small amount of feces, sometimes containing blood or mucus, and some flatus. Because of the sense of incomplete evacuation, the patient returns to defecate on several occasions, sometimes with tenesmus and the desire to strain.

As the cancer invades locally, urinary or gynecological symptoms, or pelvic pain may occur.

American Cancer Society figures suggest that approximately 40% of colorectal cancers are localized at presentation, 40% are confined to the region of the primary tumor, and 20% present with distant metastases.

Obstruction

Fifteen to 20% of patients with colorectal cancer present with an acute obstruction. The symptoms are often insidious in onset, beginning with a period of increasing constipation. Patients frequently feel the need for increasing doses of aperients, with little effect other than the production of abdominal pain. Carcinomas of the right side are less likely to present with obstructive symptoms, presumably because of the nature of the tumors, the larger size of the lumen on the right, and the fact that the intestinal contents are more fluid. Obstructing symptoms are more common with rectosigmoid carcinomas than with those in the ampulla of the rectum.

With a chronic obstruction, the colon proximal to the cancer can become dilated and thick-walled. In an acute obstruction, the proximal dilatation may be sufficient to interfere with arterial blood flow leading to ischemic perforation, usually in the cecum, particularly in patients with a competent ileocecal valve.

The abdomen may be distended, but visible peristalsis is unusual. Usually the rectum will be empty and diagnosis will be made on plain abdominal X-ray. Where there is difficulty in distinguishing a mechanical from an adynamic obstruction, examination by water-soluble contrast enema may provide a diagnosis.

Perforation

Approximately 5% of patients present with perforation. This may be as a result of stercoral ulceration and ischemia proximal to an obstructing carcinoma, or local perforation of the tumor. Abscess formation or diffuse spreading peritonitis may result from necrosis of a full thickness carcinoma.

DIAGNOSIS AND INVESTIGATION

Some of the symptoms of carcinoma of the colon may be vague, mimicking those of upper gastrointestinal problems and functional bowel disease, so the possibility of carcinoma of the colon should be considered in anyone over the age of 40 with abdominal symptoms. Investigation is mandatory in any patient who has a persistent change in bowel habit, or is passing mucus or altered blood.

Abdominal examination is often unrewarding but the presence of a mass, signs of acute or subacute obstruction or perforation and the presence of hepatic enlargement should be sought.

Digital rectal examination, which detects 50% of rectal cancers, is mandatory in all patients with altered bowel habit or the passage of blood or mucus per rectum. The typical rectal carcinoma feels indurated and is either a polypoid lesion or has a raised, firm edge. Altered blood may be seen on the examining finger. Factors that may be important in determining treatment, such as mobility of the tumor, degree of spread though the rectal wall and fixation to extrarectal tissues and organs, may be assessed by rectal examination. Sigmoidoscopy should be performed, preferably after bowel preparation. Rigid sigmoidoscopy provides the best assessment of the distance of the lower margin from the dentate line of a rectal cancer, but flexible sigmoidoscopy allows examination of more of the left colon.

CT scan and MRI have a resolution of between 1 and 2 cm in the abdomen, and are therefore not particularly useful for detection of early disease or for the staging of primary tumors. Contrast-enhanced CT is of greater use in diagnosis and assessment of liver metastases.

Abdominal ultrasound has less resolution than CT and is seldom used for these purposes.

Rectal ultrasound may allow identification of those patients who are suitable for local treatment, or who are likely to benefit from pre-operative radiotherapy. This modality is at least 80% accurate in determining the level of invasion of the rectal wall, and almost 80% accurate in the diagnosis of nodal involvement. Ultrasound-guided aspiration cytology of enlarged nodes is a promising development in the staging of rectal cancers.

Radioimmunoscintigraphy has been used for staging of disease and for detection and localization of recurrence, sometimes as a pre-operative measure, but is of limited resolution, and its place is not yet established.

Pre-operative chest X-Ray should be performed: cancer of the rectum is more likely to produce pulmonary metastases than of the colon.

PRE-OPERATIVE ASSESSMENT

On the perioperative period, preferably pre-operatively, colonoscopy should be performed, as there will be synchronous carcinomas in up to 3% of patients and polyps in up to 30%. The presence of multiple polyps or cancers may dictate a more radical resection.

STAGING SYSTEMS

The purposes of a staging system are to provide a prognosis for the patient, to allocate patients to a treatment regime, and to allow comparison of results of treatment.

Dukes in 1932 categorized cancers on the basis of histological features such as depth of tumor penetration of the bowel wall and presence of lymph nodes metastases.

The Astler–Coller system developed in the United

States is also based on histological features. Clinicopathological staging was introduced by Turnbull, and included a "D" classification to include the presence of adjacent organ involvement and distant metastases, and this concept has been extended with systems such as the Australian Clinicopathological Staging System and that of the American Joint Committee on Cancer.

PROGNOSTIC FACTORS

Clinical

Rectal tumors generally have a poorer prognosis than colonic tumors, perhaps because of technical factors sometimes limiting effectiveness of local clearance.

Other adverse prognostic factors include bowel obstruction or perforation, the presence of distant metastases at presentation, tethering of the tumor, tumor perforation or residual tumor at operation, and possibly the use of blood transfusion during surgery. Invasion of adjacent organs does not appear to be of significance unless en-bloc resection is not possible.

Local perforation at operation adversely affects local recurrence, independent of tumor stage of fixity, perhaps due to implantation of exfoliated cells. In the rectum, adverse features include local spread to peritoneum and parietes, tumor size > 3 cm and ulceration.

Biologic and other features

The most accurate histological predictor of outcome is nodal status. Involvement of nodes along major named vessels and of apical nodes carries a poor prognosis. In rectal carcinoma, patients with 1–4 nodes involved have survival rates of 50–55%, which fall to 20–30% with involvement of five or more nodes.

Microscopic features such as depth of penetration, extensive stromal fibrosis and a positive resection margin carry a poor prognosis.

Cell type, tumor grade and ploidy have been suggested as possible indicators of prognosis but, once correction for other variables is made, the evidence of independent prognostic value is weak.

Microscopic perineural, venous and lymphatic invasion are subject to observer variation and have not been confirmed as having independent prognostic significance. It appears that the lack of an inflammatory cell (lymphocyte) infiltrate around the tumor may confer a worse prognosis, as may a margin that is infiltrating rather than expanding.

Depth of rectal wall invasion correlates with metastasis, which is seen in 5–10% with tumors confined to the submucosa, 10–20% with penetration of the muscularis propria, and 30–60% with involvement of perirectal fat. The lower the cancer in the rectum, the greater the likelihood of local recurrence, perhaps due to the limited operating space in the lower pelvis.

TREATMENT

The standard treatment for colorectal cancer is surgical excision. Twenty-five to 30% of potentially curable patients will have lymph node involvement, so removal of the draining lymph nodes is standard treatment when a cure is sought. Involvement of adjacent organs such as the uterus or bladder occurs in approximately 6%.

GENERAL PRINCIPLES OF PREPARATION

A stoma therapist should be consulted pre-operatively if either a permanent left iliac fossa stoma, or a defunctioning ileostomy or colostomy, usually in the right iliac fossa or right upper quadrant of the abdomen respectively is a possibility, so that the appropriate site can be marked with the patient awake and able to stand.

Thromboembolic prophylaxis

Patients with colorectal cancer are at high risk of thromboembolic complications, and measures such as subcutaneous heparin, compression stockings and intraoperative sequential compression devices should be used.

Mechanical cleansing

For elective surgery, the colon is cleansed mechanically pre-operatively. Traditionally, this has been done by a combination of fasting and bowel washouts but orthograde lavage with sodium phosphate or polyethylene-glycol based solutions have been found to be more effective, although often less well tolerated by patients.

Perioperative antibiotics

The use of antibiotics in the perioperative period significantly decreases the likelihood of wound infection which is one of the major causes of morbidity and prolonged hospital stay. It appears that optimum results are obtained by high blood levels of broad spectrum antibiotics in the perioperative period, usually as an intravenous bolus at the commencement of the procedure, repeated if necessary during a prolonged operation. There appears to be no benefit in the continuation of antibiotics beyond the perioperative period in most circumstances although they are frequently used for 24 hours postoperatively.

Indwelling urethral catheter

For rectal excision in particular, an indwelling urethral catheter should be placed immediately prior to surgery. There is a significant incidence of postoperative urinary problems following pelvic surgery and the catheter should therefore be left in place post-operatively, particularly in middle-aged and elderly males.

Use of a suprapubic catheter for the post-operative period results in less urinary problems.

GENERAL PRINCIPLES OF RESECTION

The basic principle of curative resection is adequate removal of the primary tumor including local extensions and likely lymphatic drainage. The right colon is supplied by the superior mesenteric artery, and removal of cancers of this part of the bowel is described as right hemicolectomy. (See Figure 18.1.)

The left colon derives its blood supply from the inferior mesenteric artery and a cancer in that area is usually treated by the resection indicated in Figure 18.2.

Rectum

The treatment of middle and lower third rectal tumors in particular has progressed considerably in the past three decades and methods of removing rectal tumors

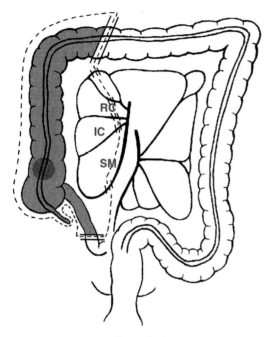

Figure 18.1.

without a permanent stoma are increasing in number. Surgical stapling devices are used as an aid to low pelvic anastomosis but techniques also include very low anterior resection with coloanal anastomosis, abdominoperineal excision of the rectum with

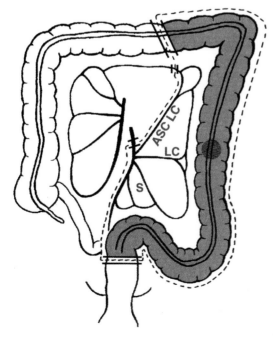

Figure 18.2.

perineal colostomy and gracilis neosphincter, trans-sphincteric resection, and local ablation by surgery, electrocoagulation or radiotherapy.

Local excision of rectal tumors

Rectal cancers may be removed by local excision through the anal canal or by a number of perineal or parasacral approaches, and the results may match those of the more standard surgical approaches in selected patients, but are suitable only for a limited number of patients without spread, and may be technically demanding.

Transanal intrarectal ultrasound can assess the extent of the primary lesion and the possibility of lymph node involvement more accurately than rectal examination. This may enable the primary tumor to be staged with a sufficient degree of accuracy to allow local excision as an acceptable alternative in some patients.

In general, if a rectal carcinoma is small ($\leq$ 4 cm, $\leq$ 30% circumferential), well differentiated and has not extended beyond the submucosa, treatment by local excision, together with post-operative radiotherapy in all but the most early tumors, should be adequate.

Rectal excision

Resections for carcinoma may be for palliative reasons, usually because of distant spread, or as an attempt to cure the patient when there is no evidence of spread of the disease.

The extent of the resection proximal to the tumor is the same for abdominoperineal excision or restorative resection (Figure 18.3).

Sphincter-saving (restorative) resections

Anterior resection involves resection of the rectum and rectosigmoid, mobilization of the left colon including the splenic flexure, followed by an end-to-end anastomosis. This technique is suitable for resections in which sufficient rectal stump is left for an anastomosis, that is to within 1–2 cm of the pelvic floor (Figure 18.3).

In general, it is possible to restore intestinal continuity with tumors as low as 6 cm from the anal verge. These procedures can be technically difficult, are more prone to post-operative complications and may not be advisable with high grade or

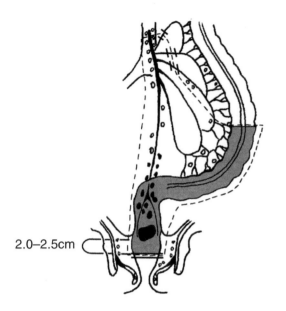

2.0–2.5cm

Figure 18.3.

locally advanced tumors, in patients in poor physical condition, or with the limited access sometimes found in the male pelvis in particular.

Anterior resection with coloanal anastomosis is an operation in which the bowel is mobilized sufficiently to allow an anastomosis to the anal canal from below. The level of resection can therefore be lower than for the standard anterior resection. A temporary diverting stoma is usually required because of the high rate of anastomotic complications. Incontinence for flatus or a minor fecal leak may result, occasionally requiring the patient to wear a pad on a regular basis.

Abdominoperineal excision of the rectum

Combined abdominoperineal excision of the rectum was at one time the standard operation for most rectal cancers. The procedure as described by Miles involved a single surgeon performing the dissections consecutively. It is now considered preferable to have two surgeons performing the procedure synchronously.

Generally, carcinomas with their lower margin within 5 cm of the anal verge are unsuitable for sphincter preservation and the appropriate procedure is abdominoperineal excision of the rectum.

The anal canal is sutured to avoid spillage of malignant cells with manipulation of the rectum, which is removed together with the anal sphincters.

A permanent end colostomy is established, usually in the left iliac fossa. The use of modern stomal appliances produces little interference with lifestyle, and this can be reduced further by regular irrigation, thus avoiding the need to wear a colostomy bag.

The development of sphincter-saving resections has reduced the rate of abdominoperineal excision from approximately 40% in 1970 to less than 20% of all rectal cancers in 1995.

Carcinomas with the lower margins between 5 and 8 cm may be treated in either way, depending upon operative factors. In general, it is easier to operate in the female pelvis because of its shape, and access is better in patients who are thin. With the circular stapler, it is sometimes possible to achieve an anastomosis in patients in whom problems with access may preclude a handsewn anastomosis.

The same basic principles apply to all anastomoses: the mucosa should be inverted, rather than everted, with serosal and muscle apposition externally; the blood supply must be adequate and there should be no tension on the anastomosis. The number of layers in the anastomosis and the choice of material is generally of less consequence.

Circular staplers generally decrease operative time, but may produce a higher incidence of anastomotic stricture, particularly in the intraperitoneal rectum or colon.

PALLIATIVE SURGERY

When the effects of secondary spread of colonic carcinoma are such that the primary lesion is unlikely to cause problems within the expected life of the patient, supportive treatment only may be warranted. In all other circumstances, optimal palliation is obtained by excision of the primary tumor.

Defunctioning colostomy or ileostomy alone seldom offer adequate palliation for rectal carcinoma. Although they may avoid an obstruction, they do little to alleviate the symptoms arising from the presence of the carcinoma in the rectum, such as spurious diarrhea, hemorrhage, local discomfort or development of fistulas. If a rectal tumor is unresectable and fecal diversion is required to avoid obstructive symptoms, it should be accompanied by treatment of the luminal component of the carcinoma, either by radiotherapy or local diathermy fulguration.

DRAINAGE

Drainage of the abdomen after resection has not been shown to influence the post-operative course, but drainage of the pelvis, with or without irrigation, may be beneficial.

DEFUNCTIONING STOMA

A defunctioning stoma does not seem to decrease the likelihood of anastomotic breakdown but, should it occur, may lessen the effects. Defunctioning loop ileostomy appears more effective than the loop colostomy, and closure produces fewer complications. There is, however, a greater likelihood of small bowel obstruction with defunctioning ileostomy.

Assuming there is no evidence of an anastomotic leak, defunctioning stomas may be closed as early as three weeks after operation.

AVOIDANCE OF ANASTOMOTIC RECURRENCE/IMPLANTATION

Intraoperative lavage of the lumen with cytocidal agents such as mercuric perchloride has been shown to reduce the incidence of local recurrence which is only a problem with removal of rectal carcinoma. There is increasing evidence that total mesorectal excision significantly decreases local recurrence following surgical treatment of rectal carcinoma.

POST-OPERATIVE CARE

Oral fluids are usually commenced within 24–36 hours of operation, and then gradually increased. Should an ileus develop, nasogastric suction should be used. Flatus is usually passed on the second or third day, at which time a light diet can be commenced, with progression to a normal diet as quickly as the patient will tolerate.

Complications include those seen after any abdominal surgery, pulmonary atelectasis and infection, intra-abdominal sepsis, thromboembolic complications, paralytic ileus, and urinary infection, usually related to catheterization.

The major specific complication is anastomotic leak, which can be relatively minor, indicated on the second or third post-perative day by a low-grade fever, ileus and general lack of progress. Small anastomotic dehiscences do not necessarily need further surgery and may resolve spontaneously with cessation of oral intake, intravenous infusions, and administration of antibiotics if there is any suggestion of continuing sepsis.

Pus initially, and then flatus and fecal material may discharge if a drain is in place. The drain should then remain at least until a drainage track is established.

If more major leakage results in localized and then diffuse peritonitis, the anastomosis should be taken down, peritoneal lavage performed, the distal bowel oversewn and a proximal end colostomy fashioned. If the fecal leakage is contained, particularly in a rectal anastomosis, it may be enough to drain the collection and establish a proximal diversion.

TREATMENT OF OBSTRUCTED CARCINOMA

Patients with obstructed colon cancer may be in poor condition as a result of the obstruction and will have a bowel full of feces and which may be edematous, friable or ischemic. Proximal fecal diversion is traditionally the surgical response to bowel obstruction due to carcinoma but better overall long-term results are obtained with resection of the tumor at presentation.

In patients with subacute obstruction, particularly on the left side of the colon, conservative management with cessation of oral intake, nasogastric suction, intravenous therapy, and distal washouts may allow resolution of the obstruction, eventual preparation of the bowel and a one-stage surgical procedure during the same admission. Where that is not possible, primary resection should be attempted, with or without a diverting stoma.

Most right-sided or transverse colon tumors presenting with obstruction can be treated with right hemicolectomy, extended to include the transverse or left colon if necessary.

Left-sided tumors presenting with obstruction but no proximal necrosis can be managed by resection of the primary tumor and on-table lavage, through a small bowel enterotomy or the appendiceal stump, to clean and decompress the proximal colon, followed by primary anastomosis.

The options for management of obstructing rectosigmoid tumors, particularly if there is local perforation or any reason for concern about anastomotic integrity are resection and anastomosis with a defunctioning ileostomy or Hartmann's procedure. This entails oversewing of the rectal stump and an end left iliac fossa colostomy, followed some months later by restoration of intestinal continuity.

Vigorous peritoneal lavage is mandatory in the presence of local or free perforation.

COMPLETENESS OF LOCAL EXCISION/ LOCAL MARGINS

Other than in the presence of extensive lymphatic involvement, usually with poorly differentiated tumors when cure by surgery is unlikely, microscopic submucosal spread seems limited to less than 1 cm. Several studies have not shown any relationship between frequency of local recurrence and margin of clearance with well-differentiated tumors provided the clearance is > 1 cm in the fresh specimen. Gaining an adequate margin of excision seems seldom a problem in the colon and intraperitoneal rectum.

Complete mesorectal excision produces local recurrence rates in curative resections as low as 4%, as opposed to 20–35% with standard dissection and seems superior to standard surgery plus adjuvant chemo/radiotherapy.

If there is doubt about local clearance, consideration must be given to an abdominoperineal excision. This does not provide greater lateral or perirectal clearance and has the disadvantage of opening new tissue planes, but it does avoid the significant morbidity associated with pelvic anastomotic recurrence, which frequently leads to a proximal stoma or further resection for palliative reasons. It allows the use of post-operative radiotherapy without producing some of the severe side effects of radiotherapy following anterior resection.

FUNCTIONAL RESULTS

The functional results of anterior resection are worse the lower the level of the anastomosis. Results are further compromised by pelvic sepsis, following an anastomotic leak for example, presumably because of the resulting loss of compliance of the neorectum. Function generally improves for 18 months after operation.

Construction of a colonic J-pouch reconstruction after anterior resection may alleviate the problems of urgency of defecation, increased stool frequency and nocturnal incontinence thought to result from the loss of rectal reservoir capacity.

Disorders of sexual function

Sexual function may be seriously disturbed due to autonomic nerve injury during excision of the rectum. Approximately two-thirds of male patients retain normal potency after operation but only half of these are able to ejaculate. The likelihood of sexual dysfunction increases with increasing age at operation.

ADJUVANT THERAPY

Approximately 80% of colorectal cancer may be potentially curable at the time of presentation. Recurrence after apparently successful removal of colorectal cancer is due to occult residual carcinoma which may be amenable to adjuvant therapy.

Colon

Chemotherapy

Use of 5-Fluorouracil and an immune stimulant, levamisole post-operatively has produced improvement in survival in colon cancer patients with nodal involvement but without obvious metastatic disease. Post-operative 5-Fluorouracil and folinic acid for six months has been shown to produce a significant prolongation of disease-free interval, and some survival benefit with primary colon cancer.

Rectum

Radiotherapy and chemotherapy

Adjuvant radiotherapy is delivered by external beam and may be given pre-operatively, post-operatively, or by a combination of both ("sandwich" technique).

Post-operative radiotherapy combined with 5-Fluorouracil based chemotherapy decreases local recurrence rates and prolongs survival after surgery, but perioperative radiotherapy alone has not been shown to produce a significant improvement in survival.

Pre-operative radiotherapy for rectal cancer produces very much less morbidity than when given post-operatively, but only patients with more advanced local disease should be so treated.

Radiotherapy after anterior resection may have a profound adverse effect on bowel function.

Endocavitary radiotherapy is suitable as a primary treatment in patients with small (< 5 cm) rectal tumors without transmural involvement within 11–12 cm of the anal verge. As this modality does not deal with proximal nodal spread, it is reserved for those unfit for operative removal of the rectum in most centers.

Palliative treatment

Radiotherapy is occasionally used after incomplete resection for locally advanced disease. Morbidity is relatively high because of the difficulty in shielding the small bowel. There is no prospective data showing survival benefit for this form of treatment.

Preoperative chemoradiotherapy

The use of preoperative chemotherapy and radiotherapy for advanced disease may increase the prospect of successful local surgical treatment.

TREATMENT OF THE MALIGNANT POLYP

If a cancer within a polyp is anaplastic or excision is incomplete, bowel resection is indicated.

When a polyp removed endoscopically or peranally is found to contain invasive carcinoma, the risks of surgery must be weighed against the likelihood of residual carcinoma, at the site of excision or in lymph nodes in determining the need for resection.

Carcinoma *in situ*, or intraepithelial or intramucosal carcinoma (without penetration of the basement membrane) in a polyp only requires adequate excision of the polyp.

Metastases occur earlier in sessile than in pedunculated polyps, and in less well-differentiated tumors, and where there is submucosal lymphatic or vascular invasion.

LAPAROSCOPIC COLECTOMY FOR CANCER

Study of resected specimens indicates that laparoscopic or laparoscopically- assisted colectomy may produce a similar degree of lymph node and local clearance to open operation. There appears little difference in perioperative morbidity or mortality, although return of bowel function may be faster and hospital stay may be shorter, with perhaps a quicker return to normal activity. There is, however, no detailed prospective analysis of the suggested benefits.

There is anecdotal evidence of a greater likelihood of port site seeding and a theoretical possibility of enhancement of lymphatic and venous spread and pulmonary embolism as a result of the pneumoperitoneum necessary for the procedure.

The technique should be regarded as unproven, in the treatment of colon cancer, and should only be used in the context of a prospective randomized trial to assess its adequacy as a cancer operation.

POST-OPERATIVE MORBIDITY AND MORTALITY

Mortality

The overall operative mortality is less than 3% for elective surgical treatment, doubling for emergency and palliative surgery.

One-third of deaths are due to surgical complications, usually related to anastomotic failure, and the remainder to cardiac, respiratory and thromboembolic problems.

Anastomotic leaks should occur in less than 5% of patients with modern techniques.

Up to 40% of patients have a complication after colorectal resection, usually respiratory or wound-related, with 5–7% having deep vein thrombosis, with or without pulmonary embolus.

RESULTS OF TREATMENT

Colon cancer has a better prognosis than rectal, which has a higher incidence of local recurrence. Hepatic recurrence occurs in one-third, pulmonary, abdominal and locoregional recurrence in one-fifth each, and isolated retroperitoneal or peripheral recurrence less commonly.

Table 18.1. Survival of colorectal cancer.

Stage		Dukes	Five-year survival
1	Invasion to M. propria	A + B1	90%
2	Invasion into or through the serosa or to the pericolic tissue	B2	75%
3	Lymph Node metastases	C	35%
		D	5%

Survival is stage-related, and advances in treatment have not materially affected overall survival, which is shown in Table 18.1.

Approximately a quarter of patients present with incurable disease.

Survival following acute obstruction

Overall survival is less, as these patients generally have more advanced disease and a higher mortality of initial treatment, but remains stage-related.

Recurrent colorectal cancer

Recurrence after local excision

With local excision and post-operative radiotherapy, the local failure rate is between 3 and 24% depending on tumor stage.

Locally recurrent colon cancer

Local or abdominal recurrent cancer is rarely curable, as it is usually retroperitoneal or multifocal throughout the peritoneal cavity.

Locally recurrent rectal cancer

Local recurrence following "curative" surgery occurs in up to 35%, depending on operative technique, and appears to be surgeon- as well as stage-dependent. Local recurrence rates are of the order of 10% for Dukes'A cancers, 15% for Dukes' B and 30% for Dukes'C. Mortality and morbidity of re-excision is significantly greater than with primary resection, and five-year survival is no more than 10–25%. Involvement of the pelvic wall is the usual reason for incurability.

Fifty percent of local rectal recurrences occur without distant metastases whereas nearly all colonic local recurrences are associated with disseminated disease.

Liver recurrence

Approximately 15% of colorectal cancers develop isolated liver metastases, of which 25% are resectable. Recent advances in imaging and therapy have improved the selection for treatment, perioperative mortality and results of resection. Five-year survivals of 25–35% have been reported for treatment of isolated metastases.

Pulmonary recurrence

Solitary lung metastasis as an isolated recurrence is unusual, but five-year survivals of 30% have been reported for resection in such circumstances.

FOLLOW-UP

Of all patients who present with colorectal cancer, approximately 75% will undergo resection with curative intent. Of these, more than 33% will develop recurrence. Follow-up has two purposes, the prevention or detection of metachronous tumors, and the reduction of mortality by early detection of recurrent disease.

The majority of recurrences, perhaps 80%, occur within the first two years and any follow-up should be at its most intense in that period.

Only a small minority of local recurrences are detected at routine clinical follow-up, with a high proportion of such patients already having disseminated disease.

The value of radiology in detection of curable recurrence is debatable, and endoscopy would appear to be of little or no value in this regard.

Carcinoembryonic antigen (CEA) estimation, in particular the analysis of the trend of any elevation, is the most reliable marker of recurrent disease. CEA is produced in large amounts by normal fetal cells and over 90% of primary colorectal cancers, but only in trace amounts by normal adult cells.

CEA is also produced in some disease states including inflammatory conditions, and is moderately elevated in smokers, but not at progressively increasing levels. Less than half the patients with primary colorectal cancer have elevated CEA levels at presentation due to its metabolisation in the liver.

With complete excision of a colorectal cancer, CEA usually returns to normal within four weeks, and subsequent progressive elevation usually indicates hepatic or parietal recurrences. CEA-directed laparotomies for non-hepatic recurrence do not appear to improve survival, but CEA is at its most sensitive in the presence of liver metastases, where it rises before the development of symptoms. It is more sensitive than radiological or nuclear medicine investigations for the detection of such recurrence.

Although estimates every four weeks are optimal for trend analysis, most suggest three-monthly use in the first two years and sixth-monthly thereafter.

Imaging techniques

On the basis that liver recurrence is the type most likely to be amenable to treatment, perioperative ultrasound or CT, with a repeat at one year, is used in some centers.

Endorectal ultrasound seems effective in the detection of pelvic recurrences. Radioimmunoguided surgery (RIGS) using monoclonal antibody markers may improve detection of local recurrence although results of treatment are poor.

CARCINOMA OF THE ANAL CANAL AND ANUS

Carcinomas of the anal canal and anus comprise 3–4% of all large bowel carcinomas and are equally distributed between men and women, with carcinoma of the anus more common in males and of the anal canal more common in females. Predisposing factors include local radiotherapy, smoking, a history of anogenital warts and sexual promiscuity, particularly anal intercourse.

There is a strong association between anorectal and cervical cancer, suggesting a common etiological factor, probably human papilloma-virus (HPV) which occurs in 90% of anal warts and approximately 70% of squamous carcinomas of the anus.

The forms of carcinoma of the anal canal and anus include squamous and basal cell carcinoma, melanoma, and primary adenocarcinoma of the anal canal and perianal tissues.

There are subgroups of squamous carcinoma, which comprises up to 80% of tumors of this region, including basaloid, transitional cell, cloacogenic, basisquamous and mucoepidermoid, all of which arise in the transitional zone.

Squamous cell carcinomas of the anal canal and anus are similar in general appearance to squamous cell carcinoma elsewhere, that is, they are firm lesions, usually with an ulcerated surface, and present either as exophytic growth or as ulcers with firm, everted edges.

Endoluminal ultrasonography appears to be the most accurate method of assessing depth of tumor penetration prior to treatment, and response to treatment.

The possibility of inguinal lymph node spread needs to be considered with all carcinomas of the anal canal and anus but they may also be enlarged because of superficial sepsis within the ulcerated part of the carcinoma.

The usual presentation is with bleeding, local discomfort and pruritus and the presence of a lump.

There may be incontinence due to involvement of the sphincters, and formation of a rectovaginal fistula in advanced cases. Perineal pain occurs with extensive local infiltration.

There may be symptoms similar to those seen with low rectal carcinoma if the tumor is large, particularly if it spreads proximally to involve the rectum.

Diagnosis may not always be easy, as a number of other anal and perianal conditions may present with similar macroscopic findings, including the anal ulceration of Crohn's Disease, perianal warts, anal fissure or a prolapsed, thrombosed, ulcerated hemorrhoid. Biopsy is required for confirmation.

Local excision may be adequate for small well-differentiated distal tumors. For the remainder, the optimum treatment for squamous carcinoma of the anus and anal canal is radiotherapy alone or in combination with chemotherapy. Radiotherapy may be administered by external beam, intraluminal or implantation techniques. Abdominoperineal excision is reserved for failures of chemo-radiotherapy regimes, which occur in 10–25% of patients.

If the inguinal nodes are involved, block dissection may be necessary. Prophylactic dissection of the nodes has not been shown to be of benefit. Anal canal tumors have a poorer prognosis than those of the anal margin.

RESULTS OF TREATMENT OF ANAL CANCER

Anal canal tumors

With radiotherapy alone to anal canal, the perineum and inguinal nodes, 90% local control is achieved, with 75–85% of patients retaining anal sphincter function. More extensive surgery is required in approximately 10%.

Local excision of tumors < 2 cm results in loco-regional control in 90%. Five-year survival is 75% for tumors less than 4 cm and 40–70% for larger tumors. Nodal involvement decreases five-year survival to 25%. Fifty to 80% of local failures can be salvaged surgically.

The addition of chemotherapy improves local control significantly overall, but may not influence survival.

Anal margin tumors

Up to 60% may be successfully treated by local excision. Adjuvant radiotherapy is used with larger tumors, which may require abdominoperineal excision if more than half the circumference is involved. Radiochemotherapy achieves local control in 80–100%, depending on patient selection, but larger tumors have a five-year survival rate of < 50% and a 30% local recurrence rate. Half of these can be salvaged surgically.

Inguinal node metastases

Prophylactic node dissection does not improve survival. Therapeutic dissection of nodes involved secondary to anal canal tumors achieves up to 70% five-year survival if combined with chemoradio-therapy.

Metachronous nodal involvement by anal margin tumors has a universally poor prognosis, and only palliative treatment is warranted.

Anorectal melanoma

Anorectal melanoma accounts for < 0.5% of ano-rectal tumours, usually presenting late, and often resembling a hemorrhoid. Patients are more likely to have mesenteric node metastases and less likely to have inguinal node involvement than squamous cell cancer. Overall results are very poor, but some long-term survivals have followed APE with or without inguinal node dissection for tumours < 2 mm in depth. Malignant melanoma is not generally radiosensitive.

References

Abulafi, A.M. and Williams, N.S. (1994). Local recurrence of colorectal cancer: the problems, mechanisms, management and adjuvant therapy. (Review) *British Journal of Surgery*, **81**, 7–19.

Banerjee, A.K., Jehle, E.C., Shorthouse, A.J. and Buess, G. (1994). Local excision of rectal tumours. (Review) *British Journal of Surgery*, **82**, 1165–1173.

Brady, M.S., Kavolius, J.P. and Quan, S.H.Q. (1995). Anorectal melanoma. A 64-year experience at Memorial Sloan-Kettering Cancer Center. *Diseases of the Colon and Rectum*, **38**, 146–151.

Deans, G.T., McAleer, J.J.A. and Spence, R.A.J. (1994), Malignant anal tumours. (Review) *British Journal of Surgery*, **81**, 500–508.

Fearon, E.R. (1994). Molecular genetic studies of the adenoma-carcinoma sequence. *Advances in Internal Medicine*, **39**, 123–147.

Fielding, L.P., Arsenault, P.A., Chapuis, P.H. *et al.* (1991). Clinicopathological staging for colorectal cancer: An international documentation system (IDS) and an international comprehensive anatomical terminology (ICAT). *Journal of Gastroenterology and Hepatology*, **6**, 325–344.

Fuchs, C.S. and Mayer, R.J. (1995). Adjuvant Chemotherapy for Colon & Rectal 10, Cancer. *Seminars in Oncology*, **22**(5), 472–487.

Jass, J.R. (1989). Do all colorectal carcinomas arise in pre-existing adenomas? *World Journal of Surgery*, **13**, 45–51.

Lynch, H.T., Smyrk, T.C., Watson, P., Lanspa, S.J., Lynch, J.F., Lynch, P.M. *et al.* (1993). Genetics, natural history, tumor spectrum, and pathology of hereditary nonpolyposis colorectal cancer: An updated review. *Gastroenterology*, **104**, 1535–1549.

Moertel, C.G. (1994). Chemotherapy for colorectal cancer. *New England Journal of Medicine*, **330**(16), 1136–1142.

Weinberg, D.S. and Strom, B.L. (1995). Screening for Colorectal Cancer: A Review of Current & Future Strategies. *Seminars in Oncology*, **22**(5), 533–447.

Winawer *et al.* (1995). Prevention of colorectal cancer: guidelines based on new data. WHO Collaborative Center for the Prevention of Colorectal Cancer: Bulletin World Health Organization, **73**(1), 7–10.

Colorectal Cancer

Worldwide: 2nd most frequent cancer in developed countries

Lifetime risk
in USA whites:
  M   1 in 16
  F   1 in 17

Relative five-year survival in 1983–87
in USA whites:
  M   60.8%
  F   58.9%

Risk factors
Hereditary bowel disease
Inflammatory bowel disease
High fat/low fibre/low vegetable diet thought to increase risk.
Some studies have linked rectal cancer and beer drinking.

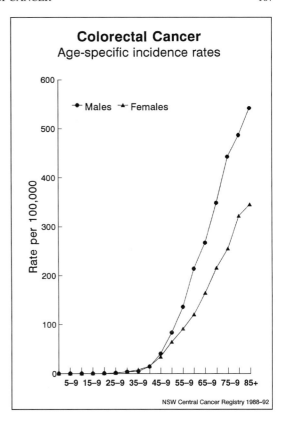

Colorectal Cancer
Age-specific incidence rates

NSW Central Cancer Registry 1988–92

Geographical variation in 1983–87

Highest rate
M: 28.0–57.4 per 100,000 in USA
F: 42.0 per 100,000 in Bermuda, blacks

Lowest rate
M: 1.3 per 100,000 in The Gambia
F: 2.3 per 100,000 in Algeria, Setif

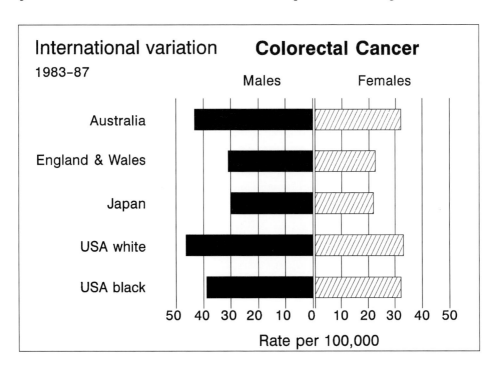

International variation
1983–87
Colorectal Cancer

19. Hepatobiliary Carcinoma

PHILIP R. CLINGAN

Illawarra Area Health Services, Cancer Care Centre, Wollongong, Australia

HEPATOCELLULAR CARCINOMA

Epidemiology

There is strong epidemiological evidence of a close association between chronic infection with Hepatitis B and C and the development of hepatocellular carcinoma. The relative risks for a patient who is a chronic Hepatitis B carrier has been calculated to be in the vicinity of 14 and for a Hepatitis C carrier has been estimated as 27. Chronic Hepatitis of whatever course progressing to cirrhosis remains the most important causal factor for liver cancer. (It has been proposed that during the course of Hepatitis B the virus DNA is integrated into the host DNA accompanied by chromosomal deletions and translocations. The exact mechanism whereby the hepatitis virus leads to the development of cancer is unknown.) The incidence of hepatocellular carcinoma varies markedly worldwide.

PREDISPOSING AND RISK FACTORS

Cirrhosis, from whatever cause, is regarded as a precancerous condition. The main risk factors for the development of hepatocellular carcinoma are Hepatitis B and Hepatitis C infection. Chronic alcohol abuse is a common cause of cirrhosis in low incidence area. Alcohol may act as a cocarcinogen with other agents, notably Hepatitis B virus infection, Aflatoxins and smoking. Individuals consuming more than 20 g of alcohol and 4 mcg of Aflatoxin per day have a 35-fold increase in the relative risk of hepatocellular carcinoma. Between 2.2 and 5.5% of cirrhotics have hepatocellular carcinoma at autopsy. About 80% of patients with hepatocellular carcinoma have associated cirrhosis. Once cirrhosis has developed, continued consumption of alcohol is not necessary for the development of liver cell carcinoma; the risk actually increases with time.

There are a number of other diseases associated with the development of hepatocellular carcinoma.

Hemochromatosis, Wilson's disease, glycogen storage disease and alpha-one antitrypsin deficiency have also been associated with the development of hepatocellular carcinoma. Aflatoxins are a group of mycotoxins derived from the fungus *Aspergillus flavus* found in peanut, soya bean, corn, rice, wheat, barley and cotton seed. These toxins may produce a mutation of the P53 tumor suppressor gene in hepatocellular carcinoma. Heavy exposure to the Aflatoxin is associated with an increased risk of hepatocellular carcinoma.

Hepatocellular carcinoma is known to have androgen receptors and it has been suggested that the tumor may be androgen dependent. There are reports that use of Cipropterone may increase the risk of developing hepatocellular carcinoma. Other drugs such as the contraceptive pill have also been implicated in increasing the risk of hepatocellular carcinoma, particularly of the fibrolamellar variety. After five years of oral contraceptive use, the risk of hepatocellular carcinoma is increased by five times.

PATHOLOGY

Malignant tumors of the liver are primary adeno-carcinoma with two major cell types; hepatocellular and cholangiocellular. Histological classification is as follows:

- Hepatocellular carcinoma
- Hepatocellular carcinoma fibrolamellar variant
- Cholangio carcinoma (central or peripheral)
- Hepatoblastoma (which occurs rarely in adults).

Fibrolamellar carcinoma is an important variant as it has a higher cure rate compared to the normal variant, when surgically resected.

Macroscopic

The tumor is often divided up into three main types of carcinoma:

1. the multinodular tumor
2. the massive solitary mass (fibrolamellar)
3. diffuse small tumors

Alpha Feta Protein (AFP)

Alpha feta protein staining is highly specific for hepatocellular carcinoma but it has a relatively low sensitivity; it is used as a serum tumor marker and can also be detected by histochemistry.

Special subtypes

Fibrolamellar carcinoma may constitute up to 5% of cases but rises up to 15–40% in children and adolescents. Over 90% of these carcinomas occur in patients under 25 years of age. Females are affected more commonly than males. The patient frequently presents with abdominal pain, malaise and weight loss. Alpha feta protein level is seldom raised. There is no association with Hepatitis B infection or cirrhosis. They are usually large and solitary tumors. The majority of tumors arise in the left lobe of the liver. The surgical resectability rate is high. Macroscopically, the tumor is well defined and may show a lobular arrangement with interconnecting fibrosis septa. Smaller satellite nodules may be seen adjacent to the main tumor mass. An abundant fibrous stroma is characteristic. The tumor may show positive staining for neuroendocrine differentiation.

The most common means of the spread of hepato-cellular carcinoma is via the intravascular extension with involvement of major hepatic vessels and portal veins. Dissemination within the peritoneal cavity is uncommon. However, dissemination to the lymphatics, namely the porta hepatis, pancreatic and coeliac axis nodes does occur in a large percentage of cases. This is often underestimated in the preoperative workup.

PREVENTION

The most important methods of preventing hepato-cellular carcinoma is likely to be by the prevention of Hepatitis B and C infections. In areas where there is a high incidence of Hepatitis B, vaccination of newborns with Hepatitis B vaccine may prove to be the most effective way to prevent development of this disease. Avoidance of a flatoxin and alcohol may reduce risk.

The spread of Hepatitis B and C by needle sharing (either recreational or vacination) and the sexual spread of Hepatitis B are clearly potentially avoidable.

SCREENING

Screening for hepatocellular carcinoma has been used in several high incidence areas using ultrasound and serum AFP levels. Subclinical lesions may be detected allowing potentially curative surgery. The five-year survival of HCC is stage dependent and screening-detected cases have a considerably better survival than in symtomatic disease (although such observation are subject to several types of bias (see Chapter 2 on screening).

Use of AFP levels as a diagnostic tool is limited by the fact that up to one-third of small HCC and 10% of advanced HCC will not have an elevated level. Patients with cirrhosis may be offered surveillance based on ultrasound/αFP to attempt to achieve early diagnosis.

CLINICAL PRESENTATION

The tumor may present with a sudden illness, with pain, weight loss and fever. Hepatic decompensation with jaundice, ascites and encephalopathy is com-

Table 19.1. Prognostic variables for hepatocellular carcinoma.

AFP level (high)
    tumor size (> 5 cm poor prognosis)
    number of tumors (> 3 poor prognosis)
    age
    stage of cirrhosis
    surgical resectability
    portal involvement
    Hepatitis antigen positivity (liver transplantation)

mon. Physical examination may reveal a large mass in the liver and 25% of cases will have an hepatic friction rub. The tumor may present with sudden rupture or bleeding from esophageal varices.

There have been a number of paraneoplastic syndromes associated with the development of hepatocellular carcinoma, including hypoglycemia, hypercalcemia and erthrocytosis.

INVESTIGATIONS

Preoperative investigations of hepatocellular carcinoma fulfill several functions. The fitness of the patient to undergo the recommended treatment is measured (full blood count coagulation studies, liver function tests, albumin, perhaps indocyanin green retention test). Other tests are important to detect distant spread (lung CT, bone scan) CT and US scans are used to measure number, size and side of lesions. Angiography may help in the diagnosis and assessment of resectability. Lipidol when given intra-arterially is usually taken up actively by the hepatocytes and may demonstrate multifocal disease.

PROGNOSTIC FACTORS (Table 19.1)

One of the most important factors in deciding the prognosis of patients with hepatocellular carcinoma is the associated degree of hepatic disease which complicates the patient's ability to withstand any further treatment. All patients should be classified by either the Okuda or Stillwagon prognostic criteria.

The Okuda prognostic staging system defines four adverse criteria:

1. Tumor burden greater than 50% of the liver.
2. Ascites.
3. Albumin < 3 g/dl.
4. Serum bilirubin > 3 ng.

Okuda Stage 1 is defined as having no adverse criteria.
Okuda Stage 2 has 1 or 2 adverse criteria.
Okuda Stage 3 has 3 or 4 adverse criteria.

Patients with an unfavourable Stillwagon criteria or Okuda class 3 are not suitable for either surgical resection or for most intra-arterial and radiotherapy treatment.

TREATMENT

The type of treatment for liver cancer depends on presence or absence of cirrhosis and whether the disease is localized to the liver; whether it is locally resectable or locally advanced. Surgery provides the only potentially curative treatment for hepatocellular carcinoma. Only 10–15% of patients are suitable for surgery. The major determinant of resectability is the presence of and severity of cirrhosis. Cirrhosis results in a limited functional reserve.

If tumors are confined to a solitary mass and are anatomically placed in the liver to allow resection, the preferred treatment is local resection of the tumor.

Some locally unresectable tumors may be rendered resectable by perioperative treatment with chemotherapy or radiation.

Patients with unresectable fibrolamellar hepatocellular carcinomas should be considered for liver transplantation.

RESULTS OF SURGICAL TREATMENT

Liver resection has resulted in five year survival rates of 10–40%. Tumor diameter affects the outcome, in patients with tumors < 5 cm a five year survival of upto 75% has been reported.

LIVER TRANSPLANTATION

Only a small number of patients are suitable for liver transplantation. These principally include the fibrolamellar type and hepatoblastomas although small good prognosis lesion which are unresectable because of cirrhosis could be considered. Intrahepatic bile duct carcinoma, larger HCCs and those with lymph node or other spread should be excluded from liver transplantation programs.

Three and five-year survival rates of liver transplant for hepatocellular carcinoma have been reported between 16–56% and 19–36% respectively.

The presence of Hepatitis surface antigen positivity has been shown to have a negative impact on liver transplant and patients with Hepatitis B antigen positivity. There was a three year survival of 69% in Hepatitis antigen negative patients versus 18% in those patients who underwent liver transplant who were Hepatitis antigen positive.

MULTIMODALITY TREATMENT

The untreated patient with symtomatic HCC will be fortunate to survived six months. Regional chemotherapy or radiation therapeutic treatment may prolong survival to an average of 18–24 months.

PERCUTANEOUS INTRATUMORAL ALCOHOL INJECTION

Percutaneous intratumoral injection of ethyl alcohol of 95% concentration produces cellular dehydration and intracellular coagulation. Alcohol also causes vascular injury with resulting ischemia of the tumor. Percutaneous ethanol injection is usually performed under ultrasonography and between 1–8 ml of 95% ethanol are injected into the lesion. The patient needs to have a platelet count above 40,000 and a prothrombin time of 40 to make them suitable for treatment. Treatment can be repeated as an outpatient and is often given weekly. The technique is well tolerated by most patients. The major reported complications of this treatment include intraperitoneal hemorrhage, right sided pleural effusion, cholangitis or jaundice secondary to injury of the bile ducts and liver abscess. Survival following percutaneous alcohol injection is again dependent on the tumor diameter, and the best results are acheived in small (< 2 cm) tumor. Five-year survival rates of ~40% have been described, very similar to the results of liver resection.

CRYOSURGERY

Cryosurgery involves the localized destruction of tumor by using cryo probes with liquid nitrogen (–196°C). The procedure require a laparotomy but is less likely to lead to liver failure in cirrhosis from resection. Similar survival data to resection have been reported by a Chinese group.

LIPIODOL-BASED THERAPY

Lipiodol (iodized poppy seed oil) is taken up avidly by many HCCs and some other liver tumours; this can be used to selectively deliver a cytotoxic or radioactive iodine bound to the lipiodal, to the HCC. The response rate using intra-arterial Lipiodol/I131 has been reported as high as 50%. This is particularly well tolerated in patients with portal vein thrombosis as arterial flow is not altered. Long-term survival of our three-year is seen in some patients.

EXTERNAL RADIATION

General radiation can also be used to treat hepatocellular carcinoma but doses > 2500 cgy will induce radiation hepatitis which is frequently lethal. A 2500 cgy dose can induce 15–30% response rate in most hepatomas.

REGIONAL CHEMOTHERAPY

Use of regional chemotherapy produces response rates between 8–40% using Adriamycin or 5-Fluorouracil (5-FU). Neither of these agents shows an improvement in survival above those patients receiving no treatment.

Intra-arterial Cis-Platinum is currently reported to give response rates between 50–60% and remains the most active agent in the treatment of hepatocellular carcinoma.

In an effort to improve the response from chemotherapy in patients, chemoembolization has been undertaken using a number of agents including starch, microspheres, macroagulated albumin, cryogranulate, gelfoam impregnated with the drug or Lipiodol. The partial response rate using chemoembolization has been reported as high as 50%. Chemoembolization carries a risk of producing massive tumor or hepatic necrosis or duodenal perforation or if Lipiodol is used there is a small risk of pulmonary injury.

ADVANCED HEPATOCELLULAR CARCINOMA

Advanced hepatocellular carcinoma is cancer that has spread through much of the liver or to distant metastatic sites. Median survival is usually 2–4 months. The most common metastatic sites for hepatocellular cancer are the lungs and bone. Multifocal disease in the liver is common, particularly when cirrhosis or chronic Hepatitis is present. The treatment of these patients is palliative. Chemotherapy used systemically has very little effect upon survival or response in this group of patients. These patients also respond poorly to local regional therapy. The median survival in patients selected for chemotherapy trials is reported as six months. The most effective drug is Doxorubicin with a 20% response rate. Other drugs with activity in this disease include Etoposide, Mitozantrone and Cis-Platinum.

ADJUVANT THERAPY

In separate studies adjuvant doxorubicin, infusion of 5-FU and intravenous Mitozantrone have reported improvement in survival over historical controls. As yet there is not enough data to support routine use of adjuvant treatment in these patients.

FOLLOW-UP

As well as clinical examination use of AFP and CT scans at three monthly intervals in potentially curable patients is usual. The aim of follow-up is to detect local recuitent tumors in patients who had prior resection so that further local treatment can be undertaken. In patients who have widespread disease, follow-up should be limited to clinical examination and institution of the appropriate palliative measures.

CHOLANGIOCARCINOMA

Bile duct carcinoma is much less common than liver cancer. Cholangiocarcinoma affects both sexes equally and is more prevalent in individuals aged from 50–70. Association with many other diseases is known, in particular with primary sclerosing cholangitis and parasitic infections particularly liver fluke seen is SE-Asian Countries. About 95% are histopathologically classified as adenocarcinoma. Localization of the tumor determines clinical course and prognosis. If the tumor is located above the hepatic duct bifurcation only one side of the biliary tree may be obstructed resulting in silent atrophy of the corresponding liver lobe with later clinical presentation. When the remaining liver becomes obstructed, cholongitis/abscess in the obstructed biliary tree may occur. Obstructive jaundice is the characteristic symptom of hilar tumors. Laboratory examination shows hyperbilirubinemia and liver enzymes indicating cholestasis are elevated. Pathological elevation of serum tumor markers, particularly CEA, CA19.9 are frequently found. Treatment consists of curative resection or palliative decompression to relieve jaundice. The prognosis is poor and only a few patients survive more than six months after diagnosis. If possible the tumor should undergo local resection with adequate surgical margins. Perhaps 25% will enjoy survival for more than a few years. Liver transplantation has not been a useful form of treatment for patients with cholangiocarcinoma. Many patients will be unresectable because of invasion of the portal veins or significant liver involvement; palliation of jaundice may be achieved by placement of an intraluminal stent either placed at GDCP or PTC. Surgical bypass procedures have the advantage of avoiding stent blockage but the disadvantage of requiring a laporotomy an ill, jaundiced incurable patient. Peripheral cholongiocarcinoma can produce a large HCC-like tumor; it has relatively good programs.

GALLBLADDER CANCER

Cancer which arises in the gallbladder is uncommon and accounts for < 4% of all gastrointestinal cancers in the United States. In areas of Pakistan and Peru considerably higher incidence is seen. Cholelithiasis is an associated finding in the majority of cases but fewer than 1% of patients with cholelithiasis develop this cancer. The most common symptoms caused by gallbladder cancer are jaundice, pain and fever. The histological types of gallbladder cancers include the following: carcinoma *in situ*, adenocarcinoma, papillary adenocarcinoma, adenocarcinoma intestinal, mucinous adenocarcinoma, clear cell adenocarcinoma, signet cell carcinoma, adenosquamous carcinoma, squamous cell carcinoma, small cell carcinoma, undifferentiated carcinoma. Papillary carcinoma has the best prognoses. Survival in gall bladder cancer is very stage dependent and can simply be divided into disease limited to the gall bladder wall, full thickness disease, lymph node involvement and metastase. The response rate of bile duct cancer to chemotherapy is bleak and has not shown any improvement in survival. There has been a report of improved survival using adjuvant 5-FU as a continuous infusion plus Calcium, Leucovorin, Mitomycin C and Dipyridamole. The treatment of early gall bladder cancer is undoubtedly chole-cystectomy; for patients with full thickness disease procedure to remove or destroy the gall bladder bed may improve results but have not been subjected to control trials. Regional chemotherapy is also been investigated with some encouraging results.

References

Anthony, P.P. (1994). Tumours and tumour-like lesions of the liver and biliary tract. In *Pathology of the Liver*, ed. Roderick, N.M. and MacSween, pp. 635–674. Edinburgh: Churchill Livingstone.

Chang, W.L. *et al.* (1992). The Role of Hepatitis B and C Viruses Among Chinese Patients with Hepatocellular Carcinoma in a Hepatitis B Endemic Area. *Cancer*, **69**, 2052–2054.

Mima, S., Sekiya, C., Kanagawa, H., Kokyama, H., Gotol, K., Mizuo, H., Ijiri, M., Tanase, T., Maeda, N. and Okuda, K. (1994). Mass screening for hepatocellular carcinoma: experience in Hokkaido, Japan. *Gastroenterol. Hepato.*, **1**(9), 361–365.

Alan, F. Venook (1994). *Journal of Clinical Oncology*, Vol. 12, No 6 (June), Treatment of hepatocellular carcinoma: Too many options? pp. 1323–1334.

Okuda, K., Ohtsuki, T., Obata, H., Tomimatsu, M., Okazaki, N., Hasegawa, H., Nakajima, Y. and Ohnishi, K. (1985). Natural History of Hepatocellular Carcinoma and Prognosis in Relation to treatment, Study of 850 Patients. *Cancer*, **56**, 918–928.

Stillwagon, G.B., Order, S.E., Guse, C., Leibel, S.A., Asbell, S.O., Klein, J.L. and Leichner, P.K. (1991). Prognostic Factors in Unresectable Hepatocellular Cancer: Radiation Therapy Oncology Group Study 83–01. *I.J Radiation Oncology, Biology, Physics, Phase !/!! Clinical Trials*, 65–71.

Pichlmayr, R., Weimann, A., Oldhafer, K.J., Schlitt, H.J., Klempnauer, J., Bomscheuer, A., Chavan, A., Schmoll, E., Lang, H., Tusch, G. and Ringe, B. (1995). Role of Liver Transplantation in the Treatment of Unresectable Liver Cancer. *World Journal of Surgery*, **19**, 807–813.

Sitzmann, J.V. and Abrams, R. (1993). Improved Survival for Hepatocellular Cancer with Combination Surgery and Multimodality Treatment. *Annals of Surgery*, **2**, 1490154.

Livraghi, T., Lazzaroni, S., Meloni, F., Torzilli, G. and Vettori, C. (1995). Intralesional Ethanol in the Treatment of Unresectable Liver Cancer. *World Journal of Surgery*, **19**, 801–806.

Farmer, D.G. and Busuttil, R.W. (1994) The Role of Multimodeal Therapy in the Treatment of Hepatocellular Carcinoma. *Cancer*, June 1, **73**(11), 2669–2670.

Groupe d'Etude et de Traitement du Carcinome Hepatocellulaire. (1995). A Comparison of Lipiodol Chemoembolization and Conservative Treatment for Unresectable Hepatocellular Carcinoma, *The New England Journal of Medicine*, **332**(19), 1256–1260.

Liver Cancer

More common in males in high-risk populations

Worldwide: Mainly in developing countries where 3/4 of world's total occurs

Lifetime risk
in USA whites:
  M   1 in 200
  F   1 in 400

Relative five-year survival in 1983–87
in USA whites:
  M   3.9%
  F   10.7%

Risk factors
(a) Hepatitis B virus
(b) Hepatitis C virus
(c) Alcohol
     (a)(b)(c) usually accompanied by cirrhosis
Oral contraceptive use
Aflatoxin contamination of food
Exposure to vinyl chloride monomer implicated in angiosarcoma of liver.

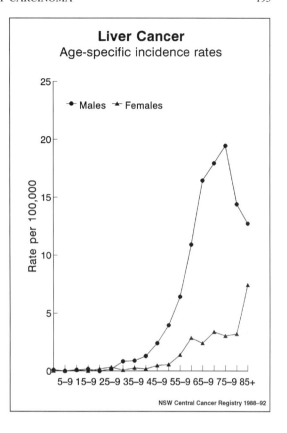

Geographical variation in 1983–87

Highest rate
M: 90.4 per 100,000 in Thailand, Khon Kaen
F: 38.3 per 100,000 in Thailand, Khon Kaen

Lowest rate
M: 1.1 per 100,000 in Southern Ireland
F: 0.4 per 100,000 in Netherlands, Eindhoven

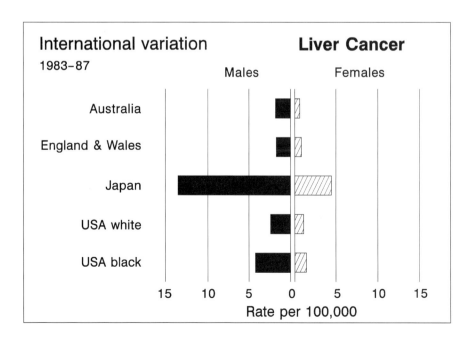

Gallbladder Cancer

More common in females than males

Worldwide: About 1% of all cancers

Lifetime risk
in New South Wales:
    M   1 in 475
    F   1 in 525

Relative five-year survival in 1977–90
in South Australia:
    M   12.6%
    F   15.5%

Risk factors
Obesity
Parity
Gallstones
Hormonal factors

Geographical variation in 1983–87
Highest rate
M: 8.0 per 100,000 in Japan, Nagasaki
F: 12.9 per 100,000 in Peru, Trujillo
Lowest rate
M: 0.4 per 100,000 in India, Ahmedabad
F: 0.4 per 100,000 in China, Qidong

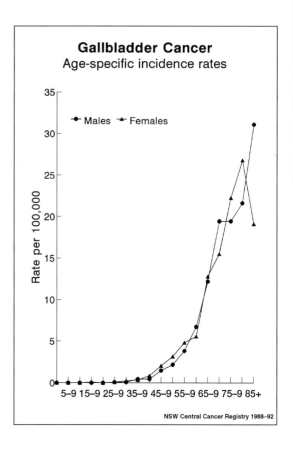

Gallbladder Cancer
Age-specific incidence rates

NSW Central Cancer Registry 1988–92

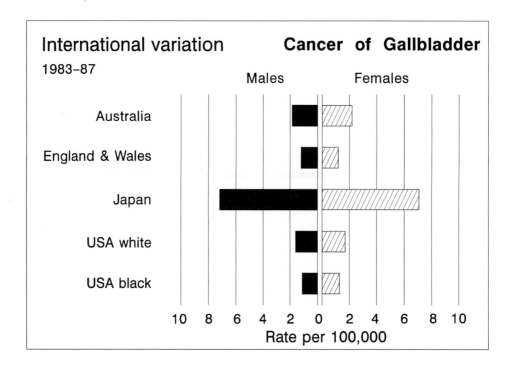

International variation   **Cancer of Gallbladder**
1983–87

20. Female Genital Cancers

MAURICE J. WEBB

Professor of Obstetrics & Gynecology, Mayo Medical School; Head, Division of Gynecologic Surgery, Mayo Clinic & Mayo Foundation, Rochester, MN 55905, USA

The incidence of gynecologic malignancies varies widely throughout the world. In Western countries, breast cancer and endometrial cancer are predominant, whereas in developing countries, cervical cancer is the major problem. Evidence indicates that decreased mortality rates for breast and cervical cancer are related to screening, but screening for other gynecologic malignancies is in its infancy. However, treatment of gynecologic cancer has led the way as far as screening is concerned: cure rates are high in cases of early stage disease, and many advanced stage gynecologic malignancies are sensitive to nonsurgical modes of therapy.

ENDOMETRIAL CANCER

Endometrial cancer is most common after menopause; the median age at onset is 60 years. The incidence has been increasing slowly during the last half century, and it is now the most common gynecologic malignancy in developed countries.

Evidence suggests that prolonged exposure to unopposed estrogen increases the risk of endometrial cancer. Proliferation of the endometrium to adenomatous hyperplasia and eventually adenocarcinoma is caused by prolonged stimulation of estrogen without the counter effect of progesterone. Obesity, hypertension, diabetes mellitus, nulliparity, and a high-fat diet are also predisposing factors. Oral contraceptives containing an estrogen progesterone combination have a protective effect.

Pathology

Adenomatous and atypical adenomatous hyperplasias are precursors of endometrial cancer. Most endometrial cancer is of the endometrioid adenocarcinoma type. Special types such as serous papillary adenosquamous and clear cell cancer have a poorer prognosis. Aneuploid tumors have a significantly worse prognosis than diploid tumors. Histologic grade is also of prognostic significance.

Screening

No effective method of mass screening is available. Endometrial sampling in high-risk patients is recommended on a regular basis (e.g. yearly).

Clinical presentation

The most common symptom of endometrial cancer is post-menopausal bleeding. However, up to 20% of patients with endometrial cancer have no symptoms.[1] All patients presenting with post-menopausal bleeding should be evaluated with dilatation and curettage to exclude endometrial cancer.

Investigations

Ultrasonography of the post-menopausal endo-metrium shows that it seldom exceeds 3 mm in thickness. Increased endometrial thickness is asso-ciated with endometrial neoplasms in post-meno-pausal patients.[2] However, regardless of endometrial thickness, endometrial biopsy is indicated if abnor-mal bleeding is present. Endometrium greater than 4-mm thick in a post-menopausal woman warrants investigation, even if there is no bleeding.

Treatment

Surgery

Precancerous lesions of the endometrium are best treated with simple hysterectomy. This can be per-formed vaginally. In younger women in whom conservation of reproductive function is desired, progesterone therapy may reverse the process.

Total abdominal hysterectomy and bilateral salpingo-oophorectomy have long been the defini-tive treatment for frank carcinoma of the endo-metrium. However, as in many other areas of oncology, individualization of therapy is impor-tant. Factors such as tumor grade, ploidy, HER-2/neu, cell type, depth of myometrial invasion, vol-ume of tumor, nodal status, stage, and extrauterine spread influence prognosis. Some of these factors are assessable preoperatively and others only after hysterectomy.

If the tumor is *in situ*, simple hysterectomy, ei-ther abdominally or vaginally, is sufficient. An invasive tumor necessitates abdominal hysterec-tomy and bilateral salpingo-oophorectomy; how-ever, with a low-grade cancer in a medically unfit patient, vaginal hysterectomy may be adequate. If the tumor involves the endocervix (stage II), radical hysterectomy with removal of the parametrium and pelvic lymphadenectomy are indicated, because the tumor spreads in a manner similar to that of cervical cancer. If the tumor is fundal and stage I, pelvic lymphadenectomy should be performed together with simple hysterectomy and bilateral salpingo-oophorectomy if the tumor is high grade, clear cell, adenosquamous or serous papillary type, or invades more than 50% of the myometrium. Para-aortic lymphadenectomy is performed if the pelvic nodes contain metastatic disease. Peritoneal washings should be collected because positive washings in-fluence prognosis. Serous papillary cancer should be managed surgically similar to ovarian carcino-mas, with peritoneal biopsies and omentectomy performed at the time of hysterectomy because this tumor type tends to spread in a similar manner to that of ovarian cancer.

Radiation

Although preoperative irradiation at one time was common in the treatment of endometrial cancer, the standard approach now is to operate and ade-quately stage the disease and use radiation therapy selectively in appropriate cases. This usually means treatment of high-risk patients with external beam radiation to the pelvis and brachytherapy to the vaginal vault, a common site of recurrence. High-risk patients are those with stage I disease with clear cell, adenosquamous or serous papillary cell types, myometrial invasion greater than 50% or a high grade histologically and all patients with stage II, III, and IV disease. However, if pelvic lymphadenectomy has been performed in a patient with stage I or III disease and the findings are negative, external irradiation is unlikely to be of benefit.[3] Disagreement exists about the indications for postoperative vaginal vault brachytherapy, which is designed to decrease the incidence of vault re-currence.

Chemotherapy

Although cytostatic agents are used in the palliative treatment of advanced disease they have not been shown to be of benefit as adjuvant therapy after primary surgery. Therapy using cisplatinum, doxo-rubicin and cyclophosphamide or a combination of methotrexate, vinblastine, doxorubicin, and cisplatin (MVAC) produces high response rates and pro-longed remissions and appears to be superior to single-agent therapy in advanced disease.

Many endometrial carcinomas contain progester-one receptors, and the response to therapy with high doses of progesterone in receptor-positive patients is about 70%, whereas it is about only 10% in receptor-negative patients. Unfortunately, most high-risk endometrial carcinomas are receptor-negative and, therefore, unlikely to respond to progesterone in either an adjuvant setting or as treatment for recurrence. Thus the clinical usefulness of proges-terone therapy is confined to the treatment of recur-rent disease in well-differentiated tumors, most of which have progesterone receptors.

Results of treatment

Changes in the FIGO staging of endometrial cancer (the most recent being a surgical/pathologic stage) make statistics on survival difficult to compare. A recent review of 1974 cases of endometrial cancer in Norway showed a five-year survival rate of 83% for stage I disease, 71% for stage II, 39% for stage III, and 27% for stage IV. Survival by histologic type at five years was 91% for adenoacanthoma, 74% for endometrioid type, 65% for adenosquamous carcinoma, 58% for undifferentiated carcinoma, 42% for clear cell type, and 27% for serous papillary carcinoma.[4]

Recurrence

More than half of the recurrences of endometrial cancer occur in the first two years postoperatively. Sites of recurrence may be locoregional (vaginal vault, suburethral area, or pelvic sidewall) or distant (lung, abdomen, liver, para-aortic nodes, brain, bones, supraclavicular nodes, or groin nodes). The location of the recurrence is of prognostic importance. Local recurrences in the vagina are more easily treatable than distant recurrences, and locally, vault recurrences have a better prognosis than suburethral recurrences. Treatment of recurrence depends on the location and the presence or absence of other disease, but it can involve surgical excision, radiation, chemotherapy or hormonal therapy, or a combination of these.

Follow-up

Postsurgical follow-up examinations are recommended every 3–4 months for the first two years, then every six months until five years and annually thereafter. Chest radiography and Papanicolaou smear should be performed at each visit together with a complete blood cell count and blood chemistry. Occasionally CA 125 may be increased with recurrence. In patients at high risk for recurrence, abdominopelvic CT should be performed regularly for the first two years, the period when most recurrences first present.

Estrogen replacement therapy may be used in patients with *in situ* disease and probably also in those with low-risk stage I tumors. In other patients, it may be prudent to wait until the period of the highest risk of recurrence is past and then weigh the risks versus the benefits with the patient.

CERVICAL CANCER

Carcinoma of the cervix is second only to breast cancer as the most common female cancer worldwide, and in developing countries, it is the most common cancer. Organized screening programs have helped to decrease the incidence of the disease in developed countries. Incidence ranges from about 8 per 100,000 women to 70 per 100,000 worldwide.

Multiple sexual partners and early age at first coitus are the most important risk factors. Other suggested factors include smoking, high parity, human papillomavirus infection (HPV 16 and 18), and herpesvirus type 2 infection.

Pathology

Cellular atypia in the cervical epithelium is termed "cervical intraepithelial neoplasia" (CIN). Mild dysplasia is referred to as "CIN I" moderate dysplasia as "CIN II," and severe dysplasia and carcinoma *in situ* as "CIN III." CIN can behave in various ways. It can regress, persist, or progress to invasive disease. The milder dysplasias are more likely to regress — whereas this is less likely for the severe forms. It is the presence of these preinvasive forms of the disease that makes mass screening for cervical cancer so worthwhile.

Adenocarcinoma *in situ* of the cervix is also a recognized entity and consists of atypia in the endocervical glandular epithelium. The disease is most common around the squamocolumnar junction but can occur anywhere along the endocervical canal.

The main invasive types of cervical cancer are squamous cell cancer and adenocarcinoma. Verrucous cancer is a well-differentiated form of squamous cell carcinoma and tends to invade locally rather than to metastasize. Adenoma malignum is a highly differentiated adenocarcinoma and is rare. Other less common cell types are adenosquamous cancer and clear cell cancer, both of which have a poor prognosis. Minimally invasive or noninvasive examples of cervical cancer occur and may be treated with less radical methods.

Screening

Cytology is the method used for screening for cervical cancer, with colposcopy used as an adjunctive diagnostic technique when abnormal cytologic findings are obtained. Because lesions can occur on the endocervix as well as on the ectocervix, it is mandatory to take an endocervical sample with a cytobrush and an ectocervical smear with an Ayre's spatula. The recommended frequency of cytologic examination is yearly from the onset of sexual activity or age 18 years. It may be reasonable in a patient at low risk to perform three-yearly screenings after negative findings on at least two yearly smears, but one must remember that the detection rate decreases with increasing screening intervals.

False-negative rates range from 15% to 30% and are most frequent in the presence of clinical carcinoma.[5] Therefore, biopsy should be performed on all suspicious-appearing lesions regardless of the results of the Papanicolaou smear.

Clinical presentation

Early stages of cervical cancer may produce no symptoms at all, thus emphasizing the importance of regular screening. Intermenstrual bleeding and postcoital bleeding in conjunction with vaginal discharge are common as the disease progresses. Sciatic nerve pain, leg edema, and flank pain from ureteric obstruction are symptoms of advanced disease.

Investigations

Colposcopy is used to diagnose and locate the site of the abnormality detected by a Papanicolaou smear. Biopsy can be performed specifically on abnormal-appearing epithelium to obtain specimens for histologic examination. Colposcopy can also be used to inspect and to perform biopsy on an abnormal-appearing cervix, even in the presence of normal cytologic results. A colposcopically directed biopsy of the most abnormal part of the lesion has proved to be highly accurate for diagnosing cervical lesions and it helps avoid the need for conization of the cervix. However, to avoid a false result, rules related to what constitutes a satisfactory colposcopic examination must be adhered to and cone biopsy must be performed if the colposcopic examination is deemed unsatisfactory. Modern practice involves a "see and treat" approach to CIN. The abnormal area is removed with an electrocautery wire loop electrode under colposcopic guidance. This both removes the abnormal epithelium in its entirety and provides a specimen for histologic examination.

Where a clinical cancer is apparent, a punch biopsy specimen from the lesion is evaluated histologically. If invasive disease is confirmed, the appropriate investigations are performed to rule out metastatic disease and accurately stage the disease.

These investigations include chest radiography, complete blood cell count, and serum chemistry. Intravenous pyelography is necessary to exclude ureteric obstruction from paracervical infiltration. Abdominopelvic CT gives added evidence of spread beyond the cervix. MRI of the tumor can provide an accurate estimation of its volume and measurements, giving a more objective assessment than possible with clinical examination. If the tumor appears to be spreading anteriorly toward the bladder or posteriorly toward the rectum, cystoscopy and sigmoidoscopy are necessary. Evaluation under anesthesia may be necessary in some patients to stage the disease clinically.

Treatment

Surgery

Treatment of CIN involves local excision or destruction of the lesion. Excisional techniques include wire loop electrode and conization either with a scalpel or laser. Destructive techniques include laser vaporization, radical diathermy, and cryocautery. Conization of the cervix must always be performed if colposcopy is thought to be unsatisfactory, or if the biopsy results suggest invasive disease; it is also needed to treat microinvasive disease in women who wish to preserve reproductive function.

Invasive cervical cancer may be treated with radiotherapy or surgically. Surgical therapy is performed if the cancer is confined to the cervix (stage Ib) or has spread to the upper vagina (stage IIa). Surgical treatment involves radical hysterectomy, upper vaginectomy, and pelvic lymphadenectomy. The ovaries may or may not be conserved. Para-aortic lymphadenectomy is performed if the common iliac nodes are positive for malignancy. Surgical treatment is also used for recurrent disease, primarily with pelvic exenteration in the management of centrally recurrent cancer in the pelvis.

Radiotherapy

More advanced cervical cancer (stages IIb to IV) are usually treated with radiation therapy. Recent studies have attempted to improve survival rates by giving neoadjuvant chemotherapy primarily and following this with a radical operation if the tumor is operable and with radiotherapy if it is not operable. Radiation therapy is often given postoperatively to patients at high risk for recurrence, although survival differences have not been demonstrated between treated and nontreated patients.

Chemotherapy

Neoadjuvant chemotherapy is used to decrease the tumor volume in bulky or high-stage disease, hopefully allowing surgical extirpation in an otherwise nonoperable situation. High objective response rates of up to 80% have been reported, with occasional complete responses.

Adjuvant chemotherapy after surgical treatment in patients at high risk for recurrence has also been tried but must be regarded as experimental. In this disease most chemotherapy is given for recurrence and is palliative.

Results of treatment

Treatment of CIN should be 100% successful, but this is not so in practice. Recurrences of CIN or even invasive cancer have been reported after initial treatment of CIN. Many of these "recurrences" in fact may be persistent residual disease, as with ablative techniques of treatment of CIN, neither underlying invasive cancer nor residual CIN can definitely be ruled out. Local excisional techniques are more effective, because the margins can be checked to be certain that the lesion is completely excised and there is no invasive component. However, even after hysterectomy, recurrent CIN at the vaginal vault has been reported. This is less common after vaginal hysterectomy than after abdominal hysterectomy, presumably because a cuff of vagina is removed with the vaginal hysterectomy specimen.[6]

Microinvasive carcinomas have an extremely low incidence of pelvic nodal metastases or recurrence and usually can be managed with simple hysterectomy. In some instances in which conservation of reproductive function is desired, conization may be adequate therapy as long as the patient understands that there may be some risk, however minimal.

Five-year survival rates for early invasive cancer of the cervix are similar for patients receiving surgical treatment or irradiation, but the morbidity from surgical treatment is less. Most recent series report a five-year survival of about 85% to 90% for stage I(b) disease, 75% for stage II(a), 60% for II(b) cancers, 30% for stage III, and 10% for stage IV. The presence of positive pelvic nodes significantly alters the prognosis, decreasing the five-year survival to 50% in stage I(b) disease. Tumor volume has also been shown to significantly affect prognosis.

Recurrence

Most recurrences and deaths due to cervical cancer occur in the first two years after primary therapy.[7] More than half of the recurrences occur in the pelvis, and the prognosis of a patient with recurrent disease is poor.[8] Patients in whom a solitary central recurrence develops in the pelvis may be suitable for pelvic exenteration, with an expected 40% five-year survival. Other sites of recurrence are the para-aortic nodes, liver, abdomen, lungs, bones, central nervous system, and supraclavicular nodes. Combination chemotherapy, platinum-based, is used as palliative treatment.

Follow-up

Because about 80% of recurrences occur in the first two years after primary treatment of invasive cervical cancer, frequent follow-up is important, usually every 3–4 months for the first two years and then every six months until five years and yearly thereafter. Investigations should include chest radiography, complete blood cell count, serum chemistry, and Papanicolaou smear and a complete general examination should be performed to look for evidence of recurrence. Regular CT scans of the abdomen and pelvis are also important in the first two years.

OVARIAN CANCER

Ovarian cancer is not the most common gynecologic malignancy, but it is the most common one to cause death of the patient. Its incidence rises until the sixth decade, and there is a significantly greater incidence of the disease in Western countries. Nulliparity and infertility seem to have a relationship to ovarian cancer, and pregnancy and the use of oral contraceptives appear to have a protective effect. Ascending carcinogens via the lower genital tract such as talc, have also been implicated in the etiology of this disease. An important risk factor is a family history of ovarian cancer or a personal history of breast cancer although this accounts for only a small percentage of all ovarian malignancies. Women with two or more first-degree relatives with ovarian cancer may have a 30% lifetime risk of developing the disease, in comparison with approximately a 1 in 70 chance in the general population.

Pathology

Most ovarian malignancies are of epithelial origin. Less common types are germ cell tumors, stromal tumors, and tumors metastatic to the ovary. Specific histologic types of epithelial ovarian cancers are serous, mucinous, endometrioid and clear cell adenocarcinomas, and the rare malignant Brenner tumor. About 45% of epithelial cancers are the serous type; mixed types are common. Both the serous and mucinous cell types have a low malignant potential or "borderline" group in which there is cytologic and structural evidence of malignancy but no evidence of stromal invasion. These tumors can metastasize and can kill the patient, but the overall prognosis is excellent. They comprise about 10–15% of serous tumors of the ovary and 20% of mucinous tumors and so are not uncommon.

Tumors metastatic to the ovary most commonly are from the breast, stomach, colon, and endometrium and signify a poor prognosis.[9] Malignant germ cell tumors are uncommon, accounting for about only 3% of ovarian malignancies. Malignant teratomas, dysgerminomas, endodermal sinus tumors, choriocarcinomas, and embryonal carcinomas make up this group; there are also tumors of mixed type. Chemotherapy has greatly altered the management and prognosis of this group of ovarian tumors.

Although gonadal stromal tumors such as granulosa cell tumors and Sertoli-Leydig cell tumors generally act in a benign fashion, they have the potential for malignancy. Granulosa cell tumors may not recur until many years after primary surgery, whereas if Sertoli-Leydig cell tumors recur, they usually do so within 2–3 years postoperatively.

Screening

The methods currently available for screening for ovarian malignancy have not been shown to be of benefit. Various combinations of pelvic ultrasonography, tumor markers (CA 125), and clinical examination have not proved to be accurate enough for mass screening. Currently, these screening techniques are recommended only for patients at high risk for ovarian cancer because of their family history. This group accounts for only a very small percentage of all ovarian malignancies, and the patients may be better served by the use of prophylactic oopborectomy after reproduction is no longer an issue.

Clinical presentation

Most early stage ovarian carcinomas are discovered incidentally because they usually are asymptomatic until they metastasize. Vague abdominal symptoms, increasing abdominal girth, or the presence of a mass usually causes the patient to go to the doctor, and at the time of diagnosis, about 75% of these tumors have already spread. Other symptoms may be abnormal uterine bleeding or dyspnea due to pleural effusion.

Investigations

Although in practice most patients presenting to a gynecologic oncologist for surgical treatment will have already had CT or ultrasonography performed, scanning usually adds little to the decision regarding management of this disease. If the patient has a pelvic mass, especially with nodularity or ascites, and is in the age group in which ovarian cancer is a possibility, surgical exploration is indicated because it gives far more information than a scan. Assay for the tumor marker CA 125 should be performed together with a complete blood cell count, serum chemistry, and chest radiography. If the patient is young, and especially if the mass is solid, blood should be drawn to check for germ cell markers, (α-fetoprotein, lactate dehyrogenase, and β-human chorionic gonadotropin). These tumor markers are not used to make the diagnosis, which is made surgically, but to discover whether a marker is present that will be useful in postoperative follow-up of the patient. If the patient has a pleural effusion, it should be tapped to obtain a specimen for cytologic analysis as part of the staging process.

Treatment

Surgery

The primary aim of surgical treatment in ovarian epithelial cancer is to remove as much tumor bulk as possible. This involves performing total abdominal hysterectomy and bilateral salpingo-oophorectomy, total omentectomy, and appendectomy and collecting peritoneal samples for cytologic analysis, performing peritoneal biopsies for staging, and resecting as much tumor bulk as possible. Pelvic and aortic lymphadenectomy may be indicated for staging purposes or for removing metastatic nodes. "Optimal" debulking has occurred if all remaining tumor nodules are less than 0.5 cm in diameter.

In patients with a unilateral, intracystic, low-grade, unruptured epithelial ovarian tumor, unilateral salpingo-oophorectomy with omentectomy, appendectomy, lymphadenectomy, and staging biopsies may be performed if the patient wishes to conserve reproductive function.

Germ cell tumors and stromal tumors are usually unilateral, and if the patient desires to conserve reproductive function, unilateral oophorectomy with removal of any metastases may be fitting together with appropriate staging biopsies and cytologic examination. With practically all germ cell tumors, follow-up chemotherapy is indicated. Many patients with metastatic germ cell tumors who have received conservative surgical treatment and, subsequently, chemotherapy have gone on to have successful pregnancies.

Surgical exploration is also used for secondary debulking of recurrent disease. This is effective only if the tumor can be resected to the level of microscopic residual cancer; it is considered only in patients who have had a prolonged tumor-free interval before recurrence developed and whose tumors potentially are fully resectable.

Second-look laparotomy is undertaken in patients with epithelial cancer who have had a complete clinical response to chemotherapy. Fifty percent or more of the patients with negative findings on second-look laparotomy subsequently have recurrence.

Chemotherapy

All patients with epithelial cancer except for some patients with stage I disease receive chemotherapy postoperatively. The standard therapy is six courses of cisplatin and paclitaxel (Taxol); this has a response rate of 60–80%. Second-line chemotherapy is less effective, with response rates of only 20–30%.

Malignant germ cell tumors are very sensitive to chemotherapy, and except for a few specific instances, nearly all these tumors are treated with combination chemotherapy after primary surgery. The effectiveness of this therapy makes possible the preservation of reproductive function in these patients. Common chemotherapeutic regimes for germ cell tumors are vincristine, actinomycin, and cyclophosphamide (VAC); cisplatin, vinblastine, and bleomycin (PVB); and cisplatin, etoposide, and bleomycin (PEB). There is no unanimous opinion about what the length of a course of chemotherapy for these tumors should be.

No standard chemotherapeutic regimens are recognized for the treatment of sex-cord stromal tumors of the ovary.

Radiation

Two techniques are used to administer radiotherapy in patients with ovarian cancer: external beam and intraperitoneal radioisotopes. External beam therapy is seldom used now as primary therapy after surgery for epithelial cancers, but it still has a place as salvage therapy following chemotherapy for patients with minimal disease. Intraperitoneal radioactive colloids (^{32}p) are effective in the adjuvant treatment of some high-risk patients with early stage disease. The role of these radioactive colloids as consolidation therapy after negative findings on second-look laparotomy is being investigated.

Dysgerminoma is a particularly radiosensitive tumor, but systemic chemotherapy is replacing irradiation in the treatment of these tumors, especially if reproductive function is to be conserved.

Results of treatment

Many factors influence survival in epithelial ovarian cancer, including tumor cell type, tumor grade, stage, volume of initial disease, volume of residual disease, ploidy, nodal metastases, presence of ascites, performance status of the patient, and subsequent response to chemotherapy. At five years reported survival rates are between 75% and 90% for stage I disease, 50–75% for stage II, 10–40% for stage III, and 0–20% or stage IV. The results reported in the literature consistently support the fact that the amount of residual disease after primary surgery is one of the most important prognostic factors.[10]

Except for dysgerminoma, germ cell tumors previously had a dismal prognosis; however, in the past 20 years, chemotherapy has improved survival significantly, so that now 70–80% of patients survive. Again, survival is related to the stage of disease, residual tumor, and cell type.

Recurrence

Most ovarian epithelial cancers recur in the abdomen or pelvis within 12–24 months postoperatively. More effective treatment regimens have produced a group of patients who seem to remain tumor-free in the peritoneal cavity but in whom liver, lung, and cerebral metastases develop. However, most patients die of bowel obstruction related to recurrent intraperitoneal tumor.

Recurrence may be detected by serial measurement of CA 125 levels. Increasing levels usually predate by about three months detectable recurrence of epithelial ovarian cancer.

Serum levels of α-fetoprotein may be used to check for tumor recurrence in a patient with endodermal sinus tumor, and β-human chorionic gonadotropin levels may be increased with recurrent choriocarcinoma of the ovary. An increased serum level of LDH is a good marker for recurrent dysgerminoma. If α-fetoprotein and β-human chorionic gonadotropic are both increased, the tumor may be an embryonal cancer or a mixed type.

Follow-up

Most patients with ovarian cancer are evaluated fully each month as they initially receive chemotherapy. At each visit a complete blood cell count, serum chemistry, assays for tumor markers, and chest radiography are performed. CT should be performed every three months during the initial two-year period.

After completion of the full course of chemotherapy, the patient may be evaluated for consideration of second-look laparotomy. This operation is considered only if there is no clinical or scanning evidence of disease and effective follow-up therapy is available if disease is found. After completion of chemotherapy, evaluations are performed every three months for two years and, then, less frequently if free of disease.

CARCINOMA OF THE VULVA

Most patients with vulvar cancer are older than 60 years, but recently there has been an increase in preinvasive and invasive tumors of the vulva in young women. Vulval dystrophies are found in the skin adjacent to vulvar cancer in about 60% of patients, suggesting a link between benign vulvar epithelial disorders and the development of vulvar carcinoma. Human papillomavirus, herpes virus type 2, poor genital hygiene, diabetes mellitus, and obesity have also been linked to the development of vulvar cancer.

Pathology

Vulval intraepithelial neoplasia (VIN) is classified similar to that of CIN into VIN I, II and III. Macroscopically, the lesions are quite variable in appearance, and most of them are multifocal. Early invasive cancer (microinvasive) occurs, but a precise definition is lacking. Because nodal metastases rarely occur with invasion of 1 mm or less, a lesion of this degree of invasion is generally accepted as the cut-off point.

Most vulval cancers are the squamous cell type. Adenocarcinoma of Bartholin's gland, Paget's disease, basal cell carcinoma, malignant melanoma, and sarcoma are rare entities.

Screening

No effective screening test exists, but all patients with vulval dystrophies warrant regular observation. Colposcopy of the vulva may help to delineate lesions. The rule is that biopsy should be performed on *all* abnormal areas on the vulva before therapy is instituted. All pigmented lesions should be removed because the potential for the development of malignant melanoma is high for vulval nevi.

Clinical presentation

The most common presenting symptom is pruritis, possibly associated with discharge, bleeding, and the presence of ulceration or a lump. However, many patients have no symptoms. Because most of the patients are elderly, the lesion often is discovered by a caregiver rather than by the patient.

Investigation

Although colposcopy of the vulva is not as useful as cervical colposcopy, it can aid the clinician in choosing appropriate biopsy sites. Biopsy is easily accomplished under local anesthesia using Keye's dermal punch. Only after histologic diagnosis should treatment be given. In patients with invasive disease, chest radiography, complete blood cell count, serum chemistry, and CT of the abdomen and pelvis should be performed preoperatively.

Treatment

Surgery

For VIN, local excision is adequate. This may require skinning vulvectomy and grafting for large lesions. Laser vaporization is also used, often in combination with excision of some areas. Paget's disease needs to be excised locally with wide margins. Often, the disease extends well beyond the abnormal-appearing skin beneath normal skin, and repeated excisions to achieve a clear margin are necessary.

Radical vulvectomy with inguinofemoral lymphadenectomy is the standard treatment for invasive cancer. More recently, wide local excision or hemivulvectomy has been used for some lesions, and only unilateral groin lymphadenectomy is performed if the lesion lies laterally on the vulva. Performing vulval excision and groin node dissection through separate incisions allows for better primary healing in comparison with *en bloc* techniques.

Malignant melanoma is treated with wide local excision. The nodes are removed only if they are suspicious clinically for metastatic disease.

Occasionally exenteration is necessary for lesions involving the bladder or anus.

Chemotherapy

As well as palliative treatment of recurrent disease, chemotherapy has a place alongside radiotherapy in the initial treatment of locally advanced disease. After chemotherapy, some of these patients may require a less radical operation then they would have without chemotherapy.[11]

Radiotherapy

The main indication for radiotherapy in the treatment of vulvar cancer is treatment of the groin and pelvic nodes if the groin nodes are involved with metastatic disease at the primary operation. As mentioned above, radiation is also used in conjunction with chemotherapy, to reduce tumor bulk in extensive local disease.

Results of treatment

Survival rates are dependent mainly on the status of the groin nodes. Five-year survival rates for patients with squamous cell carcinoma with negative groin nodes are usually greater than 80%; this rate decreases to about 45% if the groin nodes are positive and to less than 20% if the pelvic nodes are positive. Melanoma has poorer results, with five-year survival rates usually reported at about 20–50%.

Recurrence

Recurrences are most common in the vulva, and with radical re-excision, cure rates are excellent. Recurrences in the groin or pelvic nodes are almost always fatal.

Follow-up

Examinations every 3–4 months are recommended for initial follow-up, with rebiopsy of any suspicious areas on the vulva or perianal area. Regular CT scans of the abdomen and pelvis may be indicated in patients with positive groin nodes, but the results of treatment of recurrent disease outside the vulva are poor.

VAGINAL CANCER

Primary vaginal cancer is uncommon. Most malignancies occurring in the vagina are metastases from other organs or direct spread of the tumor from the cervix, rectum, or vulva. Cancer in the vagina that involves the cervix is classified as cervical cancer rather than as vaginal cancer, even if it appears to have originated in the vagina.

The etiologic factors in the development of vaginal cancer are similar to those of cervical cancer and vulvar cancer. In fact, multifocal disease of the cervix, vagina, and vulva is common. Most vaginal malignancies occur in older women, usually in the seventh decade of life.

Pathology

More than 90% of vaginal malignancies are squamous cell carcinomas. Adenocarcinomas are uncommon, although the clear cell type that occurs in younger women due to exposure to diethylstilbestrol in utero has increased the incidence of adenocarcinomas.

Precursor lesions of squamous cell cancer are termed "vaginal intraepithelial neoplasia" (VAIN). However, VAIN is much less common than CIN, and in many instances, it may merely be an extension of CIN on to the vaginal fornix. Most invasive tumors occur on the posterior wall of upper third of the vagina. Metastatic tumors may commonly be located in the suburethral area as a nodule or plaque. Primary melanoma of the vagina is rare and almost always fatal.

Screening

Papanicolaou smear with follow-up colposcopy and biopsy is the only way to diagnose VAIN; therefore, vaginal cytologic examinations should continue to be performed even after hysterectomy. This is most important if the patient had a history of CIN or invasive cervical cancer before hysterectomy.[12]

Clinical presentation

Abnormal vaginal bleeding or discharge is the usual symptom of invasive cancer. Occasionally, a suburethral lesion causes urethral obstruction. Fistula formation to the bladder or rectum is also possible with advanced lesions.

Investigations

A complete blood cell count, serum chemistry, chest radiography, and CT of the abdomen and pelvis are indicated for invasive vaginal cancer. A cystoscopic examination should be performed for tumors on the anterior vaginal wall and sigmoidoscopic examination for those on the posterior wall. Colposcopically directed biopsies are used to diagnose VAIN.

Treatment

Vaginal cancer, like cervical cancer, spreads by direct extension, infiltrating the paracolpos eventually out to the pelvic sidewall, or anteriorly or posteriorly to the bladder or rectum. Spread also occurs via the lymphatics; upper vaginal tumors spread to the pelvic nodes, similar to the spread in cervical cancer, and lower vaginal tumors spread to the inguinofemoral nodes as well. This mode of spread dictates the type of treatment.

Surgery

Local excision or ablation of the lesion with laser, electrocautery, or cryocautery is used for treatment of VAIN. Excisional treatments tend to shorten or narrow the vagina. For more extensive lesions, partial or complete vaginectomy with skin grafting may occasionally be necessary.

Surgical treatment can be used for invasive vaginal cancer located in the upper third of the vagina but only if the cancer is stage I (limited to the vaginal wall) or early stage II (involving subvaginal tissues). The surgical treatment is similar to that for cervical cancer in these situations, with radical upper vaginectomy (plus hysterectomy if the uterus is present) and pelvic lymphadenectomy.

Pelvic exenteration may be performed as a primary procedure for tumors involving the bladder or rectum (stage IV) and for those cases in which radiotherapy would likely produce a vesicovaginal or rectovaginal fistula. It may also be used after irradiation for treatment of residual disease or local recurrence.

Radiation

Pelvic irradiation is the treatment of choice for vaginal cancers. Usually, a combination of external therapy and brachytherapy is used. It is also used postoperatively if the patient is at high risk for recurrence.

Chemotherapy

Regimens similar to those used in the treatment of squamous cervical cancer have been tried as palliative therapy with limited effect. Because these patients often are elderly, they do not tolerate chemotherapy well. Intravaginal 5-fluorouracil cream has been used with some success to treat VAIN.

Results

Five-year survival rates depend on the stage of the disease. Approximately 75–85% five-year survival can be expected with stage I disease, with a rapid decrease in survival rate as the disease advances.

Recurrence

Recurrences may be local in the vagina, regional at the pelvic sidewall, or distant in the para-aortic nodes, Ever, lungs, bone, and central nervous system. Only a few patients, those with central recurrence in the vagina, will be curable by means of subsequent pelvic exenteration.

Follow-up

Follow-up evaluations should be performed as outlined above for cervical cancer. Often after irradiation, the vagina is obliterated, making evaluation difficult.

FALLOPIAN TUBE CANCER

Primary cancer of the fallopian tube is a rare gynecologic malignancy accounting for less than 1% of all female genital malignancies.[13] Patients are usually in the sixth decade of life, and most of them are post-menopausal. No specific risk factors have been identified.

Pathology

The majority of fallopian tube malignancies are papillary adenocarcinomas. Rare examples of sarcomas, squamous cell cancers, and other types of adenocarcinoma occur.

Screening

No effective screening test exists. A not infrequent occurrence is a Papanicolaou smear containing adenocarcinoma cells (with negative findings on dilatation and curettage) that subsequently are shown to come from fallopian tube tumor.

Clinical presentation

The symptoms and signs of fallopian tube cancer resemble those of ovarian malignancy. The clinical triad is pelvic pain, abnormal bleeding, and profuse vaginal discharge, with the finding of a pelvic mass.

Investigation

The disease usually is diagnosed at operation rather than preoperatively. However, with symptoms and findings similar to that of ovarian cancer, the usual work-up for suspected ovarian cancer is performed, including checking for the tumor marker CA 125.

Treatment

Surgery

This is the primary therapy for fallopian tube cancer. Treatment is total abdominal hysterectomy with bilateral salpingo-oophorectomy, omentectomy, pelvic and aortic lymphadenectomy, staging biopsies, and debulking of any metastases. As with ovarian cancer, there is evidence that optimal debulking improves survival.[14]

Radiation

Whole abdominal irradiation or intraperitoneal radioactive colloids are effective as adjuvant therapy.[15] Radiation can also be given as palliation for recurrent disease.

Chemotherapy

Significant responses do occur with the use of chemotherapy combinations containing platinum, and the indications for adjuvant therapy are similar to those used in the treatment of ovarian cancer. Survival rates are best for patients who have no gross residual disease after primary surgery.

Results of treatment

Prognosis depends primarily on the extent of disease at the time of diagnosis and on the amount of surgical debulking. Survival rates at five years are reported to be about 60% for stage I disease, 40% for stage II, and less than 10% for stages III and IV. However, many of the reports in the literature are from series in which complete staging was not performed and extensive surgical treatment and effective chemotherapy were not used.

Recurrences

As in ovarian cancer, most recurrences tend to occur in the peritoneal cavity. However, in comparison with ovarian cancer, fallopian tube cancer is more likely to metastasize to the liver and lungs. The serum level of CA 125 appears to be useful in monitoring for recurrent disease. Second-look laparotomy has been used in the management of this disease, but its role has not been established.

Follow-up

Regular follow-up with a routine similar to that for ovarian cancer is recommended.

GESTATIONAL TROPHOBLASTIC DISEASE

Gestational trophoblastic disease comprizes a group of tumors of varying degrees of malignancy, ranging from hydatidiform mole, invasive mole, and placental site trophoblastic tumor, to choriocarcinoma. The incidence of this disease is greatest in Asian countries. In about 3% of patients with hydatidiform mole, choriocarcinoma subsequently develops and most choriocarcinomas come from an antecedent hydatidiform mole. Other choriocarcinomas develop from an abortion, ectopic pregnancy, or term delivery.

Pathology

Hydatidiform moles are distinguished by grape-like clusters of hydropically dilated trophoblastic villi, with hyperplastic trophoblast between the villi. Invasive moles show evidence of invasion into the myometrium. Choriocarcinoma consists of rapidly proliferating trophoblast with absence of villi. It is highly malignant and widely metastatic, especially to the lungs, liver, kidneys, and central nervous system. Placental site trophoblastic tumors are malignant and invasive but slow growing; they are distinguished by the presence of human placental lactogen in the tumor.

Clinical presentation

Hydatidiform moles usually present in the first trimester of pregnancy with vaginal bleeding, a uterus large for dates, and, often, toxemia and hyperemesis.

An invasive mole is usually discovered after evacuation of a hydatidiform mole because of persistent increased levels of β-human chorionic gonadotropin, vaginal bleeding, and a failure of the uterus to involute.

Choriocarcinoma usually presents with vaginal bleeding and pelvic pain or symptoms due to metastatic disease, for example, hemoptysis or central nervous system symptoms.

Investigation

Serum human chorionic gonadotropin is the major diagnostic test for this group of diseases, but a normal pregnancy needs to be ruled out. Ultrasonography has revolutionized the treatment of gestational trophoblastic disease, but not only can it define a mole or normal pregnancy, but it can estimate the volume of the tumor, the presence of theca lutein cysts in the ovary, and reveal metastatic disease in other abdominal or pelvic organs.

Chest radiography is important in excluding lung metastases. However, CT is more sensitive and it is useful as is MRI in assessing intra-abdominal, pulmonary, and central nervous system metastases.

Arteriography can define the vascular supply, which can be embolized if necessary to stop hemorrhage.

A complete blood cell count, blood typing, and serum chemistry are essential in management.

Treatment

Surgery

Suction curettage is used to evacuate hydatidiform moles and repeat dilatation and curettage may be necessary to evacuate completely the uterine contents. Because of the higher risk of subsequent choriocarcinoma in patients older than 40 years of age, hysterectomy is indicated for molar disease in this age group.

Radiation therapy

This therapy is used occasionally for the treatment of central nervous system metastases.

Chemotherapy

This is the primary therapy for gestational trophoblastic disease. Low-risk patients are usually administered single-agent methotrexate with folinic acid rescue.

High-risk patients receive multiple-agent chemotherapy with etoposide, actinomycin D, methotrexate with folinic acid rescue, vincristine, and cyclophosphamide (EMACO).

Intrathecal methotrexate is given for treatment of central nervous system metastases.

Results of treatment

Complete tumor eradication is usual in patients with low-risk disease, although some require a change to a multidrug regimen to effect this.

In high-risk patients, complete remission can be expected in about 90% of those not previously treated and in about 70% of those in whom chemotherapy had failed.[16]

Follow-up

It is suggested that patients avoid pregnancy for 12 months after chemotherapy so that monitoring serum levels of human chorionic gonadotropin will be effective in following the patient for recurrence. Close follow-up utilizing serial determinations of serum human chorionic gonadotropin levels is the most important aspect of follow-up. Subsequent fertility is not a problem after therapy, because more than 80% of patients wishing to conceive have done so, and there has been no increase in fetal abnormalities.

References

1. Malkasian, G.D., Annegers, J.F. and Fountain, K.S. (1980). Carcinoma of the endometrium, stage I. *American Journal of Obstetrics & Gynecology*, **136**, 872–888.
2. Chambers, C.B. and Unis, J.S. (1986). Ultrasonic evidence of uterine malignancy in the postmenopausal uterus. *American Journal of Obstetrics & Gynecology*, **155**, 1194–1199.
3. Morrow, C.P., Bundy, B.N. and Kurrman, R.J. (1991). Relationship between surgical pathologic risk and outcome in clinical stage I and II carcinoma of the, endometrium. *Gynecologic Oncology*, **40**, 55–56.
4. Abeler, V.M., Kjorstad, K.E. and Berle, E. (1992). Carcinoma of the endometrium in Norway: a histopathological and prognostic survey of a total population. *International Journal of Gynecologic Cancer*, **2**, 9–22.
5. Morell, N.D., Taylor, J.R., Snyder, R.N., Ziel, H.K., Saltz, A. and Willie, S. (1982). False negative cytology rates in patients in whom invasive cervical cancer subsequently developed. *Obstetrics & Gynecology*, **60**, 41–45.
6. Burghardt, E., and Holzer, E. (1980). Treatment of carcinoma *in situ*: evaluation of 1069 cases. *Obstetrics & Gynecology*, **55**, 539–545.
7. Di Saia, P.J. and Creasman, W.T. (1981). *Clinical Gynecologic Oncology*. St. Louis, Missouri: Mosley.
8. Webb, M.J. and Symmonds, R.E. (1980). Site of recurrence of cervical cancer after radical hysterectomy. *American Journal of Obstetrics & Gynecology*, **138**, 813–817.
9. Webb, M.J., Decker, D.G. and Mussey, E. (1975). Cancer metastatic to the ovary: Factors Influencing Survival. *Obstetrics & Gynecology*, **45**, 391–396.
10. Neijt, J.P., Huinink, W. and Van der Berg, M. (1987). Randomized trial comparing two combination chemotherapy regimens in advanced ovarian carcinoma. *Journal of Clinical Oncology*, **5**, 1157-1168.
11. Boronow, R.C. (1982). Combined therapy as an alternative to exenteration for locally advanced vulvovaginal cancer. *Cancer*, **49**, 1085–1091.
12. Dancuart, F., Delclos, L., Wharton, J.T. and Silva, E.G. (1988). Primary squamous cell carcinoma of the vagina treated by radiotherapy. *International Journal of Radiation Oncology*, **14**, 745-749.
13. McMurray, E.H., Jacobs, A.J. and Perez, C.A. (1986). Carcinoma of the fallopian tube — management and sites of failure. *Cancer*, **58**, 2070–2075.
14. Gurney, H., Murphy, D. and Crowther, D. (1990). The management of primary fallopian tube carcinoma. *British Journal of Obstetrics & Gynecology*, **97**, 822–826.
15. Schray, M.F., Podratz, K.C. and Malkasian, G.D. (1987). Fallopian tube cancer: the role of radiation therapy. *Radiotherapy Oncology*, **10**, 267-275.
16. Newlands, B.S., Bagshawe, K.D., Begent, R.H.J., Rustin, G.J.S., Holden, L. and Dent, J. (1986). Development in chemotherapy for medium-and high-risk patients with gestational trophoblastic tumors. *British Journal of Obstetrics & Gynecology*, **93**, 63–69.

Cancer of Cervix Uteri

Steadily declining in most populations in the last half century

Worldwide: Most frequent in women in nearly all developing countries; 2nd most common worldwide

Lifetime risk
in USA whites:
  1 in 110

Relative five-year survival in 1983–87
in USA whites:
  68.9%

Risk factors
Sexually transmitted infectious agents probably
Human Papilloma Virus
Tobacco smoking

Geographical variation in 1983–87
Highest rate
48.9 per 100,000 in Brazil, Goiania
Lowest rate
2.6 per 100,000 in Israel, non-Jews

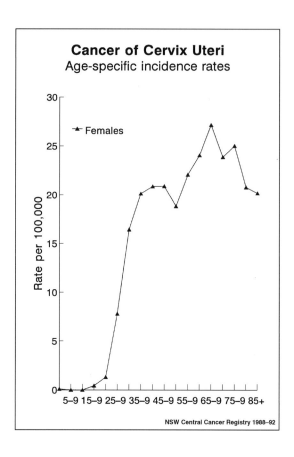

Cancer of Cervix Uteri
Age-specific incidence rates

NSW Central Cancer Registry 1988–92

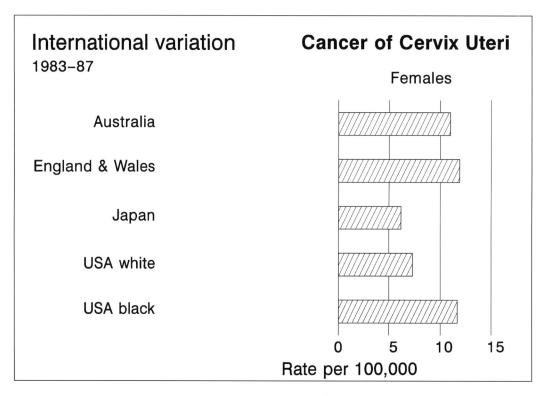

International variation
1983–87

Cancer of Cervix Uteri

Females

Australia

England & Wales

Japan

USA white

USA black

Rate per 100,000

Cancer of Corpus Uteri

Worldwide: Twice as common in developed as
developing countries;
globally one third as frequent as cervical cancer

Lifetime risk
in USA whites:
1 in 40

Relative five-year survival in 1983–87
in USA whites:
84.6%

Risk factors
Obesity
Unopposed exogenous estrogens
Nulliparity

Geographical variation in 1983–87
(corpus uteri plus uterus unspecified)
Highest rate
22.4 per 100,000 in USA, Bay Area, white
Lowest rate
1.2 per 100,000 in China, Qidong

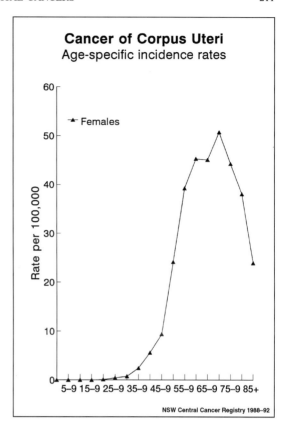

Cancer of Corpus Uteri
Age-specific incidence rates

NSW Central Cancer Registry 1988–92

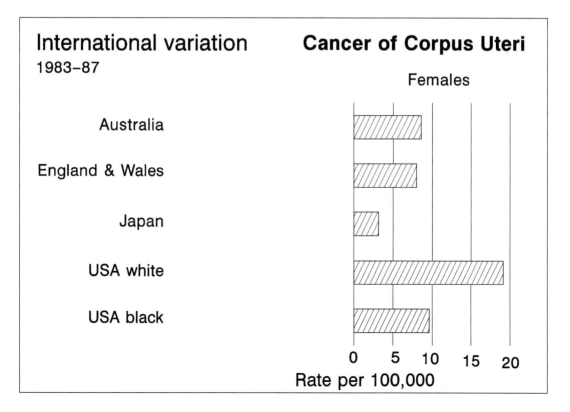

International variation
1983–87

Cancer of Corpus Uteri

Females

Rate per 100,000

Ovarian Cancer

Worldwide: Most common cause of death from gynecological cancers in western countries

Lifetime risk
in USA whites:
  1 in 55

Relative five-year survival in 1983–87
in USA whites:
  38.8%

Risk factors
Nulliparity or low parity
Ionizing radiation
Use of combined oral contraceptive confers protection

Geographical variation in 1983–87
Highest rate
17.0 per 100,000 in Switzerland, St Gall
Lowest rate
1.5 per 100,000 in China, Qidong

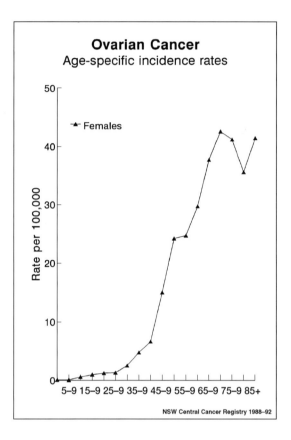

Ovarian Cancer
Age-specific incidence rates

NSW Central Cancer Registry 1988–92

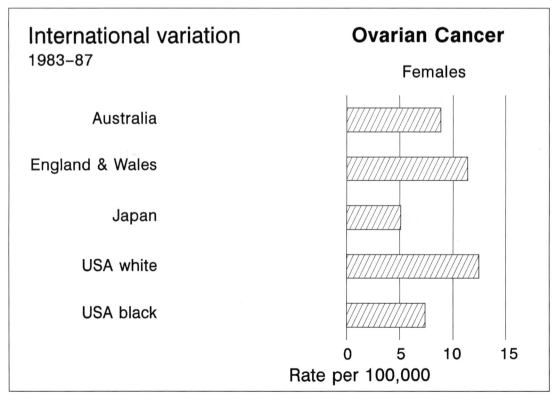

International variation
1983–87

Ovarian Cancer

Females

21. Male Urogenital Cancer

MARK NOSS and LAURENCE KLOTZ

Division of Urology, University of Toronto, Canada

PROSTATE CANCER

Incidence

Carcinoma of the prostate is currently the most common cancer affecting males in the Western world, accounting in North America for nearly 21% of all newly diagnosed cancers. The median age at diagnosis is 70 years with the incidence rising each decade after age 50. In the US, there are approximately 134,000 newly diagnosed cases each year. The incidence of the disease is 75.3/100,000.

Predisposing and risk factors

There is a higher incidence among relatives of prostate cancer patients. With two affected first-degree relatives, the relative risk is increased eight-fold. African Americans have a higher incidence of the disease compared to whites and have worse survival, stage for stage.

Eunuchs do not develop clinical prostate cancer. Androgens are necessary for prostatic growth, and likely promote growth of prostate cancer once transformation has occurred.

High dietary fat has been associated with an increased incidence of prostate cancer as have exposure to such chemical carcinogens or promoters as car exhaust, air pollution, cadmium fertilizer and industrial chemicals. Oncogenic viruses, such as SV-40, HSV-2 and CMV, have been shown to trans-form normal prostate cells *in vitro*. *In vivo*, this has not been demonstrated.

Pathology

Ninety-five percent of prostate cancers are adenocarcinomas. The remaining 5% are primarily transitional cell carcinomas (TCC). The normal prostate gland contains both acinar glands and ducts. The glands are lined with columnar epithelium one cell layer thick on a basement membrane. The ducts are lined with a single layer of cuboidal cells peripherally and transitional cells centrally. In prostate cancer there is a loss of this basal layer along with a loss of the orderly branching of the normal glands. There is also blurring of the stroma-epithelial interface.

Prostate cancer is graded by the Gleason system, based on overall cellular architecture and glandular differentiation. The most and second most predominant pattern are each graded from one to five to give a score out of ten.

Carcinoma of the prostate spreads by: (1) local invasion, (2) vascular invasion and (3) lymphatic spread. Locally, the tumor may penetrate the prostatic capsule along the perivesical sheath and bladder base, where the ureters may become obstructed. This occurs in 10–35% of patients. Metastases to bone occurs in 85% of patients dying of prostate cancer. Visceral spread occurs in 15% of patients. Lymphatic spread occurs to the perivesical, hypogastric, obturator, presacral then presciatic lymph nodes.

Screening

Screening for prostate cancer is a highly controversial issue, with substantial medical and fiscal implications. Screening is based on the serum prostate specific antigen (PSA), and digital rectal exam (DRE). PSA is an enzyme produced by prostatic epithelium whose function is to liquefy the seminal coagulum after ejaculation. Prostate cancer cells leak PSA into serum at 10 times the rate of benign prostate cells. Thus patients with prostate cancer tend to have elevated PSA. The PSA test results in detection of prostate cancer at an earlier stage, when it is more amenable to curative therapy. About 10% of men over 50 have an elevated PSA; one-third of these (3%) will be found to have prostate cancer. About 1/3 of patients with clinical prostate cancer will have a normal PSA; thus the DRE is complementary.

The controversy regarding screening is related to the slow growing nature of PC in many patients, and the tendency for the disease to occur in older men, whose life expectancy may be limited. Patients may thus be exposed to treatment which does not benefit them, and incur a reduced quality of life as a result. On the other hand, some patients, especially younger men, who are diagnosed at an earlier stage by screening and cured by definitive therapy, will have a longer survival as a result of screening. In other words, screening involves a trade-off between quality and quantity of life. Currently, several randomized trials evaluating the efficacy of screening, and radical therapy for prostate cancer, are under-way which should clarify this question.

Clinical presentation

Sixty-five percent of patients will present with localized disease. Early prostate cancer is usually asymptomatic; patients with advanced disease may have marked obstruction, urinary retention, renal failure or bony metastases.

Investigations

After confirming the diagnosis of prostate cancer, effort should be made to ascertain that the disease is confined to the prostate. Trans rectal ultrasound

Table 21.1. Prostate cancer.

TNM	
TX	Tumor cannot be evaluated
T0	Tumor cannot be identified
T1a	Occult, <=5% of total surgical specimen and of low to medium grade
T1b	Occult, > 5% of specimen, any grade or <=5% of specimen high grade
T1c	Identified by PSA
T2a	<=1/2 of one lobe, regardless of location
T2b	> 1/2 of one lobe but not > 1 lobe
T2c	> 1 lobe or bilaterally palpable cancer
T3a	Extension through prostatic capsule unilaterally
T3b	Extension through capsule bilaterally
T3c	Seminal vesicle involvement
T4	Extension into contiguous organs

Bladder

TNM		Jewett–Strong–Marshall
T0	No tumor in the specimen	0
Tis	Carcinoma *in situ*	0
Ta	Noninvasive papillary tumor	0
T1	Submucosal invasion	A
T2	Superficial muscle invasion	B1
T3a	Deep muscle invasion	B2
T3b	Invasion of perivesical fat	C
T4	Invasion of contiguous organs	D1

Testis cancer

TNM		Walter-Reed	Skinner
TX	Unknown status		
T0	No evidence of primary		
T1	Confined to testis	I	A
T2	Beyond tunica		
T3	Invasion of rete testis or epididymis		
T4a	Invasion of cord		
T4b	Invasion of scrotum		
N0	No lymph node involvement		
N1	single node ≤ 2 cm,	IIA	B1
N2	1 node, 2–5 cm or, > 1 node < 5 cm	IIB	B2
N3	Lymph nodes > 5 cm	IIC	B3
M+	Supra-diaphragmatic metastases	III	C

(TRUS) is primarily useful for aiding in the diagnosis with biopsy, and may detect extra capsular and seminal vesicle involvement.

Regional lymph nodes are assessed with CT, bone metastases by bone scans. The TNM staging systems is given in Table 21.1, a simpler system is:

A. Incidental finding
B. Palpable but inside prostate
C. Spread outside prostate capsule
D. Metastases

Treatment

The optimal management remains controversial. Patients with Tla disease usually offered surveillance as this disease is indolent (15% progression rate at 10 years). The treatment options for localized prostate cancer (stage Tlb-c, T2) are radical prostatectomy (RP), external beam irradiation, and watchful waiting. In general, the more aggressive the therapy the greater the chance of disease control and the greater the side effects. Treatment is individualized according to age, co-morbidity and personal preference.

Stage T3 patients are treated with external beam radiotherapy, androgen ablation therapy, or watchful waiting. Surgery is not an option. The patient will receive 60–70 Gy to the prostate along with the pelvic lymph nodes. Radiation is also useful in treating patients with painful bony metastases. Interstitial radiotherapy, using I-125, Iridium, or Gold seeds implanted into the prostate has been used with some success.

Androgen ablation is the treatment of choice for metastatic disease. This can be accomplished either surgically, with a bilateral orchiectomy, or medically, with drugs that reduce and/or block androgens. Orchiectomy alone will remove 90% of the circulating androgens. One can also use luteinizing hormone releasing hormone (LHRH) agonists, estrogens (DES), non-steroidal (flutamide) and steroidal (cyproterone acetate, CPA) anti-androgens. The anti-androgens block adrenal androgens as well, and are often used in conjunction with androgen ablation (i.e., orchiectomy or LHRH analogue).

There are a number of agents with activity in hormone refractory prostate cancer including Mitoxantrone, VP-16, Estramustine, Suramin. These improve quality of life but have little impact on survival.

Risks of treatment

Prostate cancer is usually a slowly progressive, chronic disease. The mortality of prostate cancer depends on the stage and grade of the disease, and the life expectancy of the patient. In a large study of 223 patients with early disease who were not treated, 29% showed evidence of progression. Nineteen percent of the deaths were due to prostate cancer. The progression rate for Tlb and T2 disease at five years were 36 and 38%, respectively.

However, patients living > 10 years have a 60% chance of dying of prostate cancer.

Radical Prostatectomy (RP) may be associated with impotence and incontinence. With the advent of nerve sparing and cavernous nerve stimulation, the incidence of impotence is lower. The generally, quoted figures for severe incontinence is 1–2% while the impotency rate varies from 30–50%. Ten to twenty percent of patients may experience mild incontinence. The 15-year survival in patients with organ confined disease treated with RP has been reported to be equivalent to age matched controls.

Radiation complications include impotence, incontinence and radiation cystitis. These have been reported as 50%, 3% and 7%, respectively. They are usually transient. Genital and leg edema have also been reported at a frequency of 1.6%.

The side effects of the hormonal therapy are related to the withdrawal of androgens and consist of hot flushes, mood swings and decreased libido. Estrogens are associated with an increased risk of thromboembolic disease.

Results of treatment

Early prostate cancer or that of low stage or grade can be managed by watchful waiting. Proponents of watchful waiting indicate that in men with a life expectancy of less than 10 years, advanced age or poor medical status, watchful waiting is a reasonable option. Although they have not been directly compared, the outcomes are similar to that of aggressive therapy.

In men who were candidates for and have undergone RP, the results are good. In one series, the five-year actuarial rate for local recurrence was 4%, distant metastases was 5%, distant metastases with local recurrence was only 2%, the rate of elevated PSA without evidence of disease was 10%. A review of the literature revealed that five-year local recurrence rate for B1 disease was 6-7%. In patients with organ confined disease, on pathological examination, 8–26% will have a local recurrence at five years. This is compared to 10–41% of patients with penetration through the capsule.

The 5- and 10-year cause-specific survival after RP for stage B disease ranges from 95–100% and 92–97%, respectively. The actuarial 5- and 10-year clinical disease-free survival for stage C disease was 39% and 9%, respectively.

It is difficult to compare results of radiation with that of RP. This is due to differences in the patient population. Radiation, however, does have excellent results. In two large studies in the USA, 10-year survivals were 63% and 57% for stage A, 47% and 45% for stage B and 33% and 35% for stage C. At 15 years, survival rates were 40%, 25% and 23%, respectively.

BLADDER CANCER

Incidence

More than 90% of bladder neoplasms are transitional cell carcinomas (TCC). Bladder cancer is 2.7 times more common in men than women. It is the fourth most common cancer in males accounting for 10% of all cancers. It is almost twice as common in whites than blacks although these tend to be non invasive tumors. Bladder cancer can occur at any age. The median age at diagnosis is 67 years of age.

Predisposing and risk factors

The bladder is an end organ for environmental carcinogens. These include industrial exposure to certain chemical, cigarette smoking, coffee drinking, analgesics, artificial sweeteners, certain infections, bladder stones and pelvic irradiation.

Aniline dyes, which have been used to color fabrics, have been shown to be carcinogens to the bladder. The latent period for the exposure to development of the tumors may be up to 50 years. Other occupational exposures include machinists, chemical workers, and those exposed to organic chemicals including benzidine, and naphthylamine.

Cigarette smoking has been shown to increase the risk of bladder cancer four fold over non-smokers. The particular carcinogen in the smoke has yet to be identified. There have been reports linking coffee and tea drinking and the use of artificial sweeteners to the development of bladder cancer. Large doses of the sweeteners saccharin and cyclamates have demonstrated malignancies in animal models, but little or no evidence exists in humans. It is likely that the association of bladder cancer with coffee, tea and sweetener is related to the cigarette smoking that it usually accompanies. The analgesic, phenacetin, consumed in quantities of 5 to 15 kg over 10 years, has been associated

with an increased incidence of bladder cancer. The latent period is up to 25 years.

Chronic infections, such as that from a chronic indwelling catheter and infection with *Schistosoma haematobium* can result in squamous cell carcinoma of the bladder. Exposure to Cyclophosphamide predisposes to bladder cancer. Women who have previously irradiated for uterine or cervical cancer are at a two- to four-fold increased risk of developing the disease.

Pathology

Ninety-five percent of bladder cancers are TCC, in the Western world. Squamous cell carcinomas account for 5% of malignancies while adenocarcinoma accounts for approximately 1%. In Egypt, where *S. haematobium* is endemic, squamous cell carcinoma constitutes 90% of bladder cancers. TCC may be considered a spectrum of disease starting with carcinoma *in situ* (CIS). CIS appears as a velvety patch of erythematous mucosa on cystoscopy. Forty to eighty percent of CIS will progress to invasive disease if untreated.

Approximately 70% of bladder tumors are papillary while 10% are nodular and 20% are mixed. Microscopically, normal bladder mucosa consists of a transitional cell layer three to seven cells thick. Beneath these cells are intermediate cells on a basement membrane. In bladder cancer, there may be an increased number of epithelial cell layers, compared to the normal bladder. There also may be loss of cell polarity, abnormal cell maturation, giant cells, prominent nucleoli, nuclear crowding, increased mitoses and an increased nuclear/cytoplasmic ratio.

Transitional cell cancer is a field change disease, with tumors arising at different sites and different times within the urothelium (polychronotropism). In addition, primary tumors implant in other areas in the bladder following resection. Both mechanisms account for the high incidence of recurrence following initial tumour resection.

Bladder cancer can spread via direct extension, lymphatic and vascular spread and wound implantation. Bladder cancer can invade by growing through the lamina propria into the submucosa and muscularis of the bladder wall. This occurs in 25% of cases; the majority remain superficial. Beneath the submucosa, the tumor cells can invade into the blood vessels and lymphatics and therefore gain access to other sites. Bladder cancer may also invade locally into the prostate, uterus, cervix, vagina, ureters and bowel. The most common site of lymph node metastases are the pelvic lymph nodes. These occur in 80% of patients. The common site of vascular spread is liver (38%), bone (27%), adrenal (21%) and intestine (13%).

Screening

Urinalysis has been used as a screening test for bladder cancer, but has never been demonstrated conclusively to reduce mortality from the disease. Its use in the general population is controversial. Certainly high risk patients, i.e. with a history of industrial carcinogen exposure, should be screened with urinalysis and urine cytology.

Clinical presentation

The most common clinical presentation of bladder cancer is painless hematuria. This occurs in approximately 85% of patients. Patients may also present with bladder irritability, as suggested by urinary frequency, urgency and dysuria. This presentation is more common in CIS. Patients may present with symptoms of urinary obstruction. They may complain of flank pain from ureteral obstruction or may have a pelvic mass.

Staging

Patients who present with gross or microscopic hematuria should be investigated with a urinalysis, imaging of their upper tracts with either ultrasound or IVP and cystoscopy. At cystoscopy, specimen of urine should be taken for culture as well as a saline bladder washing, as opposed to a voided urine for cytology. The mechanical action of the washing enhances tumor shedding and provides fresh, better preserved cells. The bladder should be carefully examined with the cystoscope and any abnormal areas should be biopsied. Lesions seen on the IVP or ultrasound can be examined more carefully using retrograde pyelography or ureteroscopy with samples obtained.

After a tumor is diagnosed, the tumor must be identified and staged. This is accomplished by a resection of all identifiable disease. At the time of transurethral resection of the bladder tumor (TURBT), the patient should undergo a pre- and post- resection, bimanual examination. Some urologists also do random or directed bladder biopsies of different sites or the prostatic urethra.

If invasive disease is identified, a CT scan is used to assess the extent of local disease as well as the presence of adenopathy. Ideally, the CT scan should be done prior to the TURBT as the resection obscures the tissue planes and reduces specificity due to edema in the bladder wall.

There are two staging systems in common use, the Jewett-Marshall classification and the TNM system (see Table 21.1).

Treatment

Superficial bladder cancer (Ta, Tl) is usually managed adequately with TURBT or fulgerization of the tumors. If following repeated resection the patient has multiple recurrences of superficial disease or has CIS, then the patient is treated with intravesical therapy. The most commonly used intravesical therapy for recurrent superficial bladder cancer is BCG.

BCG is an attenuated strain of the tuberculous bacteria *Mycobacterium bovis*. The instillation of the bacteria stimulates an immune reaction in the bladder mediated by interferon and other cytokines which have antineoplastic effects. It is administered weekly for six weeks. It may also be administered as a prophylactic agent in patients who are tumor free or for patients with CIS. Other intravesical agents commonly in use include Mitomycin C, Thiotepa, doxorubicin (Adriamycin) and etoglucid (Epodyl).

Management of invasive bladder cancer (T2, T3a,b, T4) involves radical therapy. TURBT alone is usually ineffective in rendering these patients free of disease. It is useful for patients with low volume of disease and in those who are not medically fit for major surgery. The treatment of choice for most patients with invasive bladder cancer is radical cystectomy. In most males, a new bladder can be reconstructed from bowel, permitting relatively normal voiding. In most women and some men, a pouch is constructed from bowel and brought to the skin. The opening is covered with a small gauze square and catheterized 3–4 times/day. An external appliance (e.g. a bag) is rarely required. Patient with invasive disease are also considered for radiation therapy. Patients who recur or progress after radiation therapy may be considered for a salvage cystectomy.

Patients with metastatic disease may be treated with a combination of cytotoxic chemotherapeutic agents. These include cisplatin, methotrexate and vinblastine (CMV) or the above plus Adriamycin (MVAC).

Risks of treatment

Risks of TURBT are minimal. The primary complication is bladder perforation. Although infrequent, this can usually be managed conservatively and will rarely require surgical correction. The main side effect of BCG is bladder irritability. Symptom complex includes dysuria (91%), frequency (90%), hematuria (46%), fever (24%), malaise (18%), nausea (8%), chills (8%), arthralgia (2%) and pruritis (1%). Patients have also developed granulomatous prostatitis after therapy. Six percent of patients have developed symptoms severe enough to require a course of treatment with antituberculous agents. If a patient develops an adverse reaction to BCG, then the treatment should be held until symptoms resolve.

Approximately 70% of patients treated with radiation therapy will develop temporary symptoms of bladder irritability or diarrhea. Severe or persistent complications may occur in 5–10% of patients. Complications of cystectomy are related to both bowel and pouch function. The serious complication rate is in the order of 10–15%, including intestinal obstruction and wound infections. Minor side effects from BCG are not uncommon, occurring in up to 90% of patients and include cystitis, hematuria, malaise and low grade fevers. Serious side effects are rare and require immediate treatment with antituberculous agents.

Results of treatment

Most patients presenting with superficial disease can be managed effectively with TURBT with or without intravesical therapy. Fifteen percent of patients will ultimately require radical therapy. The use of BCG has been shown to reduce tumor recurrences from 42% to 17%. Overall the response rate for BCG is 58%. BCG is effective in decreasing the rate of progression to muscle invasive disease from 36% to 9%.

In selected patients with invasive disease treated with TURBT alone, the five-year disease-free survival rate is 40%. Radiation therapy produces five-year disease-free survival rates of 35, 40, 30 and 7% for stages T2, T3a, T3b and T4, respectively. Studies have failed to demonstrate significant differences in five-year survival in patients treated with radiation plus cystectomy over those with cystectomy alone. Survival following cystectomy at five-years is 80%, 60%, 40% and 20% for each stage. The use of adjuvant chemotherapy following cystectomy for high risk TCC appears to improve survival by 10–15%.

Follow-up

Follow-up for patients following TURBT for Ta-T1 TCC consists of cystoscopies every three months for two years, then every six months for two years then yearly.

TESTIS CANCER

Incidence

Testis cancer represents approximately 1% of all cancers in males. The lifetime risk of developing a testis cancer in American white males is 1 in 500. The annual age-adjusted incidence of testis cancer in American white males is 3.7 per 100,000 and 0.9 per 100,000 in American black males.

Age

Testis cancer can occur at any age but occurs predominantly in late adolescence and early adulthood (15–35 years).

Predisposing and risk factors

A history of cryptorchidism increases the risk of testicular malignancy by 3–14 times, A history of exposure to diethylstilbestrol (DES) has been associated with an increased relative risk for testis cancer of 2.8 to 5.3 in male progeny of women exposed to DES.

Pathology

Ninety percent of malignancies arise from the germinal elements of the testis. Germinal neoplasms are classified as seminoma (40%), embryonal (20–25%), teratocarcinoma (25–30%), teratoma (5–10%) and choriocarcinoma (1%). Nongerminal tumors account for the remaining 5%. These elements include the stroma, mesenchymal structures and ducts.

Testicular cancer spreads via the lymphatics in a highly predictable fashion. The primary lymphatic drainage of the testis is related to the embryology of testicular ontogeny. Embryologically, the testis is intraabdominal, hence the lymphatic drainage is intraabdominal. Metastases usually occur initially in the ipsilateral para-aortic or paracaval nodes and interaortocaval region. Inguinal lymph nodes tend only to be involved if the tunica albuginea has been invaded or there has been previous surgery such as orchidopexy or inguinal herniorrhaphy.

Screening

The only effective screening for testis cancer is testicular self-examination. Men between the ages of 15 to 35 should be encouraged to perform this monthly.

Clinical presentation

The usual presentation of a testicular tumor is one of a painless swelling or nodule in one testis. Ten percent of patients will present with acute scrotal pain and 10% present with signs and symptoms of metastatic disease. Gynecomastia is present in up to 5% of patients.

The common differential diagnosis of a testicular mass, painful or painless, includes epididymoorchitis, hydrocele, spermatocele, hematocele, tumor, infarction, hemorrhage into a tumor and torsion. In particular, a patient diagnosed with acutc epididymoorchitis must be seen in follow-up to ensure that the testicular mass has resolved completely.

Investigations

A scrotal ultrasound is helpful in confirming the presence of a solid mass in the body of the testis. If a tumor is suspected, the diagnosis is established by inguinal orchidectomy.

Prior to orchidectomy, the patients should have serum tumor markers drawn. These include alpha-fetoprotein (AFP) and human chorionic gonadotropin (hCG). These tumor markers are elevated in 60% of patients with nonseminomas. A persistent elevation or a rising tumor marker post orchiectomy indicates residual or recurrence disease.

After radical orchidectomy, the patient is staged with a CT scan of the abdomen and chest X-ray. Abdominal CT scan allows for assessment of the retroperitoneal lymph nodes.

There are three common staging system in testis cancer (see Table 21.1).

Treatment

Primary therapy consists of inguinal orchidectomy. This provides the pathological diagnosis and local control. Seminomas are very radiosensitive tumors and stage I and IIA disease is treated with retroperitoneal irradiation (2500 cGy). For advanced seminoma (stage IIB and above), the treatment is platinum based chemotherapy (Bleomycin, VP-16 and cis-platinum).

Nonseminomatous tumors, stage I disease, is managed with surveillance or a retroperitoneal lymph node dissection (RPLND). On surveillance, 30% of patients eventually progress. However, 98% of stage I patients will eventually be cured regardless of whether surveillance of RPLND is selected initially. Stage II disease is usually treated with RPLND in combination with platinum based chemotherapy. Stage III disease is treated with combination platinum based therapy and resection of residual masses.

Risks of treatment

The main risk of chemotherapy and RPLND is infertility. Many centers therefore offer sperm banking. Following RPLND, patients may be left infertile as a result of damage to the sympathetic nerves that control seminal fluid emission. Recent advances in surgical technique have aided in the identification of the sympathetic nerves and have allowed sparing of the nerves. Mortality of RPLND is less than 1%.

Results of treatment

Testis cancer represents the greatest success of chemotherapy for solid tumors. Overall, most patients with testis cancer are cured. Virtually 100% of stage I seminoma and 98% of nonseminoma patients are cured. This drops to 65% for patients presenting with very advanced disease.

Cancer of Prostate

Incidence increasing more rapidly than mortality;
early detection likely to be responsible
Clinical and latent cancers rare before age 50
Particularly common in American blacks

Worldwide: 4th most frequent male cancer

Lifetime risk
in USA whites:
  1 in 7

Relative five-year survival in 1983–87
in USA whites:
  78.4%

Risk factors
Race
Family history of prostate cancer
Dietary factors suspected but not proven

Geographical variation in 1983–87
Highest rate
102.0 per 100,000 in USA, Atlanta, blacks
Lowest rate
0.8 per 100,000 in China, Qidong

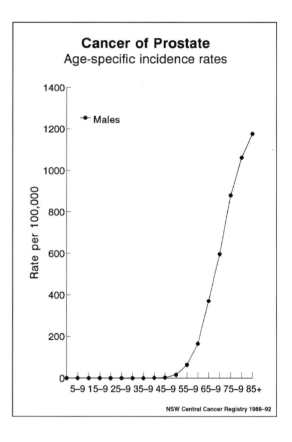

Cancer of Prostate
Age-specific incidence rates

NSW Central Cancer Registry 1988–92

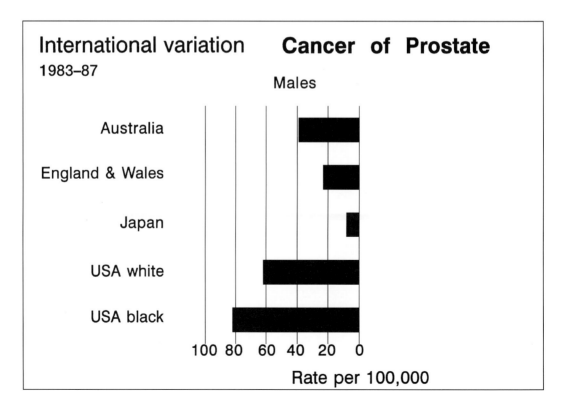

International variation **Cancer of Prostate**
1983–87

Males

Rate per 100,000

Testicular Cancer

Increasing incidence; falling mortality
Primarily in white males under age 50

Lifetime risk
in USA whites:
  1 in 250

Relative five-year survival in 1983–87
  92.8%

Risk factors
Cryptorchidism

Geographical variation in 1983–87
Highest rate
8.8 per 100,000 in Switzerland, Zurich
Lowest rate
0.4 per 100,000 in China, Qidong

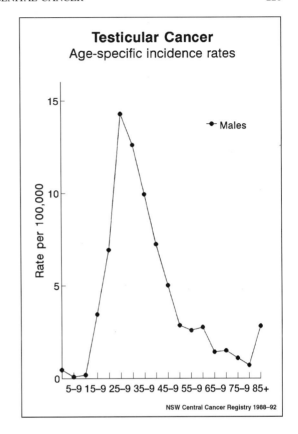

Testicular Cancer
Age-specific incidence rates

NSW Central Cancer Registry 1988–92

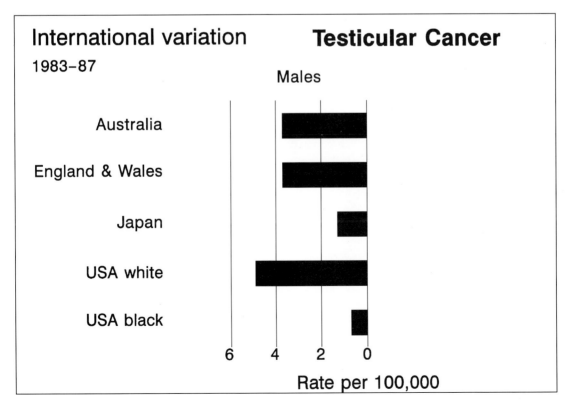

International variation
1983–87

Testicular Cancer

Males

Rate per 100,000

Bladder Cancer

More common in men by a factor of 3

Lifetime risk
in USA whites:
  M 1 in 28
  F   1 in 80

Relative five-year survival in 1983–87
in USA whites
  M 81.1%
  F   75.3%

Risk factors
Tobacco
Occupational exposure to aromatic amines
Phenacetin-containing analgesics
Schistosomiasis (in endemic areas)

Geographical variation in 1983–87
Highest rate
M: 34.0 per 100,000 in Italy, Trieste
F: 7.4 per 100,000 in USA, New Orleans, white
Lowest rate
M: 1.8 per 100,000 in India, Madras
F: 0.5 per 100,000 in India, Bangalore

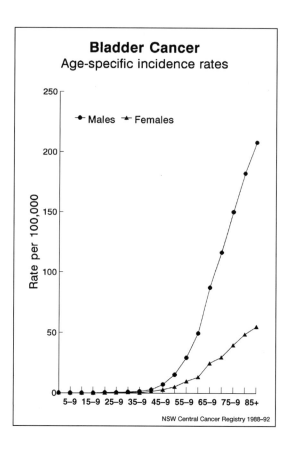

NSW Central Cancer Registry 1988–92

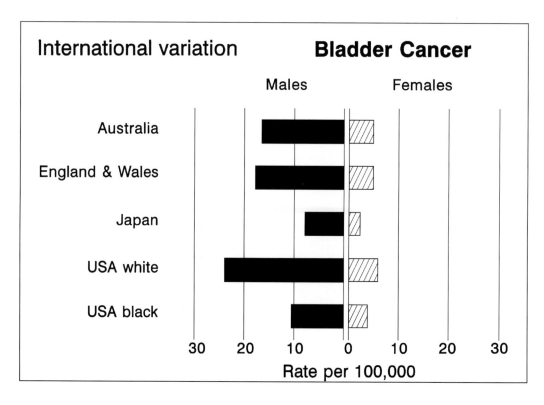

22. Renal Tumors

N.A. WATKIN and T.J. CHRISTMAS

Department of Urology, Charing Cross Hospital, London, UK

INTRODUCTION

Malignant renal tumors may occur in adults and children and originate in both the renal parenchymal and calyceal tissues. In adults, renal cell carcinoma (RCC) accounts for 85–90% of cases, transitional cell carcinoma (TCC) 5–7%, sarcoma 3%, lymphomas, squamous carcinoma and metastases account for the remainder. The principal childhood malignancy is Wilms' tumor.

RENAL CELL CARCINOMA

This is otherwise known as a hypernephroma (mistakenly thought to be adrenal in origin), and clear cell carcinoma (on the basis of the histological appearance).

Etiology

It accounts for 2–3% of adult malignancies and is commoner in men than women by a factor of 1.6:1, with a peak incidence in the 50–70 year age group. There is an increased incidence in cigarette smokers and a possible link with cadmium exposure. Patients with tuberous sclerosis, multicystic kidney disease of dialysis, adult polycystic kidney disease, and von Hippel Lindau syndrome (hereditary cerebellar and retinal haemangioblastomas), may also

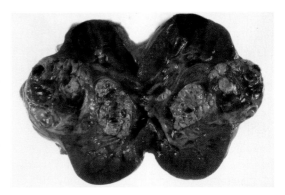

Figure 22.1. A renal cell carcinoma with the characteristic yellow cut surface.

develop RCC. Chromosomal abnormalities described in RCC most frequently involve translocations and deletions of the short arm of chromosome 3(3p).

Pathology

The tumor is an adenocarcinoma arising from renal tubules and macroscopically has a yellow cut surface (Figure 22.1). Histologically, the cells have a lipid rich cytoplasm and a small peripheral nucleus. Tumors are initially well encapsulated and tend to spread late to lymph nodes and may metastasize to the lungs, bone, brain and liver. A particular feature of RCC is the predilection for direct spread along

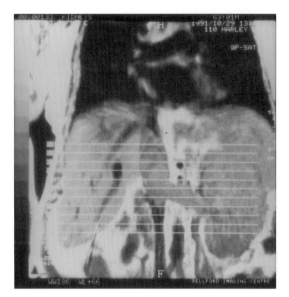

Figure 22.2. An MRI scan showing a large left upper pole renal cell carcinoma with tumor thrombus extending along the renal vein into the inferior vena cava.

the renal vein and into the inferior vena cava (IVC) (Figure 22.2). In very advanced cases, tumor can extend up into the right atrium.

Symptoms and signs

The commonest presenting features are haematuria, loin pain and a palpable abdominal mass. This triad of symptoms is present together in only 10% of patients, and generally indicates advanced disease. Patients with metastatic disease to the lungs or bone may have symptoms of dyspnoea, cough or bone pain. RCC may also present with paraneoplastic syndromes, which may delay diagnosis. These syndromes occur as a result of over-expression of proteins or hormones normally produced by the kidney, e.g. renin, erythropoeitin and prostaglandins, and those not normally produced, e.g. parathyroid hormone. This can result in hypertension, poly-cythemia, pyrexia of unknown origin, hypercal-cemia and vague constitutional upset.

Investigations

An IVU may show deformity of the calyceal system or abnormal renal outline. Ultrasound distinguishes a cystic from a solid lesion, and the size of the tumor and its possible extension into the renal vein

can also be determined. A CT scan of the abdomen and pelvis with intravenous contrast confirms the extent of the tumor, the lymph node status and the functionality of the contralateral kidney. With the widespread use of MRI, CT and ultrasound, an increasing number of asymptomatic 'incidental' tumors are being detected. A chest X-ray deter-mines if these are lung metastases and a full blood count, hepatic, renal and bone profile are performed prior to definitive treatment. Angiography is indi-cated in only a few patients in whom partial nephrectomy or pre-operative embolization is be-ing considered.

Staging system

The Robson system is simple and consists of:

Stage 1   Confined to the renal capsule
Stage 2   Extracapsular spread into the peri-nephric fat
Stage 3   Extension into the renal vein IVC or lymph nodes
Stage 4   Involvement of adjacent organs or distant metastases

The Tumor-Node-Metastasis (TNM) classification is more detailed and better reflects prognosis.

T1   Tumor < 2.5 cm diameter
T2   Tumor > 2.5 cm diameter
T3a   Extension into perinephric fat
T3b   Extension into the renal vein
T3c   Extension into the IVC
T4   Invasion of adjacent structures
N0   No nodes
N1   Single node
N2   Multiple nodes
N3   Fixed nodes
M0   No metastases
M1   Metastases

Surgical treatment

Radical nephrectomy is the treatment of choice. It involves removal of the kidney, peri-nephric fat and hilar lymph nodes. The adrenal gland is usually removed, particularly if the tumor involves the upper pole of the kidney. The therapeutic benefit of *en bloc* regional lymphadenectomy is not proven. For small tumors, a 12th rib extraperitoneal approach or anterior transperitoneal approach is used. For large upper pole tumors, a thoraco-abdominal approach provides better access to the major vessels. When caval tumor thrombus extends beyond the hepatic veins into the right atrium, thoraco-abdominal exploration is mandatory but cardio-pulmonary by-pass is rarely indicated. Pre-operative embolization of the renal artery, to reduce blood loss during excision of large vascular tumors, can be performed.

In patients with bilateral tumors, or a tumor in a solitary kidney, partial nephrectomy is considered.

Five-year survival for stage Tl, T2, N0 tumors is >80%. For T3a, T3b, N0, survival is reduced to 40–50%. The presence of tumor positive nodes is associated with a poor prognosis (0–20%).

Adjuvant treatment

The role of adjuvant treatment after surgical resection, and for patients with node positive/metastatic disease at the time of diagnosis, has been the subject of extensive research. Unfortunately no currently available treatment modality achieves a favourable response.

1. *Radiotherapy*: RCC is only poorly radiosensitive. Its use is limited to symptomatic treatment of bone pain, and treatment of refractory haematuria.
2. *Chemotherapy*: The single most active agent is vinblastine, and is associated with a 15% complete remission in node positive disease, but remission times are short (several months). Combination regimes involving vinblastine are not significantly better. The chemo-resistance appears to be due to the presence of a trans-membrane efflux PUMP (P_{170}) coded by the multi-drug resistance (MDR) gene.
3. *Hormonal therapy*: Several non-randomized studies suggest that medroxyprogesterone acetate (MPA) is associated with complete and partial response rates of 10%. The mechanism of action is unclear.
4. *Immunotherapy*: Host immune responses may play a role in tumor control, and further stimulation with adoptive immunotherapy is currently under investigation. Non-randomized studies using alpha-interferon and interleukin-2 result in a 10–15% complete response which may be more durable than for chemotherapy. The se-

vere side effects associated with intravenous therapy are diminished when the drugs are given subcutaneously without a reduction in response.

5. *Surgery for metastases*: Solitary recurrences in the renal bed, liver, lung or brain can be removed surgically with occasional cures. Resection of multiple metastases has not been shown to prolong survival.

Follow-up

Initially, surveillance is with a three-monthly chest X-ray and ultrasound or CT of the renal bed. The interval of follow-up is gradually increased to annual review. There is no evidence that this confers any survival benefit.

TRANSITIONAL CELL CARCINOMA

The renal pelvis is lined with transitional cell epithelium identical to that of the ureters and bladder. TCC of the renal pelvis accounts for 3–4% of TCC of the renal tract. Fifty percent of patients with renal TCC develop TCC of the bladder. The etiology is similar to bladder TCC. There is also increased risk in patients with renal papillary damage secondary to analgesic (phenacetin) abuse. The commonest presenting symptoms are frank hematuria (70–90%), flank pain and clot colic. A tumor may be identified as a filling defect on IVU (Figure 22.3), and occa-

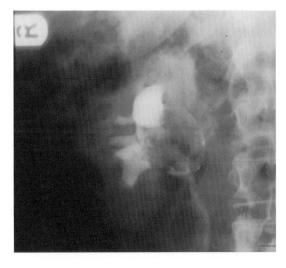

Figure 22.3. Intravenous urogram of the right pelvicalyceal system demonstrating a large filling defect within the renal pelvis. This proved to be a transitional cell carcinoma.

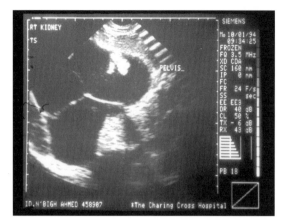

Figure 22.4. A small papillary transitional cell tumor seen during an ultrasound scan of a hydronephrotic kidney.

sionally on CT or ultrasound (Figure 22.4), and can be further evaluated with cytology and retrograde ureteropyelography. Tissue diagnosis can be obtained with brush cytology or biopsy using a ureteroscope. Staging is analogous to TCC of the bladder, with the recognition that disease progression is more rapid through the thin wall of the renal pelvis. Because of the multi-focal nature of the disease, treatment is radical nephroureterectomy including the ureteric orifice (Figure 22.5). Complete excision is associated with 70–90% five-year survival. For small, low-grade tumors, conservative therapy involving percutaneous or ureteroscpic fulguration is possible, particularly for bilateral disease. Lymph node positive and metastatic disease has a poor prognosis (0–30%). Treatment for advanced disease is based on cisplatin combination

chemotherapy such as MVAC: methotrexate, vinblastine, adriamycin and cisplatinum.

RARE MALIGNANT TUMORS

Sarcomas constitute 2–3% of malignant renal tumors, with leiomyosarcoma the most common, but virtually every other type of sarcoma has been recognized. Treatment is radical nephrectomy, but the outcome is generally worse than for RCC. Lymphomas are uncommon and generally occur as a manifestation of the systemic disease. Squamous carcinoma is associated with chronic irritation usually as a result of renal stones. Metastases may occur but are rarely symptomatic, and are most frequently discovered incidentally at autopsy.

BENIGN TUMORS MIMICKING RCC

1. *Renal adenoma*: This is a small, well-circumscribed solid tumor, which is clinically and radiologically indistinguishable from a small RCC. Most are discovered incidentally or at autopsy. Histologically it consists of uniform low grade clear cells. The relationship between adenoma and carcinoma is blurred, and some authors regard all tumors < 2 cm diameter as adenomas and all > 2 cm as carcinomas. If there is any increase in size during a period of observation, partial or radical nephrectomy is considered.

2. *Renal oncocytoma*: This is a round, tan-colored tumor comprised of polygonal cells with

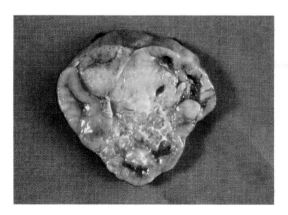

Figure 22.5. An excised transitional cell tumor obliterating the whole renal pelvis.

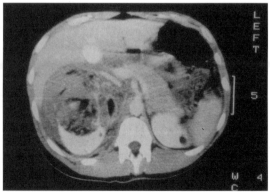

Figure 22.6. A CT scan showing a large angiomyolipoma of the right kidney. Note the low density (dark) regions which represent fat.

eosinophilic cytoplasm; it is frequently asymptomatic. The well-documented characteristic appearance of a central stellate scar on CT, or spoke wheel pattern of tumor vessels on angiography, is uncommon, and the majority are indistinguishable from RCC. Furthermore, many RCCs have oncocytic elements and biopsy is therefore unreliable. Treatment is partial or radical nephrectomy.

OTHER BENIGN TUMORS

1. *Angiomyolipoma*: The tumor contains variable amounts of blood vessels, muscle and fat. It occurs sporadically in 70% of cases, with a high female preponderance. There is also an association with tuberous sclerosis, in which the tumors are more frequently bilateral, larger, and present at an earlier age. The radiographic appearance is based on their high fat content. They are hyperechoic on ultrasound, and have heterogeneous density on CT, with the fat at around –40 Hounsfield units (Figure 22.6). Asymptomatic lesions can be observed. Large tumors may bleed and need embolization or excision by partial nephrectomy.

2. *Juxtaglomerular tumor*: These rare tumors secrete a renin-like substance resulting in severe hypertension. They are not detectable radiologically and are diagnosed by an abnormally high plasma renin. Treatment is by simple nephrectomy.

References

1. deKernion, J.B. and Belldegrun, A. (1992). Renal tumors. In *Campbell's Urology*, edited by P.C. Walsh, A.B. Retik, T.A. Stammey and E.D. Vaughan, 6th ed. Chapter 27, pp. 1053–1093. Philadelphia: W.B. Saunders.

2. Gore M.E. (1993). Advances in management of renal cell carcinoma. In *Recent advances in Urology/Andrology*, edited by W.F. Hendry and R.S. Kirby, Vol. 6. Chapter 6, pp. 81–102. Edinburgh: Churchill Livingstone.

3. Levine, E., Huntrakoon, M. and Wetzel, L.H. (1989). Small renal neoplasms: Clinical, pathological, and imaging features. *Am. J. Radiol*, **153**, 69–73.

Kidney Cancer

More common in men

Worldwide: Increasing incidence and mortality

Lifetime risk
in USA whites:
M   1 in 80
F   1 in 130

Relative five-year survival in 1983–87
in USA whites:
M   57.0%
F   54.1%

Risk factors
Renal parenchymal cancer
Tobacco
Obesity
Dietary factors
Renal pelvic cancer
Tobacco
Phenacetin-containing analgesics

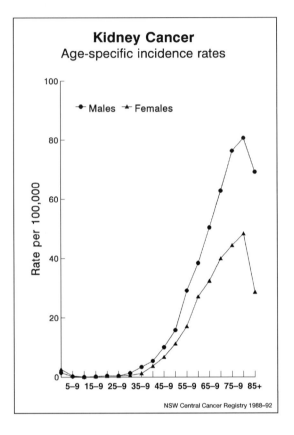

Geographical variation in 1983–87
Highest rate
M: 15.5 per 100,000 in Italy, Trieste
F: 7.8 per 100,000 in Iceland

Lowest rate
M: 0.7 per 100,000 in China, Qidong
F: 0.4 per 100,000 in China, Qidong

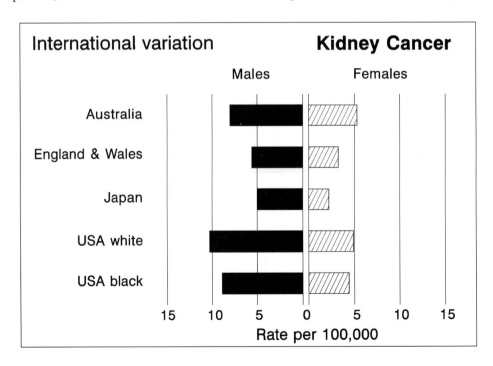

23. Bone and Soft Tissue Sarcomas

PATRICK BOLAND

Memorial Sloan-Kettering Cancer Center, New York, USA

The Greek word *Sarkoma* means fleshy growth. For the most part, sarcomas of bone and soft tissue refer to malignant tumors arising from tissues derived from the primitive mesoderm. This designation is based on embryologic rather than morphologic criteria. Therefore malignant tumors of blood vessels, although they arise from vascular endothelium, are sarcomas rather than carcinomas. Peripheral nerve sheath tumors are exceptional, since they arise in tissues derived from ectoderm. They are included because of the similarities in anatomic distribution, pathologic appearance and clinical behavior.

Most of these tissues form the supporting structures of the body. In the limbs they form the tissues of the locomotor system (bone, muscles, tendons), as well as fat and loose connective tissue. Visceral organs contain tissues of mesodermal origin in which sarcomas rarely arise.

There is thus a wide variation in the anatomic distribution and histologic appearance of these tumors which makes meaningful classification very difficult. Sarcomas are named and classified based on their histological resemblance to normal tissues. Benign tumors and well differentiated neoplasms, such as low grade chondrosarcoma or liposarcoma, present little difficulty. Poorly differentiated lesions or tumors whose cell of origin is unknown, such as epithelioid sarcoma, are much more difficult to designate. Electron microscopic examination and the use of immunohistochemical staining are employed to help better define these lesions.

While sarcomas are malignant, they vary in their aggressiveness and tendency to metastasize. At the present time, biologic behavior is best determined by the histologic grading of the tumor.[6] Grading is based on the mitotic rate, nuclear morphology, degree of cellularity, and the presence of necrosis. Low grade lesions more closely resemble normal adult tissues and have a lower tendency to metastasize. Pathologic diagnosis of bone tumors includes careful examination of their radiographic appearance in addition to the microscopic features. While histologic grading is the best predictor of biologic behavior, it has definite limitations which may be lessened with the increasing information derived from molecular biologic studies.

Most tumors of bone and soft tissue are benign. True sarcomas account for only 1% of all malignant tumors in the United States. They are relatively more common in children. This low incidence does not discount their importance to the practicing clinician since a constant awareness of these lesions will lead to early diagnosis that is critical in achieving a cure of the tumor with better possibility of limb preservation.

DIAGNOSIS AND STAGING

In addition to a pathologic diagnosis, detailed knowledge of the local extent of the tumor, and the presence or absence of distant spread, is essential prior to treatment. This information is necessary to plan treatment, provide the patient with a prognosis, and provide a uniform system for comparing results of treatment from one center to another. The performance of a detailed history and physical examination cannot be over-emphasized. A painless, mobile, subcutaneous mass present for many years indicates a benign diagnosis while the presence of a large deep immobile mass with no history of trauma, which is painful at rest, favors the diagnosis of a malignant tumor. A plain X-ray is the most useful test in the diagnosis of bone tumors. Computed axial tomography and magnetic resonance imaging are extremely useful in determining the local extent of the tumor and its relationship to adjacent neurovascular structures. A high degree of heterogeneity noted on examination of an MRI image of a tumor favors a malignant diagnosis. While these studies are good indicators of anatomic extent, they should not be relied on to provide information related to tumor biologic activity. New imaging techniques, such as Positron Emission Tomography (PET scans) measure metabolic activity and may permit assessment of biologic behavior. Bone Scintigraphy is routinely used in the staging of bone sarcomas. It outlines the extent of local bony involvement and will also demonstrate the presence of other lesions in the same bone (skip lesions), as well as distant bony lesions. Since the lung is the most frequent site of disseminated disease, chest X-ray and lung CT are essential parts of the staging process.

BIOPSY

The pathologic diagnosis can only be made by biopsy. This procedure requires careful planning and meticulous execution. It should not be performed until the other staging procedures described above are completed. The biopsy may be done with a needle or as an open operation. In general, the more tissue obtained, the more pathological examinations can be done.

Discussion of the advantages of one procedure over the other is beyond the scope of this chapter. It is essential that the biopsy tract be in a position that can be easily removed at the time of definitive surgery. In the limbs, biopsy incisions should be longitudinal. The surgeon should carefully select the portion of the tumor which is likely to be the most informative. The most lytic portion, as seen on an X-ray, of a bone tumor should be chosen. The

periphery of a growing tumor is more likely to contain viable proliferating cells than the center where necrosis is likely to be present. In distinguishing the benign condition of myositis ossificans from osteogenic sarcoma arising in soft tissues biopsy of the periphery is especially important. In the former condition, maturation occurs from outside in, while in the sarcoma, malignant growth is more vigorous at the tumor edges. Based on all these studies, the tumor is staged. Since different staging systems are used for bone and soft tissue sarcoma, they will be described under the appropriate heading.

TREATMENT

Complete surgical resection is the mainstay of treatment for local control of malignant tumors of bone and soft tissues. Up to 20 years ago most patients with extremity sarcomas underwent amputation. The dramatic improvement in imaging techniques, the use of adjuvant treatment modalities, and progress in reconstructive limb surgery have resulted in our ability to retain functional extremities in 85% of patients without compromising local control or patient survival. Surgical resection of a sarcoma requires excision of the tumor together with a surrounding cuff of normal tissue. This is referred to as a wide excision (Table 23.1). Involvement of the major neurovascular structures in a limb render wide excision impossible unless these structures are sacrificed, and is therefore usually an indication for

Table 23.1. Classification of surgical procedures*. (Enneking W.F., Shapier S.S. and Goodman, M.A. (1980). A system of surgical staging of musculoskeletal sarcoma. *Clinical Orthopaedics*, **153**, 106–120).

Margin	Local	Amputation
Intralesional	Curettage or Debulking	Debulking amputation
Marginal	Marginal excision	Marginal amputation
Wide	Wide local excision	Wide, through bone amputation
Radical	Radical local resection	Radical Disarticulation

*Classified by the type of margin they achieve and whether it is obtained by a local or ablative procedure.

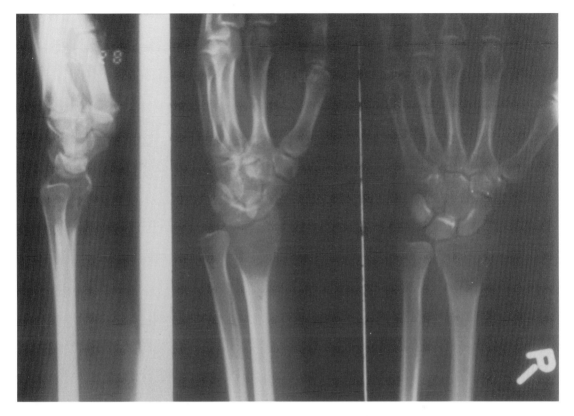

Figure 23.1.   Giant Cell Tumor of the distal radial epiphysis.

wide amputation. In tumors sensitive to chemo-therapy, e.g. osteogenic sarcoma, a good response may render surgical resection easier but does not compensate for an inadequate surgical margin. The types of surgical procedures are shown in Table 23.1.

Intralesional incisions involve cutting into the tumor leaving gross tumor behind. Marginal proce-dures shell out the tumor and therefore leave mi-croscopic tumor behind. Neither of these procedures are cancer operations, but are employed when doing a biopsy or treating benign tumors. Physical adjuvant treatment modalities, such as freezing surrounding tissues with liquid nitrogen, may be used in com-bination with these procedures in order to kill re-maining tumor cells in benign tumors. Such com-bined treatments are more commonly used in the management of benign aggressive bone lesions such as Giant Cell Tumors (Figure 23.1).

A radical resection is one that involves removal of the entire compartment containing the tumor. An example of this is removal of the entire femur for an intraosseous femoral lesion. Wide amputation is an amputation through normal tissue above the site

of tumor. Wide margins may be enhanced by the use of adjuvant irradiation. Radiation therapy may be administered by external beam and may be given pre-operatively or post-operatively. Advantages of pre-operative administration include:

1. A smaller radiation field is possible when tis-sues have not been surgically manipulated.
2. Tumor cells will be inactivated and therefore reduce the risk of implantation.
3. Reduction in tumor size may render an un-resectable tumor operable.

The use of surgery and pre-operative irradiation has been reported to achieve satisfactory rates of local control in the management of soft tissue sar-comas.[8] The rate is similar to that obtained by post-operative external beam radiation therapy. The theoretic advantages of pre-operative radiation therapy, however, are somewhat offset by the high rate of post-operative wound complications.

Adjuvant radiation can also be delivered using the brachytherapy technique.[7] Catheters are placed in the tumor bed at the time of surgery and are

Table 23.2.

Tissue cell of origin	Benign	Malignant
Bone	Osteoma Osteoid Osteoma Osteoblastoma	Osteogenic Sarcoma
Cartilage	Osteochondroma Enchondroma Chondroblastoma Chondro myxoid Fibroma	Chondrosarcoma
Fibrous	Benign Fibrous Histiocytoma Desmoplastic Fibroma	Fibrosarcoma Malignant Fibrous Histiocytoma
Vascular	Hemangioma	Hemangioendothelioma Hemangiopericytoma
Notochord	—	Chordoma
Unknown	Giant Cell Tumor	Ewings Sarcoma Adamantinoma Malignant Giant Cell Tumor

Table 23.3. Surgical staging for bone sarcomas. (Enneking W.F., Shapier S.S. and Goodman, M.A. (1980). A system of surgical staging of musculoskeletal sarcoma. *Clinical Orthopaedics*, **153**, 106–120).

Stage	Grade	Site	Metastases
1A	G1	T1	M0
1B	G1	T2	M0
IIA	G2	T1	M0
IIB	G2	T2	M0
III	G1 or 2	T1 or T2	M1

loaded five days later with Iridium 192. This will deliver 40–60 Gy over 4–6 days. Excellent results have been reported using this form of adjuvant radiation therapy in the treatment of high grade soft sarcomas with a low complication rate.[3] As with adjuvant chemotherapy, the use of adjuvant radiation therapy should not give the surgeon a false sense of security leading to inadequate surgical resection.

SARCOMAS OF BONE

The overwhelming majority of malignant tumors of bone are metastatic carcinomas and most primary tumors are benign. Approximately 2000 new cases of primary bone sarcomas occur annually in the United States. The incidence is highest in children and adolescents since the most common sarcomas, Osteogenic and Ewings, occur in this age group. Tumors, both benign and malignant, arise from any of the tissues which constitute bony tissue and are named accordingly. The cell of origin of some tumors is unknown.

The staging system for bone sarcoma was designed by Enneking and Associates and adapted by

the Musculoskeletal Tumor Society in 1980. The system is based on:

1. the histologic grade of the tumor — low grade G1, high grade G2.
2. the site of the tumor. A tumor enclosed within an anatomic space surrounded by a natural barrier, i.e. within a bone or fascial compartment, is said to be intracompartmental T1. A tumor which has extended through a natural barrier into another space or exists in a space without natural barriers, e.g. popliteal space, is designated T2. The tumor site is determined by examination of the pre-operative radiographic studies.
3. the presence or absence of metastases. M0 indicates no metastases, while the presence of metastases is indicated by M1.

Table 23.3 shows the Enneking staging system.

BENIGN BONE TUMORS

Since these are not sarcomas there will be but brief mention of them in this chapter. Many of them are developmental abnormalities and don't require treatment. Symptomatic lesions, such as osteoid osteoma or osteoblastoma, are treated with marginal surgical excision. Giant Cell tumors of bone deserve special mention (Figure 23.1). While it is benign, it tends to be locally aggressive and on rare occasions can metastasize to the lung ("benign metastases").

Epidemiology

Giant Cell tumors of bone represent 5% of all primary bone tumors. Its highest incidence is in the third decade and it is extremely rare before skeletal maturity. Unlike most bone tumors, it is more common in females.

Etiology

The cause is unknown. Giant Cell tumors of bone occasionally arise in Paget's disease.

Location

The epiphysial regions of the distal femur, proximal tibia, and distal radius are the most frequently involved areas. In the spine, the sacrum is the most common site.

Radiographic features

Typical lesions are purely lytic and are epiphysial in location (Figure 23.1). The bony cortex is thin and often expanded. Cortical erosion and extension into adjacent soft tissues may be seen.

Pathology

Grossly, the tissue is soft and is typically yellow and brown in color. Microscopically, the tumor consists of multinucleated cells whose nuclei are similar to the stromal cells.

Treatment

Surgical excision is the primary treatment modality. Its proximity to the subchondral bone of major weight-bearing joints renders effective joint sparing surgery difficult. Traditionally, Giant Cell tumors were treated with intralesional excision alone. This was associated with a 50–70% local recurrence rate. Curettage with bone grafting reduces this rate. Unacceptably high rates of recurrence prompted Marcove to add cryosurgery, using liquid nitrogen to curettage as a physical adjuvant.[5] The freezing causes necrosis of surrounding bone which may contain microscopic tumor. The procedure, therefore, increases the margin of excision. This treatment achieved a cure rate of 88% with preservation of the adjacent joint. Methyl methacrytate may be used instead of bone graft in order to reconstruct the bone. This achieves immediate stabilization and permits early radiographic detection of recurrence. For extensive lesions or in cases of multiple recurrences, wide excision and joint reconstruction or fusion is indicated. Radiation therapy should be avoided, since its use is associated with malignant transformation in a significant number of cases.

OSTEOGENIC SARCOMA

Osteogenic sarcoma is a primary malignant tumor of bone in which the malignant proliferating spindle cell stroma directly produces osteoid.[4] (Osteogenic sarcoma in childhood is covered in Chapter 24.)

Epidemiology

Osteogenic sarcoma is the most common primary malignant bone tumor. The estimated incidence is approximately two new cases per million per year. The tumor occurs most frequently in the second decade especially during the adolescent growth spurt. Ten percent of tumors occur in the over 60 years age group and are usually associated with a pre-existing condition, such as Paget's disease. Males are affected more frequently than females.

Etiology

No recognizable etiological factor is known for the vast majority of cases. Paget's disease may be predisposed to the development of the sarcoma in the older age group. It may also arise in other benign conditions, such as bone infarction or Fibrous Dysplasia. Post-radiation osteogenic sarcoma may arise as a late complication in normal bone exposed to ionizing radiation for the treatment of non-osseous tumors. It may also occur following radiation of benign bone tumors and Ewing sarcoma of bone. Abnormal functioning of the Rb suppressor gene located on the long arm of chromosome 13 and of P53 gene on the short arm of chromosome 17 have been demonstrated in Osteogenic sarcoma.

Clinical features

Typically, the patient is a teenager and presents with pain and swelling around the knee. A history of recent trauma is usually proffered; however, on closer questioning one can usually elicit a history of discomfort over several weeks. The area involved is swollen and the overlying skin is hot and often contains dilated veins. A pathologic fracture is the presenting feature in some cases.

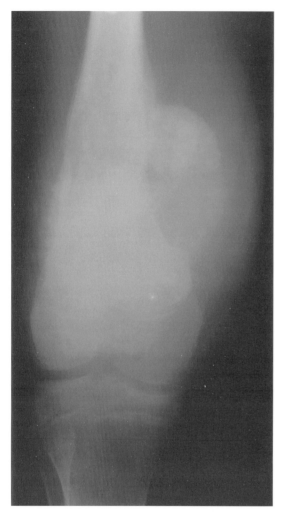

Figure 23.2. Osteogenic sarcoma involving the distal femoral metaphysis. Note the typical sunburst spiculation laterally and a Codman's triangle supromedially.

Radiographic features

The lesion is most commonly situated in the metaphysis of a long bone and may be lytic, blastic or mixed. It is poorly marginated and associated with cortical destruction and soft tissue invasion. Periosteal new bone formation in the form of a Codman's triangle and sunburst spiculation is common (Figure 23.2).

Pathology

The essential histological feature is that the sarcomatous stroma produces osteoid. Based on the predominant cell present, the tumor is divided into fibroblastic, chondroblastic, osteoblastic, and small cell osteogenic sarcomas. A small percentage of osteogenic sarcomas are low grade and usually arise in a juxta-cortical site.

Treatment

The tumor is staged based on the histology and radiographic studies. Most osteogenic sarcomas as Stage IIB at the time of presentation. The use of chemotherapy has dramatically improved survival in this disease. In non-metastatic osteogenic sarcoma, amputation alone achieves a cure rate of less than 20% while surgery with adjuvant chemotherapy has achieved survival rates approaching 80%. Treatment usually commences with pre-operative chemotherapy followed in 8–12 weeks by local treatment of the tumor. A wide excision is essential and in some cases this will require amputation. Following excision, reconstruction is carried out if necessary. Resection of bones, such as the clavicle and rib, require no reconstruction. Larger resections, which include joints, are reconstructed with custom joint replacement, insertion of allograft or arthrodeses.

If pulmonary metastases are present, every attempt should be made to resect them. High dose methotrexate-based chemotherapy protocols have proven very successful at the author's institution. Ifosfamide-based protocols are also effective. The use of biologic agents such as muramyl tripephlide phosphoethorelamine, which stimulates macrophage activity and is an extremely active agent in the treatment of canine osteogenic sarcoma, have recently been added to protocols. It is hoped that such agents will further increase survival. Patients with low-grade osteogenic sarcoma are treated with wide resection or amputation and do not require chemotherapy.

CHONDROSARCOMA

Chondrosarcomas represent a heterogenous group of tumors in which the basic neoplastic tissue is cartilaginous without direct osteoid formation.

Epidemiology

It is the second most common primary malignant bone tumor, accounting for about 20% of the total.

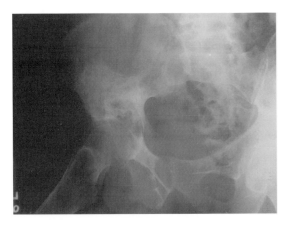

Figure 23.3. Chondrosarcoma of the pelvis.

While it may occur at any age, it most frequently occurs in the fourth, fifth and sixth decades. Males are more commonly affected. The pelvis and proximal femur are the favored sites of origin.

Etiology

Chondrosarcomas are divided into primary and secondary tumors. Primary, or central, chondrosarcomas arise in normal-appearing bone while secondary malignancies arise in pre-existing benign cartilage tumors. Pre-existing benign cartilage lesions include solitary or multiple hereditary osteochondromas, solitary or multiple enchondromas (Olliers disease) and Moffucci's syndrome (multiple enchondromas and soft tissue hemangiomas). Multiple hereditary osteochondromatosis is transmitted as an autosomal dominant trait with a high degree of penetrance. Secondary chondrosarcomas can also occur following irradiation and in Paget's disease.

Clinical features

Pain and the presence of a hard mass are the most common findings. Sciatica is not uncommon in large pelvic tumors. Chondrosarcoma most commonly occurs in the pelvis and femur. Patients with chondrosarcoma often have an abnormal glucose tolerance test.

Radiographic features

Central chondrosarcomas commonly occur in flat bone (Figure 23.3). In long bone, they occur in the metaphysis. Partial calcification with endosteal or full thickness cortical erosion is common. Extensive lysis is seen in high grade lesions. In secondary chondrosarcoma arising in an osteochondroma, the catilaginous caps is greater than 2 cms in thickness in skeletally mature individuals. Magnetic resonance imaging is used to assess the cap thickness. Clear cell chondrosarcoma is a histologic subdivision. It is lytic and occurs in the epiphysis of the femur or humerus.

Pathology

Tumors show abundant blue-gray chondroid matrix. They vary in cellularity depending on the grade. Binucleate cells are frequent. Chondrosarcomas are graded from I to III. Mesenchymal chondrosarcoma is a rare sub-type which has a bimorphic pattern consisting of cartilage cells surrounded by areas of highly cellular round cells. A particularly aggressive sub-type chondrosarcoma is dedifferentiated chondrosarcoma, in which a benign, or low grade, cartilaginous tumor is associated with a high grade spindle cell component.

Treatment

Wide surgical excision is the primary treatment modality for all chondrosarcomas with the exception of very low grade lesions where marginal excision or intralesional excision with adjuvant cryosurgery may suffice. Mesenchymal and differentiated chondrosarcomas have a particularly poor prognosis and should receive adjuvant chemotherapy.

CHORDOMA

Chordoma is a rare spinal tumor arising from remnants of the notochord. Fifty percent arise in the sacrum, 35% in the spheno-occipital region and the remaining 15% are scattered throughout the mobile spine. Wide surgical excision offers the best chance of cure. Radiation therapy is reserved for patients with surgically inaccessible lesions and patients with inadequate surgical resections.

SOFT TISSUE SARCOMA

Epidemiology

As in the bone, the majority of tumors of soft tissue are benign. The annual incidence of true sarcomas is 6000 per year in the United States of America.

Etiology

No specific etiologic agent is identified in the majority of cases. As in bone sarcomas, multiple genetic abnormalities have been shown to be associated with the development of these tumors. These abnormalities include allele loss, point mutations, and chromosome translocations. Inherited syndromes, which predispose to cancer, with demonstrable genetic abnormalities are described. Familial neurofribromatosis is associated with the development of malignant neurofribrosarcoma in 10% of cases. Mutations in the NFI gene and P53 gene are found. The Li-Fraumani syndrome is associated with germ line P53 mutations. Family members with this abnormality have an increased incidence of pediatric soft tissue sarcomas, pre-menopausal breast cancer, brain tumors and leukemia.

Environmental factors have been associated with the development of soft tissue sarcomas. Exposure to ionizing radiation has resulted in the development of both bone and soft tissue osteogenic sarcoma, malignant fibrous histiocytoma and others. It has been suggested that exposure to chemical agents such as phenxyacetic acids can result in the development of sarcomas. Lymphangiosarcoma can arise secondary to long-standing lymphedema. Sarcomas have been reported around foreign bodies implants, including orthopaedic hardware, but causal relationship is difficult to prove.

Diagnosis

Most patients present with an enlarging mass in a limb. They usually attribute the onset to a traumatic incident which may lead the unwary physician to diagnose a muscle rupture or hematoma. The depth, size, and mobility of the tumor should be assessed and a search made for enlarged regional lymph nodes. While sarcomas usually metastasize by the hematogenous route to the lung, lymphatic spread occurs in 3% of tumors. Hepatomegaly due to metastases from gastro intestinal metastases may also occur.

Imaging studies are similar to those described for staging bone sarcomas. Finally, a carefully executed biopsy is carried out.

Pathology

Soft tissue sarcomas have been described in almost every anatomic site. Visceral sarcomas arise in the gastro intestinal and genito urinary tracts. The majority of these lesions are leiomyosarcomas. In the retroperitoneum, liposarcomas and leiomyosarcomas are most common. Over 50% of soft tissue sarcomas occur in the extremities where the most common histopathologies are liposarcomas and malignant fibrous histiocytoma.

Classification of tumors is based on the histogenesis and has already been discussed. This can be extremely difficult in poorly differentiated sarcomas. However, since at this time virtually all these lesions are treated in a similar fashion, this is not a major problem. The histologic grade can be determined and this is a most useful prognostic determinant.

Staging

In order to fully evaluate the patient, estimate a prognosis, and plan treatment, the tumor must be staged. Several staging systems are available, none entirely satisfactory. The Enneking (Musculo Skeletal Tumor Society) system has already been described (Table 23.1). Since sarcomas rarely metastasize to lymph nodes, the TNM system used in carcinomas is not satisfactory, and because of this, the American Joint Committee on Sarcoma Staging developed a system which incorporates the histologic grade as well as the size of the tumor and the presence or absence of metastases.[1] A staging system used at Memorial Sloan-Kettering employs known prognostic factors.[2]

Adverse prognostic factors include:

1. lesions over 5 cms
2. lesions lying deep to the deep fascia
3. high grade histology
4. presence of metastases.

The tumor is staged 0–IV based on the number of adverse factors present. A tumor with metastases, irrespective of other factors, is Stage IV.

Treatment

Surgery is the primary modality of treatment for all patients. Resections must be wide. Intralesional and marginal excision are associated with extremely high rates of local recurrence. With improved staging studies and the use of adjuvant therapies, most extremity tumors are now treated with limb saving surgery and studies have shown that local control and disease related survival are comparable to those achieved with wide amputation.

Adjuvant radiation therapy may be used pre-operatively or post-operatively. It may also be given intra-operatively or as brachytherapy over a short period in the early post-operative period. Adjuvant radiation therapy has been shown to decrease the rate of local recurrence. When delivered using the brachytherapy technique, it is only effective in reducing recurrence in patients with high grade lesions. This improvement in local control, however, does not translate to improved survival. Effective adjuvant chemotherapy is clearly needed to improve survival. Administration of Doxirubicin-based chemotherapy protocols have been shown to reduce the size of the tumor, but studies have failed to prove a definite impact on long-term disease-free survival. Patients with resectable pulmonary metastases should be treated with surgical excision. A three-year survival rate of 25% has been reported in these patients.

References

1. Beahrs, O.H., Henson, D.E., Hutter, R.V.P. and Kennedy, B.J. (1992). *Soft tissue: American Joint Committee in Cancer manual for staging of cancer*, p. 131. Philadelphia: J.B. Lippincott.

2. Gaynor, J.J., Tan, C.C., Casper, E.S., *et al.* (1992). Refinement of clinicopathologic staging for localized soft tissue sarcoma of the extremity: a study of 423 adults. *J Clin Oncol*, **10**, 1317–1329.

3. Harrison, L.B., Franzesi, F., Gaynor, J.J. and Brennan, M.F. (1993). Long term results of a prospective trial of adjuvant brachytherapy in the management of completely resected soft tissue sarcoma of the extremity and superficial trunk. *Int J Radiat Oncol Bio Phys*, **27**, 259–265.

4. Huvos, A.G. (1991). Bone tumors: Diagnosis, Treatment and Prognosis. 2nd Edition, p. 85. Philadelphia: W.B. Saunders.

5. Marcove, R.C., Weis, L.D., Vagharwoller, M.R., *et al.* (1978). Cryosurgery in the treatment of Giant Cell tumors of bone. A report of 52 consecutive cases. *Cancer*, **41**, 957–969.

6. Russell, W.O., Cohen, J., Enzinger, F., *et al.* A clinical and pathological staging system of soft tissue sarcomas. *Cancer*, **4**, 1562–1570.

7. Shiu, M.H., Hilaris, B.S., Harrison, L.B. and Brennan, M.F. (1992). Brachytherapy and function-saving resection of soft tissue sarcoma of the extremity in adults. *Surg Gynecol Obstet*, **175**, 389–396.

8. Sielt, H.D., Mankin, J.J. and Schiller, A.L. (1985). Results of treatment of sarcoma of soft tissue by radiation and surgery at the Massachusetts General Hospital. *Cancer Treatment Symp*, **3**, 33–47.

Bone Cancer

More common in men and has comparatively young age distribution

Accounts for ≈ 0.5% of all cancers

Lifetime risk
in New South Wales:
  M   1 in 1525
  F   1 in 1900

Relative five-year survival in 1977–90
in South Australia:
  M   53.5%
  F   55.4%

Risk factors
Ionizing radiation

Geographical variation in 1983–87
Highest rate
M: 2.4 per 100,000 in Poland, Lower Silesia
F: 2.1 per 100,000 in Thailand, Khon Kaen
Lowest rate
M: 0.4 per 100,000 in Japan, Yamagata
F: 0.4 per 100,000 in Poland, Cracow

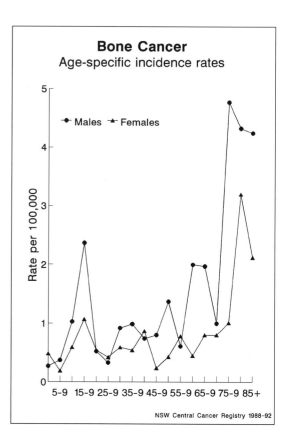

Bone Cancer
Age-specific incidence rates

NSW Central Cancer Registry 1988-92

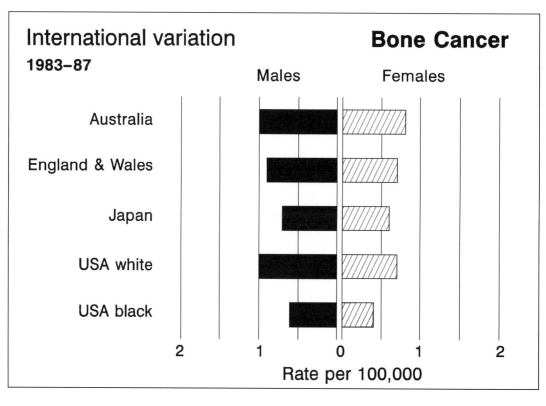

International variation
1983–87

Bone Cancer

Males   Females

Australia
England & Wales
Japan
USA white
USA black

Rate per 100,000

Cancer of Soft Tissue

Slight male excess
Increase with age is slight
Occur at relatively young ages
Relatively rare, incidence rates between countries
do not differ significantly

Lifetime risk
in New South Wales:
   M   1 in 375
   F   1 in 600

Relative five-year survival in 1977–90
in South Australia:
   M   62.3%
   F   63.8%

Risk factors
Ionizing radiation
HIV infection: for Kaposi's sarcoma

Geographical variation in 1983–87
Highest rate
M: 4.3 per 100,000 in New Zealand, Maoris
F: 2.5 per 100,000 in France, Martinique
Lowest rate
M: 0.4 per 100,000 in Kuwait, non-Kuwaitis
F: 0.6 per 100,000 in Kuwait, non-Kuwaitis

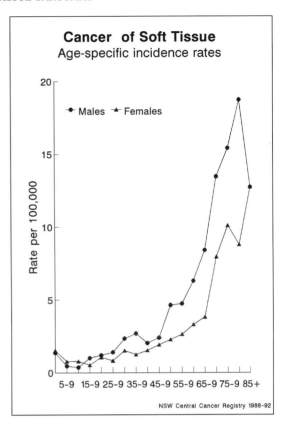

Cancer of Soft Tissue
Age-specific incidence rates

NSW Central Cancer Registry 1988–92

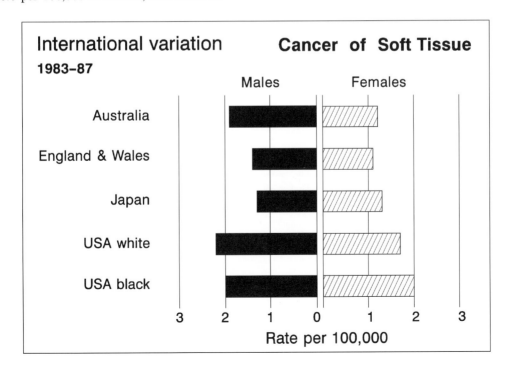

International variation 1983–87 — Cancer of Soft Tissue
Rate per 100,000

24. Hodgkin's Disease and Non-Hodgkin's Lymphoma

HELEN COLLINS and SANDRA J. HORNING

HODGKIN'S DISEASE

Hodgkin's disease is a disease of the lymph nodes characterized by the presence of multinucleated giant or Reed-Sternberg cells and a background of normal reactive cells.

Epidemiology

The incidence of Hodgkin's disease in developed countries is 3/100,000. In developed countries there is a bimodal distribution with the first peak of occurrence between the ages of 15–34 and a second peak in patients over the age of 55. The disease is slightly more common in men.

Predisposing and risk factors

The risk factors for Hodgkin's disease suggest both genetic and environmental factors. A small family size, early birth order, fewer neighborhood playmates and higher parental economic class are associated with the development of disease in patients who are between the ages of 15 and 34. These risk factors (which are similar to those for clinical Epstein-Barr infection) have led to the hypotheses that Hodgkin's disease may be caused by a common virus, if the initial infection occurs at an older age. There is also a correlation with certain human histocompatibility antigens, suggesting a genetic component to susceptibility. Patients with the human immunodeficiency virus infection are at a slightly increased risk of Hodgkin's disease.

Table 24.1. Rye classification.

Histology subgroup	Incidence
Lymphocyte predominant	15%
Nodular Sclerosis	70%
Mixed Cellularity	10%
Lymphocyte depleted	5%

Pathology

The diagnosis of Hodgkin's disease generally requires the presence of Reed-Sternberg cells, which are large cells with two or more nuclei, each with distinct nucleoli. The frequency of Reed-Sternberg (R-S) cells and the type of background cellular proliferation determine the subtype of Hodgkin's disease (Table 24.1). The pathologic diagnosis of Hodgkin's disease can be difficult as there are mononuclear variants of the R-S cell; R-S cells are not absolutely necessary for the diagnosis; and they can occasionally be seen in other diseases such as mononucleosis and non-Hodgkin's lymphoma.

Clinical presentation

Ninety percent of patients present with palpable peripheral lymph nodes that are firm, moveable and nontender. Approximately three quarters of patients present with cervical or supraclavicular adenopathy. Complaints of fever, drenching night sweats, and a weight loss of more than 10% confer a worse prognosis and are designated as "B symptoms." Other constitutional symptoms are fatigue, malaise, weak-

Table 24.2.   Ann Arbor/Cotswold staging system.

Stage I	Single lymph node region or lymphoid structure
Stage II	Two or more lymph node regions on the same side of the diaphragm
Stage III	Lymph node regions on both sides of the diaphragm
Stage IV	Disseminated to extra lymphatic organs, bone marrow, or liver
Subscript E	Direct extension from a lymph node into an extra lymphatic site
Subscript S	Splenic involvement
Subscript X	Tumor mass greater than 10 cm in diameter or greater than 1/3 of the width of the mediastinum

ness, and pruritis. Two to three percent of patients will complain of pain in their lymph nodes when they drink alcohol, a pathognomonic symptom of Hodgkin's disease. It is rare for patients to present exclusively with extranodal disease.

Investigations

Any lymph node larger than 1.0 cm and present for four to six weeks should be biopsied. A needle aspiration is not adequate for pathological evaluation. Once the diagnosis is made, a complete staging evaluation is extremely important because the treatment of Hodgkin's disease is determined by the stage at presentation (Table 24.2).

The staging evaluation includes a full physical examination, paying particular attention to the lymph node areas. Serum laboratory tests include a complete blood cell count, liver function (transaminases), renal function (creatinine), and alkaline phosphatase. The complete blood cell count may show a mild eosinophilia, a monocytosis, lymphocytopenia, a moderate leukemoid reaction and/or a normochromic, normocytic anemia. Nonspecific acute phase reactants, such as the erythrocyte sedimentation rate (ESR) and copper, will frequently be elevated. Patients with bulky disease, systemic symptoms or clinical Stage III or IV disease should undergo a unilateral bone marrow biopsy.

Radiographic evaluation includes a chest X-ray and computerized tomography (CT scan) of the chest, abdomen and pelvis. The lymphangiogram (LAG), which is a useful but technically demanding exam, is more sensitive and specific than a CT scan at evaluating the paraortic, internal and external iliac nodes and can detect abnormalities in lymph nodes even if the nodes are not enlarged. The CT

scan is more sensitive at evaluating porta hepatic, mesenteric, celiac and retrocrural lymph nodes.

A staging laparotomy was once performed on nearly all patients to determine the extent of disease below the diaphragm. However, now that combined modality therapies are used more frequently and the risk of subdiaphragmatic disease is more predictable, it is rarely necessary to perform this procedure.

Although it is not usually tested, there is also a cellular immune deficiency in patients with Hodgkin's disease, with impaired cutaneous hypersensitivity (anergy) seen. Humoral immunity is normal.

Prognostic factors

Stage, performance status, histological subtype, elevated lactate dehydrogenase, the presence of B symptoms, age, rapidity of complete response with treatment, ESR, the number of sites and bulk of disease are all prognostic factors.

Treatment

All patients should be treated with curative intent and the choice of treatment is primarily based upon the stage of the disease at presentation. The types of treatments available are radiation, chemotherapy or combined radiation and chemotherapy.

Radiation therapy

Hodgkin's disease usually disseminates by contiguous spread from lymph node area to lymph node area. Radiation therapy is, therefore, divided into "fields" that are designed to encompass involved and adjacent groups of lymph nodes (Table 24.3). The advantage of radiation is that it achieves better

Table 24.3.   Common radiation fields.

Mantle	Submandibular, cervical, supraclavicular, infraclavicular, axillary, mediastinal and hilar lymph nodes
Paraaortic	Spleen (if intact) or splenic hilum and the abdominal lymph nodes between the transverse processes of the abdominal vertebral bodies to the pelvic brim
Pelvic	Common iliac, external iliac and inguinal lymph nodes
Inverted Y	Paraaortic and pelvic fields
Subtotal Lymphoid Irradiation	Mantle and para-aortic fields

local control of Hodgkin's disease. There are few acute side effects, and the possibility of salvage chemotherapy remains if the patient relapses.

Chemotherapy

There are many active chemotherapy drugs in Hodgkin's disease, but the most widely used are MOPP (mechlorethamine, vincristine, procarbazine and prednisone), ABVD (doxorubicin, bleomycin, vinblastine, and dacarbazine), or a combination of MOPP and ABVD (either as an alternating or a hybrid regimen). The chemotherapy is given in cycles over six to eight months.

Other drugs that have known efficacy and have been used successfully in combination regimens include etoposide, cisplatin, Ara-C, methotrexate, CCNU, chlorambucil, BCNU, cyclophosphamide, and melphalan.

Treatment by stage

- *Stage I (above the diaphragm, not bulky).* Conventional therapy is radiotherapy of involved lymph node regions and adjacent nodal groups. Selected patients with very favorable clinical features and/or a negative laparotomy may receive supradiaphragmatic radiotherapy (mantle) only. Others should receive radiation above and below the diaphragm (subtotal lymphoid irradiation). Current clinical investigations are exploring the use of abbreviated chemotherapy and involved field irradiation in favorable clinical Stage I and II patients.
- *Stage II (nonbulky, asymptomatic).* Patients with favorable Stage II disease have traditionally been treated with subtotal lymphoid irradiation. As noted above, current studies are exploring the use of abbreviated chemotherapy and involved field irradiation.
- *Stage II (bulky or B symptoms).* Patients with bulky mediastinal disease should receive combination chemotherapy and consolidative irradiation.
- *Stage III and IV.* Chemotherapy alone or chemotherapy combined with radiation therapy to involved fields if there is bulky disease, particularly nodular sclerosing subtype, is recommended.

Note. In children, there is an attempt to limit the dose of radiation therapy to 25 Gy or less because of the effects on soft tissue and bone growth.

Risks of treatment

As the cure rate for Hodgkin's disease improves, the long-term side effects of treatment become increasingly important. These long-term sequelae depend upon the modality used.

For radiation, the complications are related to the technique, the total dose, the volume treated and the organs treated. It is estimated that 13% of radiation therapy patients develop a secondary solid tumor (particularly lung, melanoma, breast, thyroid, sarcoma and gastric). Radiation pneumonitis occurs in approximately 5% of patients who receive mantle radiotherapy and is manifest by symptoms of shortness of breath, cough and fever. Careful pulmonary function testing will show that nearly all patients have permanent subclinical effects. Cardiac complications also occur with mantle radiation including carditis, pericarditis and an increased risk of coronary artery disease. Other complications of mantle field radiation are hypothyroidism (30% of patients) and a transitory Lhermitte's sign (15% of patients) which is manifested by numbness, tingling, and electric sensations when the head is flexed. If the gonads are not properly shielded, radiation of the pelvic lymph nodes field leads to infertility in males and, even with shielding, results in infertility in females over 25 years of age.

The primary side effect of MOPP chemotherapy is sterility and an increased risk of second malignancy; in particular, there is a 3–4% risk of acute myelogenous leukemia (AML) over 10 years which is related to the cumulative dose of mechlorethamine received. With the ABVD regimen there is less infertility and no definite increase in risk of AML, but there are potential cardiac (doxorubicin) and pulmonary (bleomycin) toxicities, especially if the patient also receives radiotherapy to the mediastinum.

Results of treatment

The overall five-year survival is about 80%. Limited stage disease (I & II) has approximately a 90% five-year survival, and advanced stage disease (III and IV) has a 65–70% five-year survival.

Salvage therapy

If patients relapse, their chances of obtaining second remissions are affected by the primary treatment and, if chemotherapy was given, by lengths of their first remissions. If the first remission after chemotherapy is greater than one year, there is a 95% chance of achieving a second remission and a 45% chance of achieving five-year survival. If the first remission is less than one year, the five-year survival declines to 25%. Therefore, poor prognosis patients who never achieve a complete response, or relapse within the first year after completing therapy, should undergo high dose chemotherapy and autologous bone marrow transplantation if their performance status will allow it. Whether optimal treatment for patients who relapse more than one year later is standard chemotherapy or high dose chemotherapy with autologous transplantation has not been adequately studied.

Follow-up

If patients relapse, it will generally be during the first two to three years after diagnosis. The survival curve plateaus at eight years. The usual follow-up studies are careful physical examination, complete blood count, serum chemistries and chest X-ray. When clinically indicated, a plain film of the abdomen (if the patient has had a LAG) or a CT scan may be warranted. At five years, the risk of relapse is small, and follow-up is focused on screening for, and treating, the long-term side effects. Mammogram screening should start after 10 years for women who have received mantle radiation therapy, regardless of age. Because of the increased incidence of coronary artery disease, the importance of minimizing other cardiac risk factors (such as smoking or hypertension) is important. Patients who will undergo a splenectomy or splenic radiation should receive the pneumococcal vaccine pre-operatively or before treatment, but they remain at high risk for certain bacterial infections. Thyroid function tests should be checked yearly if patients received radiation therapy to the neck, and hormone replacement may be indicated for women who have undergone early menopause.

NON-HODGKIN'S LYMPHOMA

Non-Hodgkin's lymphoma (NHL) is a disease of the lymphatic system. The numerous subtypes are based upon histopathological appearance and immunohistochemical staining. Each subtype tends to have a characteristic presentation and course. As opposed to Hodgkin's disease, where stage is the most important prognostic indicator, in NHL the pathology is the primary determinant of prognosis and treatment.

Epidemiology

Approximately 20/100,000 people develop NHL each year. Patients develop NHL at all ages. Non-Hodgkin's lymphoma is slightly more common in men. The overall incidence and various histologic subtypes differ throughout the world.

The incidence of NHL has increased markedly in the United States over the past decade. A large part of that increase is seen in patients over age 60.

Predisposing and risk factors

The cause of NHL is unknown. There is an association with deficiencies of the immune system such as the acquired immune deficiency syndrome, organ transplantation, congenital immune deficiencies, autoimmune illnesses, and previous treatment with chemotherapy or radiotherapy. Viruses are closely related to certain NHL subtypes. The Epstein-Barr virus (EBV) is associated with nearly all transplant related lymphomas and 98% of endemic (African) Burkitt's lymphomas. The RNA virus HTLV 1 is associated with adult T cell lymphomas. There is also an association with certain chromosomal rearrangements such as t(8;14) in 90% of Burkitt's and t(14;18) in 80% of follicular lymphomas. Environmental exposure to certain herbicides increases the risk up to fivefold. Other industrial exposures such as grain mills have also been implicated. Recently, an association with ingestion of red meat has been suggested.

Pathology

There have been many classification schemas for NHL including those of Rappaport, Kiel, Lukes-Collins, and the Working Formulation. In 1994, a consortium of pathologists from the United States and Europe developed a new classification, the REAL (Revised European and American Lymphoma) system, which incorporates cell surface markers as well as histologic appearance to classify the NHLs (Table 24.4).

Clinical presentation

Although there are approximately 20 lymphoma subtypes in the REAL classification system, clini-

Table 24.4. The Revised American–European Lymphoma Classification.

Precursor B-Cell Neoplasm
Precursor B-lymphoblastic leukemia/lymphoma

Peripheral B-Cell Neoplasms
B-cell chronic lymphocytic leukemia (CLL)
Lymphoplasmacytoid lymphoma
Mantle cell lymphoma
Follicle center lymphoma
Marginal zone B-cell lymphoma — extranodal (MALT)
Hairy cell leukemia
Splenic marginal zone lymphoma
Plasmacytoma/plasma cell myeloma
Diffuse large B-cell lymphoma
Burkitt's lymphoma
High grade B-cell lymphoma — Burkitt's-like

T-Cell Precursor Neoplasm
Precursor T-lymphoblastic lymphoma/leukemia

Peripheral T-Cell And Nk-Cell Neoplasms
T-cell chronic lymphocytic leukemia
Large granular lymphocyte leukemia
Mycosis fungoides/Sezary syndrome
Peripheral T-cell lymphomas, unspecified
Angioimmunoblastic T-cell lymphoma (AILD)
Angiocentric lymphoma
Intestinal T-cell lymphoma
Adult T-cell lymphoma/leukemia
Anaplastic large cell lymphoma

cally it is useful to divide the lymphomas into low grade, intermediate grade and high grade as they are classified in the Working Formulation.

The low grade lymphomas tend to occur in older patients and are disseminated at presentation. They are an eclectic group in terms of their natural history and presentation, but the most common low grade lymphomas are generally indolent, with patients providing a history of months to years of waxing and waning adenopathy. Although low grade lymphomas usually respond to initial treatment, they eventually relapse and are considered to be incurable. The follicle center cell lymphomas (which comprise 40% of adult NHL) and chronic lymphocytic leukemia (CLL)/small lymphocytic lymphoma are the most common types of low grade lymphomas. These diseases remain confined to the lymph nodes, spleen, and bone marrow for long periods of time.

The intermediate grade lymphomas typically present in patients in their 50s as a rapidly enlarging mass over a period of weeks. Diffuse large cell and anaplastic large cell lymphomas are the most com-mon types (30–40% of all adult NHL). About 60% of intermediate grade lymphomas are nodal, whereas 40% are extra-nodal. These lymphomas are potentially curable with aggressive chemotherapy alone or in combination with radiation therapy. They tend to disseminate and grow rapidly and may be accompanied by constitutional symptoms such as fevers, night sweats or weight loss.

High grade lymphomas occur most commonly in adolescents and young adults. They rapidly proliferate, growing over days to weeks. Burkitt's, non-Burkitt's, and precursor B and T cell lymphoma/leukemia (also known as lymphoblastic lymphoma) are the diseases included in this group. Frequently, they involve the bone marrow or the central nervous system (CNS). T-cell precursor lymphoma/leukemia presents in children and young men with a rapidly enlarging mediastinal mass, circulating peripheral tumor cells and bone marrow involvement. The Burkitt's lymphomas are divided into the endemic (African) form which is EBV-associated and typically presents with jaw masses, and the non-endemic (non African) form which commonly presents as an abdominal mass and is less frequently EBV-associated (15–20%). The high grade lymphomas are potentially curable with intensive combination chemotherapy.

Investigations

Any rapidly enlarging lymph node or any lymph node larger than 1.0 cm and present for 4–6 weeks should be biopsied. A needle aspiration is generally not adequate for pathological evaluation because the architecture and pattern of lymph node involvement as well as cytologic features are needed for diagnosis. A careful physical exam and serum laboratory tests including a complete blood cell count, liver function, renal function, alkaline phosphatase and lactate dehydrogenase (LDH) should be performed. Bilateral bone marrow biopsies are recommended.

Radiographic evaluation should include a chest X-ray and a CT scan of the chest, abdomen and pelvis. In certain circumstances (such as indolent low grade lymphomas) a lymphangiogram can be helpful to diagnose and follow disease. Gallium scanning may be useful to monitor disease. In addition to the Ann Arbor staging system (Table 24.2), the Murphy staging system for pediatric lymphomas is sometimes employed in adult patients with high grade lymphoma.

Prognostic factors

The primary prognostic factors are the subtype of NHL as well as the patient's performance status, age and extent of disease. There is no internationally recognized prognostic factors scheme for indolent lymphoma. For the intermediate and high grade lymphomas, an international consensus, the International Prognostic Factors Index (IPFI), has been reached, where age > 60, elevated LDH, Stage III or IV disease, nonambulatory performance status and more than one extranodal site are considered to be poor prognostic factors. Stage IV disease, and in particular CNS involvement, together with elevated LDH are poor prognostic factors in high grade lymphoma.

Treatment

Low grade lymphomas

As 85% of these lymphomas are Stage III or IV at presentation, systemic management is indicated for most patients. Since low grade lymphomas are traditionally thought to be incurable, the treatment goal is to minimize symptomatic disease for as long as possible. If patients have a small tumor burden and are asymptomatic, treatment may be delayed until there is a clinical reason to treat; the policy has been called no initial therapy, or "watchful waiting." Alkylating agents like chlorambucil and cyclophosphamide with prednisone are first line treatments. Other active agents include the vinca alkyloids, doxorubicin, bleomycin, mitoxantrone, etoposide, ifosfamide, and procarbazine. The purine analogs, 2-chlorodeoxy-adenosine and fludarabine, are also active. The exceptions to this nonaggressive approach are the 10–15% Stage I or II patients who enjoy prolonged remissions and potential cure with involved or extended field radiation therapy.

Recent attempts have be made to cure follicular low grade lymphomas with high dose chemotherapy and bone marrow transplantation, but the preliminary data from these approaches suggest a prolongation of remission without an actual improvement in survival. Secondary myelodysplasias/leukemias are complicating this approach. Biological therapies with monoclonal antibodies and interferon are also being evaluated.

The length of remission in low grade lymphomas after initial treatment is approximately two years. Unfortunately, the remission intervals between relapses become shorter over time as the disease becomes resistant to chemotherapy. Also, 30% or more of follicular lymphomas and 1% of CLL will transform to a higher grade lymphoma (usually diffuse large cell), with a more aggressive course.

Intermediate grade lymphomas

These lymphomas are more aggressive than the indolent lymphomas, but they may be cured with chemotherapy. Patients with good prognosis (low or low intermediate risk on the IPFI) receive combination chemotherapy alone or with radiation therapy consolidation in Stage I or II disease. The most commonly used chemotherapy regimen is CHOP (cyclophosphamide, doxorubicin, vincristine, prednisone); however, there are several alternative, effective regimens using additional drugs or a more intensive treatment schedule for the same drugs listed above for low grade lymphomas. Studied in a large, randomized trial, none of these regimens was found to be superior to CHOP. Patients with either bone marrow, epidural, testicular or sinus involvement should undergo a lumbar puncture and receive prophylactic intrathecal chemotherapy because of the 10%–20% risk of CNS lymphoma. If patients relapse and their performance status allows it, they may be potentially cured with intensive chemotherapy and bone marrow/stem cell transplantation. A randomized trial has recently demonstrated the superiority of this approach over conventional salvage therapy.

High grade lymphomas

The lymphoblastic lymphomas/leukemias require aggressive treatment, very similar to acute leukemia regimens. The most successful treatments for high grade lymphoma have been borrowed from the pediatric experience with these diseases. All patients should receive prophylactic intrathecal chemotherapy and whole brain radiation indicated for lymphoblastic lymphoma. Consideration may be given to consolidative, preferably allogeneic transplantation, in suitable patients with Stage IV disease and an elevated LDH as they continue to be a high risk of failure.

Risks of treatment

The acute risks and long-term sequelae depend upon the modality used. The primary side effects of

Table 24.5. International prognostic factors index.

Risk group	N risk factors[a]	% cases	Relapse-free survival % at 5 years	Overall survival
Low	0, 1	35	70	73
Low intermediate	2	27	50	51
High intermediate	3	22	49	43
High	4, 5	16	40	26

[a]age > 60, elevated LDH, nonambulatory performance status 2–4, advanced stage (III, IV), > 1 extranodal disease site

chemotherapy are related to choice of regimen. Because there are so many active drugs in lymphoma, the choice of regimen can be tailored to avoid specific toxicities in patients who already have an underlying medical problem (such as avoiding doxorubicin in a patient with a history of congestive heart failure or bleomycin in a patient with pulmonary disease).

Complications of radiation therapy are outlined under the Hodgkin's disease section and are related to technical factors, total dose, and the treatment volume.

Results

With the follicle center cell low grade lymphomas, the median survival is approximately 10 years with a 70% five-year survival. In intermediate grade lymphomas (Table 24.5), the five-year survival of patients with no IPFI risk factors is 69%, but with three risk factors it is only 32%. High grade lymphomas have a five-year survival of 65–70% with aggressive treatment.

Follow-up

Low grade lymphomas

Because these tend to be chronic diseases, follow-up should be geared towards the individual circumstances of the patient. Generally, patients who are not on active treatment are seen several times a year with a physical examination, serum chemistries and a complete blood count. Radiological imaging studies also have to be individualized.

Intermediate and high grade lymphomas

If these patients relapse, it will generally be during the first one to two years after diagnosis. The usual follow-up studies are a careful physical examina-

tion, complete blood count, serum chemistries and a chest X-ray. Relapses are most frequently handled by patient observation and/or an elevated serum LDH. When clinically indicated, a CT scan may be warranted. At five years, the risk of relapse is small, and follow-up is focused on screening for and treating the long-term side effects induced by the treatment.

References

Horning, S.J. (1994). Hodgkin's Disease. In *Williams Hematology, Fifth Edition*, edited by E. Beutler, M.A. Lichtman, B.S. Coller and T.J. Kipps, pp. 1057–1075. Philadelphia: W.B. Saunders.

Diehl, V. and Engert, A. (1996). Proceedings of the Third International Symposium on Hodgkin's Lymphoma. *Annals of Oncology*, **77**, Supplement 4, 1–143.

Mauch, P.M. (1994). Controversies in the management of early stage Hodgkin's disease. *Blood*, **83**(2), 318–29.

Carde, P., Hagenbeek, A., Hayat, M., Monconduit, M., Thomas, J., Burgers, M.J., Noordijk, E.M., Tanguy, A., Meerwaldt, J.H. Le Fur, R., *et al.* (1993). Clinical staging versus laparotomy and combined modality with MOPP versus ABVD in early-stage Hodgkin's disease: the H6 twin randomized trials from the European Organization for Research and Treatment of Cancer Lymphoma Cooperative Group. *Journal of Clinical Oncology*, **11**(11), 2258–2272.

Canellos, G.P., Anderson, J.R., Propert, K.J., Nissen, N., Cooper, M.R., Henderson, E.S., Green, M.R., Gottlieb, A. and Peterson, B.A. (1992). Chemotherapy of advanced Hodgkin's disease with MOPP, ABVD, or MOPP alternating with ABVD. *New England Journal of Medicine*, **327**(21), 1478–1484.

Chopra, R., McMillan, A.K., Linch, D.C., Yuklea, S., Taghipour, G., Pearce, R., Patterson, K.G. and Goldstone, A.H. (1993). The place of high-dose BEAM therapy and autologous bone marrow transplantation in poor-risk Hodgkin's disease. A single-center eight-year study of 155 patients. *Blood*, **81**(5), 1137–1145.

Harris, N.L., Jaffe, E.S., Stein, H., Banks, P.M., Chan, J.K., Cleary, M.L., Delsol, G., DeWolf-Peeters, C., Falini, B., Gatter, K.C., *et al.* (1994). A revised European-American classification of lymphoid neoplasms: a proposal from the International Lymphoma Study Group. *Blood*, **84**(5), 1361–1392.

Horning, S.J. (1993). Natural history of and therapy for the indolent non-Hodgkin's lymphomas. *Seminars in Oncology*, **20**(5 Suppl 5), 75–88.

The International Non-Hodgkin's Lymphoma Prognostic Factors Project. (1993). A predictive model for aggressive non-Hodgkin's lymphoma. *New England Journal of Medicine*, **329**(14), 987–994.

Fisher, R.I., Gaynor, E.R., Dahlberg, S., Oken, M.M., Grogan, T.M., Mize, E.M., Glick, J.H., Coltman, C.A. Jr. and Miller, T.P. (1993). Comparison of a standard regimen (CHOP) with three intensive chemotherapy regimens for advanced non-Hodgkin's lymphoma. *New England Journal of Medicine*, **328**(14), 1002–1006.

Philip, T.C. Guglielmi, Hagenbeek, A., Somers, R., Van der Lelie, H., Bron, D., Sonneveld, P., Gisselbrecht, C., Cahn, J.Y., Harousseau, J.L., *et al.* (1995). Autologous bone marrow transplantation as compared with salvage chemotherapy in relapses of chemotherapy-sensitive non-Hodgkin's lymphoma. *New England Journal of Medicine*, **333**(23), 1540–1545.

Rohatiner, A.Z., Johnson, P.W., Price, C.G., Arnott, S.J., Amess, J.A., Norton, A.J., Dorey, E., Adams, K., Whelan, J.S. Matthews, J., *et al.* (1994). Myeloablative therapy with autologous bone marrow transplantation as consolidation therapy for recurrent follicular lymphoma. *Journal of Clinical Oncology*, **12**(6), 1177–1184.

Magrath, I., Adde, M., Shad, A., Venzon, D., Seibel, J.N., Gootenberg, J., Neely, J., Arndt, C., Nieder, M., Jaffe, E., *et al.* (1996). Adults and children with small non-cleaved-cell lymphoma have a similar excellent outcome when treated with the same chemotherapy regimen. *Journal of Clinical Oncology*, **14**(3), 925–934.

Soussain, C., Patte, C., Ostronoff, M., Delmer, A., Rigal-Huguet, F., Cambier, N., Leprise, L.Y., Francois, S., Cony-Makhoul, P., Harousseau, J.L., *et al.* (1995). Small noncleaved cell lymphoma and leukemia in adults. A retrospective study of 65 adults treated with the LMB pediatric protocols. *Blood*, **85**(3), 664–674.

Non-Hodgkin's Lymphomas

Slightly more common in men

Worldwide: Increasing incidence and mortality

Lifetime risk
in USA whites
M   1 in 55
F   1 in 60

Relative five-year survival in 1983–87
in USA whites:
M   50.8%
F   71.1%

Risk factors
Immunodeficiency

Geographical variation in 1983–87
Highest rate
M: 17.4 per 100,000 in USA, Bay Area, whites
F: 10.6 per 100,000 in Canada, Manitoba
Lowest rate
M: 2.4 per 100,000 in Poland, rural Warsaw
F: 1.1 per 100,000 in Romania, County Cluj

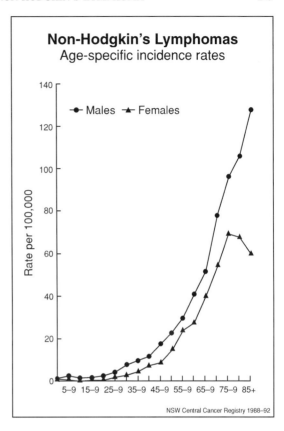

NSW Central Cancer Registry 1988–92

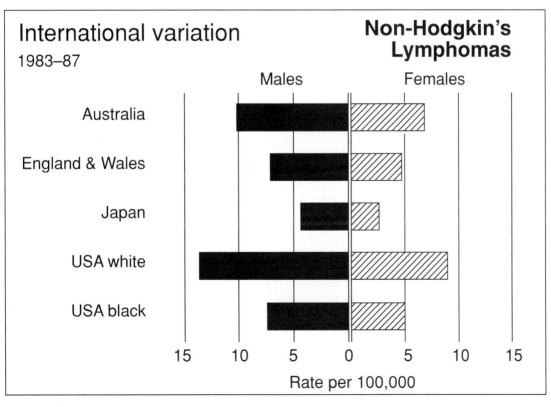

Hodgkin's Disease

More common in men

Worldwide: Decreasing mortality due to improved treatment

Lifetime risk
in USA whites
   M   1 in 350
   F   1 in 425

Relative five-year survival in 1983–87
in USA whites:
   M   83.1%
   F   90.3%

Risk factors
Sex and age patterns suggest infectious etiology
Epstein-Barr Virus is strongly suspected

Geographical variation in 1983–87
Highest rate
M: 4.4 per 100,000 in USA Connecticut, whites
F: 4.4 per 100,000 in UK, North Scotland
Lowest rate
M: 0.4 per 100,000 in China, Shanghai
F: 0.2 per 100,000 in Japan, Miyagi

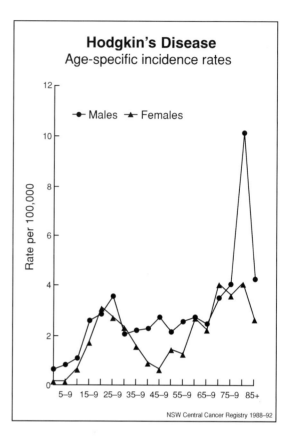

Hodgkin's Disease
Age-specific incidence rates

NSW Central Cancer Registry 1988–92

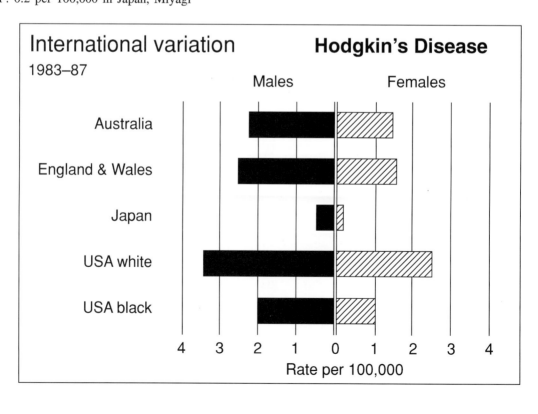

International variation   **Hodgkin's Disease**
1983–87

Rate per 100,000

25. Malignancy of Endocrine Glands

TOM S. REEVE

Emeritus Professor of Surgery, University of Sydney at Royal North Shore Hospital, Executive Officer, Australian Cancer Network

THYROID GLAND

While thyroid nodules are common, thyroid cancer is uncommon, accounting for approximately 1.5% of all malignancy and 0.5% of all cancer deaths. Of the large number of thyroid nodules occurring annually (15 million in the USA) only about 5% prove to be malignant.[1]

It is important for the clinician to appropriately evaluate thyroid nodules, as malignant lesions will almost invariably need surgery as the basis of treatment but some benign nodules will be able to be managed conservatively.

Nodules present clinically in one of three forms, as a distinct solitary nodule in an otherwise normal (not palpable) gland, as a nodule in a diffusely enlarged thyroid gland or as a gland in which multiple nodules can be felt, one of which may be dominant. If a thyroid gland containing a single nodule is submitted to imaging by ultrasound other nodules are likely to be found, which are impalpable and usually not of clinical significance. The great majority of nodules are benign; it is important, however, to identify and treat those 5% that are malignant.

Clinical features of the nodule which is either colloid, cystic, follicular adenoma, part of a multinodular goitre or cancer provide the clue to the diagnosis. Other factors such as age, sex, family history, previous irradiation and size are also important.

Age

Age is important; a thyroid nodule in a child has close to 50% risk of malignancy but in adults the risk diminishes to less than 10%, rising again after 60 years. Thyroid carcinoma is therefore a disease of the young and the elderly. In patients aged less than 14 years or those over 70 years 50% of clinical lesions are malignant.

Sex

It is widely held that thyroid nodules in males are more likely to be malignant; however, thyroid nodules, both benign and malignant, are more common in females.

Family history

A comprehensive history should elicit the existence of a relative with thyroid cancer, or a family history of Gardiner's syndrome. Medullary thyroid cancer (MTC) has a familial incidence of 25% and accounts for 5% of thyroid malignancy. It is transmitted as an autosomal dominant. When MTC is familial it may be associated with phaeochromocytoma and hyperparathyroidism. This is the multiple endocrine neoplasia Type II (MEN II) syndrome. The patient may prove to be an index case, or may have other family members with the same problem. The families of all patients with MEN II should be carefully screened.

Other contributing factors

Exposure to radiation at high or low doses increases the risk of thyroid cancer developing. Nuclear fallout has also been observed to play a part in thyroid neoplasia, with drastic effects of this following the Chernobyl tragedy. Living in an endemic or iodine deficient goitre area increases the frequency of follicular carcinoma. There is a growing body of information on the molecular genetics of thyroid cancer and it is expected that this will assist clinicians in planning their strategies and evaluating their patients prognosis.[2] Clinicians will be expected to better understand DNA technology and incorporate relevant aspects into practice.

Size

A sudden enlargement in the thyroid gland, particularly if associated with discomfort, is usually caused by hemorrhage into a cyst. Growth over a few months without pain or discomfort is most likely due to a neoplasm. These lesions usually have abnormal (atypical) cytology and 20–25% will be malignant at thyroidectomy. Nodules that increase in size while the patient is taking suppressive thyroid therapy are suspect for malignancy. Very rapid growth of the thyroid gland is usually malignant and if growth is uncontrolled, anaplasia must be suspected.

Physical examination

A number of physical characteristics of the thyroid are recognized as possibly being associated with malignancy.

About two-thirds of goitres are found to be multinodular when operated upon for a clinically single nodule. There is some argument as to the actual incidence of carcinoma in single nodules or in multinodular goitre with approximately 5% being an acceptable figure.

The nature of the gland and its *topography* and its *consistency* are important factors in clinical examination. Cancer is usually firm to hard, but some malignant thyroid lesions are soft and cystic, particularly when exhibiting moderately rapid growth. Stony hard lesions are usually calcified, benign nodules within a multinodular goitre or part of a degenerative process in a colloid nodule.

Goitres are usually mobile and should move on deglutition. When densely attached, "fixed", to surrounding structures the lesion is more likely to be malignant.

Significant cervical lymphadenopathy may indicate malignancy. It is not common in adults, occurring in only 15% of patients but it can reach 85% in children with thyroid malignancy.

Examination of the vocal cords by indirect laryngoscopy is an important component of physical examination of a patient who is hoarse or for whom thyroid surgery is planned. In a patient who has not undergone previous surgery in the neck and who has a fixed vocal cord together with a thyroid lesion, cancer of the thyroid is to be expected.

Clinical examination

The patient may be examined either facing the examiner or from behind. Either way the neck should be inspected with patient facing the examiner regardless of how the remainder of the examination is conducted; the thyroid cannot be visualized when the examiner faces the occiput. While the author prefers to examine the patient from anteriorly, many clinicians prefer the posterior approach.

Investigations

Thyroid function

It is important to determine the status of thyroid function for two reasons. Firstly, unsuspected thyrotoxicosis, especially in the elderly, must be excluded. Second, an autonomous or toxic nodule must be diagnosed at this stage otherwise FNB may give misleading results due to high cellularity (Figure 25.1). If the patient is clinically euthyroid, a serum thyroid stimulating hormone (TSH) level is usually sufficient. Free T4 and Free T3 levels can be ascertained if felt helpful, as can antibody studies. The determination of serum calcitonin levels is reserved for patients in whom medullary thyroid carcinoma is suspected.

Fine needle biopsy

Fine needle biopsy is a reliable diagnostic method for assessing thyroid nodules. The method is safe and can be performed in the consulting room. It causes minimal discomfort and does not require local anesthetic. The only significant complication occurs on rare occasions when aspiration may

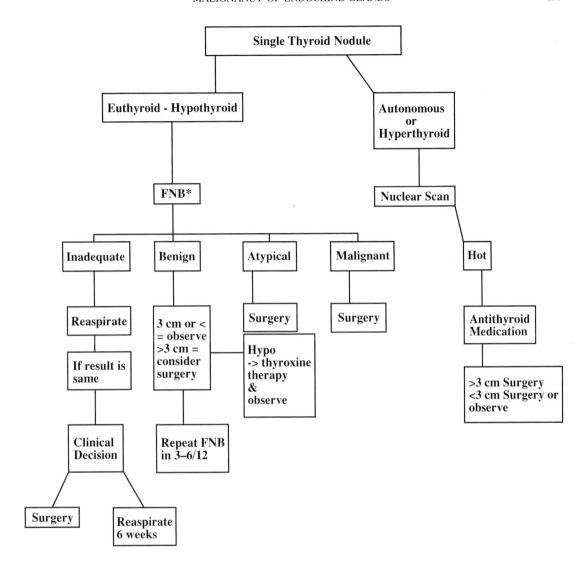

* FNB = Fine Needle Biopsy

Figure 25.1.

cause intraglandular bleeding which can be controlled by local pressure of a few minutes duration. The technique and its accuracy have been widely reported.[3] An essential component of this diagnostic process is that all slides, which need to be carefully prepared, are reviewed by an experienced cytologist.

FNB reports will be either inadequate, benign, atypical or malignant. An inadequate aspirate requires re-aspiration and, if still inadequate, treatment on clinical grounds. A benign aspirate is 98% accurate and the patient can be reassured, and treated conservatively with a repeat aspirate in six months. Papillary, medullary, anaplastic cancers and lymphomas can be clearly diagnosed on the basis of a malignant aspirate. Follicular carcinoma is difficult to differentiate on FNB and will fall into the atypical category, of which 20–25% will be found to be malignant and these malignancies are usually follicular in nature.

It is clear that sampling is an important factor in the process, as sampling inaccuracy may occur in small or large lesions. Adequate specimens obtained by guided needle biopsy under ultrasound control can assist in reducing inadequate smears after aspiration. An inadequate result should lead to re-aspiration. When cysts are encountered they should be drained and the aspirate examined cytologically, 70% are managed satisfactorily by aspiration. Large and complex cysts may be associated with a cystic papillary carcinoma and thyroidectomy should be considered.

Thyroid imaging

Radioisotopes, radionuclides
The thyroid can be scanned by nuclear medicine or ultrasonic methods. It has been customary to scan the thyroid with radioactive Iodine (^{131}I) or the radionuclide technetium (Tc99m). The scans are useful in revealing thyroid function or lack of it. A "cold" scan has been regarded as being more likely to indicate malignancy, although mildly or moderately functional lesions may also be malignant, while hyperfunctional "hot" lesions are much less likely to be malignant. The discrimination available with nuclear medicine scanning, however, is usually not helpful in clinical decision making.

Ultrasound
Ultrasonic scanning can show that a nodule is solid or cystic in nature and may demonstrate background nodularity. It can also reveal the presence of calcium, such as may be seen in papillary thyroid cancer. Once again, however, such information is generally not helpful in clinical decision making.

In most Units, fine needle biopsy has now become the first line step in diagnosis, reserving nuclear scanning and ultrasound evaluation for special situations.

Surgical treatment

Surgical treatment is determined by the pathological diagnosis. Well differentiated cancers, such as papillary and follicular, can be successfully treated by surgery in the majority of patients.

The minimum surgical treatment for a single thyroid nodule suspected of malignancy is total lobectomy, with preservation of recurrent laryngeal nerve and parathyroids. If pathological examination of the tumor, either by frozen section at the time or subsequently on paraffin section, confirms the diagnosis of thyroid carcinoma, further excision is generally warranted except for impalpable incidental papillary carcinoma where lobectomy is generally sufficient treatment provided life long thyroxine suppression is employed.

Papillary carcinoma

Papillary carcinoma is regarded by some clinicians as being a much less aggressive tumor and hence they offer minimal surgery. As better than 80% of patients do well, this approach has been in vogue for a long time. It must be said that those with recurrence and those who die of the disease are certainly out of agreement with the approach.

When a papillary cancer is clearly palpable, the favored treatment is total thyroidectomy. This procedure allows the use of radioiodine to ablate residual cells without imposing a high body burden of radiation. It removes multiple microscopic foci of cancer in the thyroid, observed in up to 75% of glands, and prevents recurrence in the contralateral lobe which has an incidence of 7% and subsequent 50% mortality. Removal also essentially eliminates the risk of a differentiated cancer becoming anaplastic. Furthermore, when the whole thyroid is removed serum thyroglobulin becomes a more sensitive indicator of tumor recurrence and thyroxine can be used in replacement rather than suppressive doses, thus avoiding the risks of osteoporosis.

While lymph node involvement with papillary carcinoma is high, local involvement has minimal effect on prognosis. It is imperative that all lymph nodes and lymph node bearing tissue in the tracheo-oesophageal groove is cleared. When nodes are palpable they should be excised and radioiodine should not be relied upon to treat them. External irradiation is rarely effective. Selective neck dissection of nodal levels III, IV and V with preservation of internal jugular vein, sternomastoid muscle and spinal accessory nerve is the recommended approach.

Follicular carcinoma

This neoplasm comprises about 10% of thyroid malignancies, presents more frequently in women and usually as a single nodule. About 60% are asymptomatic. Follicular carcinoma metastasises via the blood stream and may do this before becoming palpable. The tumors are readily differentiated from papillary carcinoma on microscopy. The lesion is virtually impossible to diagnose on FNA cytology as follicular or atypical cells indicate a follicular neoplasm predicating the need for treatment. Capsular and vascular invasion determine the diagnosis on histological examination. Older age, angioinvasion and distant metastases predicate a poor prognosis.

Total thyroidectomy and radioiodine ablation is the optimal treatment. The presence or absence of metastases is best determined by I^{131} scanning and the presence of elevated serum thyroglobulin in the presence of an elevated TSH. Lifelong thyroxine therapy is required, with serum TSH maintained at a sufficiently low level to avoid stimulation of any residual cells.

Lymphoma

Primary malignant lymphoma of the thyroid is uncommon. The number of cases, however, has been reported to be rising. Lymphoma is usually coincident with Hashimoto's disease in the thyroid gland and this finding has suggested that lymphoma arises from Hashimotos.

The disease usually occurs in elderly women, is diffuse or nodular on clinical presentation and lacks the hard consistency and invasiveness of anaplastic carcinoma with which it can be difficult to differentiate on microscopy.

While surgery was used as moderately successful treatment over many years, the only place for surgery now lies in biopsy of the gland to establish diagnosis. In practice, fine needle biopsy will usually establish the diagnosis and provide material for immunophenotyping and clinching the diagnosis.

In general radiotherapy, chemotherapy or a combination of the two is very effective for lymphoma confined to the neck. Surgical extirpation may rarely be necessary when acute mechanical obstruction of the trachea is present.

Anaplastic carcinoma of the thyroid

This is among the most lethal tumors known to man and there is little opportunity to undertake curative treatment at the time of presentation. It accounts for approximately 10% of all cancer and the incidence would appear to be slowly decreasing, but there is some geographic discrepancy in incidence. The disease occurs in the sixth and seventh decades and is frequently associated with long-standing goitre.

It is rare to have the opportunity to be able to clear the neck of tumor surgically and when done local and distant recurrence follows quickly, but it may avoid death from local causes.

There are two main cell types, large cell, resulting in early death and small cell which may result in longer survival but may in fact be inappropriately diagnosed lymphoma.

Total thyroidectomy, local debulking, radiation therapy and chemotherapy have all been advised to treat anaplastic carcinoma of the thyroid, an occasional longer term survival is reported, but most patients have rapidly progressing disease and are dead within 12 months of diagnosis.

Medullary thyroid carcinoma (MTC)

Ten percent of thyroid malignancies are medullary cancer. Medullary carcinoma is fundamentally a malignancy of neuroectoderm from cells known as C-cells entering the thyroid from the neural crest during fetal development.

Medullary carcinoma of thyroid (MTC) is found as a sporadic event in 75% of patients with the disease. Another group is comprised of those with familial medullary thyroid carcinoma (FMTC) in which medullary cancer occurs alone in a familial form, and multiple endocrine neoplasia (MEN); these constitute 25% of patients with medullary carcinoma. When medullary carcinoma of thyroid is associated with abnormalities in other endocrine glands, e.g. neoplasia or hyperplasia of the adrenal medulla as well as the parathyroid glands, it is classified as MEN II. MEN II is divided into two groups, MEN 11b in which group patients are marfanoid and have ganglioneuromata of lips, eyelids and gastrointestinal tract, and MEN IIa in which group patients lack these features. Thirty per cent of MEN II gene carriers will not develop clinical features of the disease.

As in other malignancies, early treatment of medullary carcinoma of the thyroid gives best results. Families with the genetic predisposition should be screened for plasma calcitonin, calcitonin being a tumor marker for MTC; this may be raised before metastases have developed. As the family history may be sketchy, it is probably wise to screen all families when MTC is diagnosed in a family member. Current genetic testing can give quite precise information regarding the familial or sporadic nature of MTC in any given patient.

Diagnosis

MTC can be diagnosed clinically in many instances. The thyroid lesion is usually hard and attached to surrounding structures. The lesion is usually bilateral and clinical lymph node involvement is a frequent finding. The lesion has usually been present for a few months. The lesion resembles anaplastic carcinoma clinically; however, the time interval of its presence is not consistent with that diagnosis which is usually associated with early fatality. MEN 11b is readily recognized by the associated physical changes coincident with MTC. Genetic testing of relatives is available if familial medullary thyroid carcinoma MEN IIa or MEN IIb is diagnosed.

The serum calcium should always be assessed and tests for adrenal medullary and cortical activity instituted where clinically appropriate. Biochemical and humoral markers including calcitonin and Carcino Embryonic Antigen (CEA) are diagnostic guides.[131]I-MIBG ([131]meta-iodabenzylguanadine) may be helpful in elucidating the presence of pheochromocytoma by nuclear scanning.

Fine needle aspiration cytology is a useful diagnostic aid where cytology may be enhanced with amyloid stain.

Management

Early thyroidectomy in those aged > 6 years in this situation may prevent disaster for an individual. Wells and his colleagues have used this approach and have demonstrated that detection of C-cell hyperplasia, the precursor of MTC, or MTC in its subclinical form, equates with higher rates of cure. If patients have an accompanying phaeochromocytoma, its excision should precede thyroidectomy and if parathyroid disease is present extra care and vigilance should be exercised during thyroidectomy so that parathyroid pathology can be dealt with at the same time.

A range of other syndromes can be observed in patients with MEN syndromes, e.g. carcinoid syndromes and ectopic adrencorticotropic hormone (ACTH) syndrome.

Optimal treatment for medullary carcinoma is total thyroidectomy even in the very young and appropriate management of lymph nodes if involved. Central node dissection should always accompany

thyroidectomy and modified neck dissection will be required if jugular nodes are involved; these are frequently fixed to surrounding structures.

Results of treatment when the patient receives total thyroidectomy and central lymph node clearance are much better than when corners are cut and less than total thyroidectomy or appropriate lymph node surgery is performed. Lymph node involvement adversely affects prognosis, survival being 80% at 10 years when node free, reducing to 45% when nodes are involved. The five-year survival is reduced when patients are older than 50 years, the disease is sporadic and the tumor less than 3 cm. Other growth factors and genetic diagnosis will undoubtedly prove more important in refining diagnosis and treatment as knowledge of their role increases.

CARCINOMA OF THE PARATHYROID GLANDS

Carcinoma of the parathyroid glands is a rare clinical problem. It is usually diagnosed at operation in patients with severe primary hyperparathyroidism, possibly with a parathyroid crisis,[4] although not all parathyroid carcinomata are functional.

Clinical features

There is no sexual predilection, males and females being equally affected usually aged between 45–55 years.[4] This contrasts with patients with primary hyperpara-thyroidism who are some 10–20 years older.

There is frequently a greater elevation of serum calcium than seen in benign hyperparathyroidism[4] and some patients present with hypercalcaemic crisis. The serum parathyroid hormone levels are generally high and continue to rise during the course of the disease.

The symptomatology follows that of primary hyperparathyroidism usually in a more severe form and thirst, polyuria and bone disease is featured. Bone pain and fracture are frequently seen and alkaline phosphatase elevated. Renal effects are common with nephrolithiasis and impaired renal function being major problems. Pancreatitis either in acute or recurrent form has been described, and peptic ulcer or dyspepsia is observed in approximately 10–15%.

On physical examination a mass may be felt in the neck, and this in the presence of severe hypercalcemia should arouse clinical suspicion of parathyroid carcinoma. In primary hyperparathyroidism associated with adenoma it is most unusual to palpate any tumor. Recurrent laryngeal nerve palsy has been reported.

Diagnosis

While diagnosis is infrequently made on physical examination, the clinical history and laboratory findings should provide guidance.

The diagnosis is usually suspected at operation when a large or very large gland that is very adherent to or invasive of surrounding tissue is encountered; the diagnosis is not usually made at frozen section. The gross surgical pathology features strongly in the making of the diagnosis. Histologic capsular invasion and blood vessel invasion, together with size of tumor and level of serum hypercalcemia, tend to clinch the diagnosis. DNA aneuploidy also points towards a diagnosis of malignancy. The only absolute criterion of malignancy is the presence of metastases, and these are usually seen in cervical nodes although they can occur in thoracic and abdominal viscera.

Treatment

Surgery is the only treatment that offers a chance of cure for parathyroid carcinoma. The extent of the surgery performed is dependent upon the degree of infiltration of the cancer and the presence or absence of cervical lymph node metastases.

In general the tissue associated with the embryogenesis of the parathyroid, the thyrothymic tract and the thymus can be removed transcervically. Excision of the pretracheal fascia, the ipsilateral thyroid lobe and local, modified or radical neck dissection depending on the degree of lymph node involvement completes the surgical procedure.

Long-term survival would appear to be dependent on the success of clearance of cancer from the neck. A rapid fall in serum calcium is indicative of clearance of the tumor if it is maintained.

Outcome

While 50% of patients with parathyroid cancer sustain cure, a small number — 5% — have residual disease and 40% have recurrence and are candidates for further surgery.

ADRENAL MALIGNANCY

Adrenal malignancy is rare but may occur in association with tumors of the adrenal medulla (pheochromocytoma) or tumors of the cortex (adrenocortical carcinoma).

Malignant pheochromocytoma

Pheochromocytoma represents neoplastic adrenal medulla; it is rarely malignant.

It is difficult to differentiate between benign and malignant pheochromocytoma on cytological or even histological grounds, as atypia, mitotic figures and even capsular invasion have been observed in benign tumors. When a pheochromocytoma invades sites which are free of chromaffin tissue, or metastasizes to such a site, the lesion is classified as malignant; many observers expect that metastases should retain their function if the pheochromocytoma is to qualify as a malignant tumor. Up to a third of malignant pheochromocytomata occur in the bladder wall. There is no large series to establish longevity in the presence of metastases which occur to lymph nodes, bone or brain. After initial treatment has controlled hypertension, its recurrence will usually indicate further metastases or local recurrence.

Diagnosis

This parallels the diagnosis for benign pheochromocytoma, measurement of urinary catecholamines, (Adrenaline and Noradrenaline). Localization of tumors can frequently be achieved by isotope scanning with MIBG [^{131}I] meta-iodobenzylguanidine which selectively concentrates in cells in the adrenal medulla.

These tumors occur anywhere paraganglionic tissue occurs and can be single, multiple or extraadrenal. Imaging with CT scanning or MRI can be very precise and reinforce localization with MIBG and assist materially with strategies for management.

Treatment

Treatment is surgical after the patient is carefully prepared with alpha adrenergic blockade. Anesthesia needs to be administered by an expert fully conversant with the pharmacological requirements of the patient during such surgery and in the recovery phase.

Adrenocortical carcinoma

This is again a rare disease occurring at a rate of about two per million each year. Some tumors are functioning, others are not.

Functioning adrenal cancers may produce any of the symptoms or syndromes observed in benign disease: hypercortisolism, virilizing or feminizing syndromes, hyperaldosteronism or mixed syndromes. Rapid onset of mixed syndromes in young people is highly suspicious for malignancy.[5]

It has also been observed that excretion of very high amounts of 17-K.S. (ketosteroids) accompanies adrenal cortical malignancy.

Localization

Pre-operative localization gives the best guide to treatment. CT scanning which identifies a large irregular tumor usually with greater than 7 cm diameter with varying density due to necrosis, is highly indicative of adrenal malignancy.

The vena cava may be compressed or contain propagating tumor and these features can be detected by caval venography.

Arteriography may assist in defining the vascular anatomy of the lesion.

Treatment

Treatment is surgical. When feasible, it usually needs to be radical and requires careful workup to ensure the patient will withstand the planned operation. Invasion or metastasis is common and frequently debulking alone can be achieved. This can assist in promoting the efficacy of a chemotherapeutic program.

Chemotherapy with o,p'-DDD, (mitotane) a mitochondrial poison can be effective in prolonging useful survival; it effectively reduces cortisol and adrenal androgens in 70% of patients, but reduces bulk of tumor in only 50%. Adrenal corticol carcinoma is not amenable to retroperitoneal laparoscopic surgery.

MALIGNANT ISLET CELL TUMORS OF PANCREAS — INSULINOMA

Insulinoma represents approximately 70–75% of all pancreatic endocrine tumors. The tumors are equally distributed between the sexes and the incidence is highest between the ages of 30 and 60 years. Approximately 10% are malignant.

Malignancy is difficult to diagnose histologically in endocrine tumors and even more so in pancreatic lesions, as the usual criteria for malignancy are difficult to apply. The sure evidence that a lesion is malignant is the manifestation of metastasis, the liver and local nodes being most frequently affected. Malignant insulinomas are usually larger than benign lesions and the time from onset of symptoms to diagnosis shorter.

Diagnosis

Patients with malignancy cannot be separated from benign disease by laboratory means.

The features displayed in Whipples triad remain important in making a diagnosis of insulinoma:-

1. Hypoglycemic attacks when fasting, often displayed as inappropriate behavior.
2. Blood glucose levels less than 2 mmol/L at time of episode.
3. Symptoms relieved following administration of glucose.

Tumor localization

Localization of an insulin secreting tumor is important in the approach to management and is first approached by CT with contrast and ultrasound; selective angiography is the next and most definitive imaging technique to be used if localization is not achieved by CT or ultrasound. When all three fail, portal venous sampling and measurement of insulin levels at various sites may assist in mapping the location of the tumor.

At operation the pancreas can be examined ultrasonagraphically; this assists localization and defining of tumor boundaries, and furthermore an experienced surgical finger can prove to be a very useful localizing aid.

Most malignant insulinomas occur in the body and tail of the pancreas so that biliary obstruction is rarely a problem.

Treatment

The treatment is surgical; the lesion should be excised with a margin of normal tissue when anatomically possible. This may require pancreatico-duodenectomy or distal pancreatectomy. Local nodes should be cleared where possible and liver metastases evaluated to determine their resectability.

Failure to clear the tissue secreting excessive insulin leads to other approaches as the patient has the devastating effects of persistent hyperinsulinism, diazoxide may be used to control insulin secretion and streptozotocin to treat the lesion and reduce its bulk, but it has limitations because of renal and hepatic toxicity. It can be enhanced, however by combination with 5-fluouracil. Malignant insulinoma is radioresistant.[6]

References
1. Jossart, G. and Clark, O.H. (1994). *Well differentiated thyroid cancer — Current problems in surgery*, 31. 12. pp. 944. St. Louis: Mosby — Yearbook Inc.
2. Leedman, P. (1995). Molecular genetics of thyroid cancer. *Bulletin of the Royal Australasian College of Surgeons*, **15**, 3–7.
3. Joasoo, A. (1992). Fine needle aspiration biopsy of the thyroid. (Editorial) *Medical Journal of Australia*, **156**, 675–767.
4. Sandelin, K., Auer, G. and Bondesson, L., *et al.* (1992). Prognostic factors in parathyroid cancer. A review of 95 cases. *World Journal of Surgery*, **16**, 724–731.
5. Luton, J.P., Cerdas, S. and Billard, L., *et al.* (1990). Clinical features of adrenocortical carcinoma, prognostic factors and effect of mitotane therapy. *New England Journal of Medicine*, **322**, 1195–1201.
6. Lo, C.Y., Van Heerden, J., Thompson, G.B., Grant, C.S., Söreida, J.A. and Harison, W.S. (1996). Islet Cell Carcinoma of the Pancreas. *World J Surg*, **20**, 878–884.

Thyroid Cancer

Most frequent cancer of endocrine system
Three times more common in women; female excess greater in young
Increasing incidence and falling mortality in several countries

Lifetime risk
in USA whites:
  M 1 in 425
  F 1 in 175

Relative five-year survival in 1983–87
in USA whites:
  M 91.8%
  F 94.8%

Risk factors
Ionizing radiation
In iodine-rich areas, increased risk of papillary type
In iodine-deficient areas, increased risk of follicular type

Geographical variation in 1983–87
Highest rate
M: 8.1 per 100,000 in USA, Hawaii, Chinese
F: 11.3 per 100,000 in USA, Hawaii, Chinese

Lowest rate
M: 0.6 per 100,000 in UK, South Thames
F: 1.0 per 100,000 in Poland, rural Warsaw

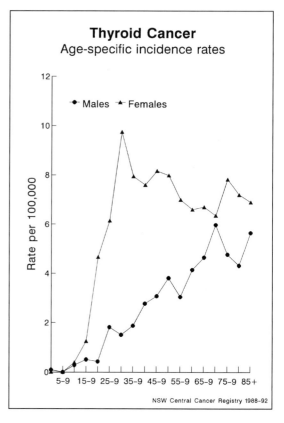

Thyroid Cancer
Age-specific incidence rates

NSW Central Cancer Registry 1988-92

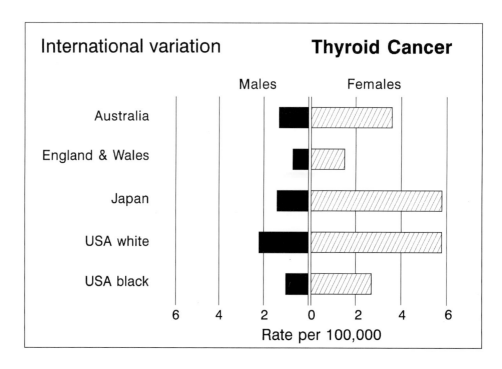

International variation   **Thyroid Cancer**

Rate per 100,000

26. Cancers of Unknown Primary

MARTIN H.N. TATTERSALL

Department of Cancer Medicine, Royal Prince Alfred Hospital, Camperdown, Australia

INTRODUCTION

Many cancer patients present with symptoms due to metastatic disease and the primary tumor site is detected by taking a careful history, clinical examination or occasionally by simple further investigations. However, a significant proportion of cancer patients, up to 8%, present with signs of metastatic cancer and detailed history, physical examination and laboratory investigations do not detect the primary tumor site. Patients who present in this way are described as having cancer from an unknown primary site. Over the past few years there has been considerable attention devoted to the characterization of this clinical syndrome and to the promulgation of strategies to identify those patients with treatable primary tumors from the majority in whom the benefits of therapy directed at the cancer are extremely limited. In this chapter, the clinical, laboratory and pathological features of patients with cancer from an unknown primary site are described, and a strategy for the efficient investigation and treatment of these patients is proposed.

INCIDENCE

Depending upon the definition used and the population of patients studied, between 0.5 and 8% of cancer patients will be diagnosed with unknown primary cancer. Unknown primary cancers are a heterogeneous group of tumors with varying natural histories. However overall, unknown primary

Table 26.1. Predominant site of metastatic disease at presentation in patients with unknown primary cancers.

Predominant site	Series (% with site involved)				
	Didolkar 1977	Osteen 1978	Stewart 1979	Kirsten 1987	Alberts 1989
Lymph node	49	16	14	14	12
Thoracic	39	11	24	29	19
Hepatic	12	19	17	18	30
Abdominopelvic	11	–	18	15	22
Bone	21	27	6	16	7
Neurological	–	9	8	8	2

cancer patients have a median survival of 3–4 months from diagnosis with fewer than 25% of patients alive one year after diagnosis. In most collected series, adenocarcinoma is the most frequent histological type followed by poorly or undifferentiated histological variants, and then by squamous carcinoma. Rare histological types include neuroendocrine carcinomas and melanoma.

CLINICAL PRESENTATIONS

Table 26.1 summarizes the major sites of disease at time of presentation in several series of patients with cancer from an unknown primary site published in the literature. Lymph node metastases are frequent, and about a third of these are located in the supraclavicular region. Thoracic and abdominal presentations are also common with skeletal and neurological presentations being less so. The wide variation of clinical presentations reflects referral sources and patterns of investigation/management.

Identification of primary site and treatable subsets

Most series report that the primary tumor site is detected before death in less than a third of patients presenting with unknown primary cancer, and in at least half the remainder, the primary tumor site is not detected if a post-mortem examination is undertaken. In those patients in whom a primary tumor site is detected during life or after death, the bulk site of disease at presentation is a useful guide to the most likely primary tumor site with by and large patients presenting with predominant infradiaphragmatic sites of disease proving to have primary tumors arising in the abdominal cavity while those presenting with supradiaphragmatic disease proving to have supradiaphragmatic tumors, most commonly lung or breast. A particular subset of patients are those who present with cervical rather than supraclavicular lymphadenopathy and these patients commonly have squamous tumors with a primary site in the oropharynx or nasopharynx. Female patients presenting with axillary lymphadenopathy not uncommonly prove to have an occult primary breast cancer or less commonly ovarian cancer. Apart from these clinical correlations, many studies report that the patterns of metastatic spread are frequently atypical for those patients in whom the primary tumor is eventually detected. Thus, for example, bony metastases are not characteristic of occult primary prostate cancer. Some authors distinguish a group of female patients with abdominal carcinomatosis which commonly has a serous histological appearance. This entity of extra ovarian serous carcinoma or coelomic cancer is recognized by many as a variant of epithelial ovarian cancer and the ovaries may be histologically clear of disease.

The pattern of disease at presentation has been noted to influence prognosis in many series. By and large patients presenting with metastatic lymphadenopathy, particularly those with cervical or axillary lymphadenopathy, have a more prolonged survival on average than those presenting with visceral disease sites. At least in some series, the better prognosis of patients with axillary lymphadenopathy has been restricted to women and presumably this subset reflects patients with occult primary breast cancer.

A diagnostic strategy in patients with cancer from an unknown primary site (CUP)

Since by definition patients have metastatic disease, in the majority the goal of investigations is to identify those patients whose disease course may be favorably influenced by local or systemic therapy, and in particular to identify those patients in whom "specific therapeutic strategies" may be effective. Thus it is important to identify patients with occult breast, prostate and thyroid cancer in whom endocrine or radioisotope therapy may be particularly effective. Rare patients with very chemosensitive tumors akin to germ cell tumors are also important since some of these patients treated with cisplatin-based therapy achieve complete remission and have a prolonged survival. As more effective systemic therapies for cancers arising in different primary sites become available, the strategy for identifying patients within the CUP category who may benefit from tumor "specific" therapy hopefully will broaden.

The need for an adequate biopsy

The initial strategy in patients presenting with apparent metastatic disease without a past history of a primary tumor is to obtain tissue on which the histological subtype of cancer can be determined, but also to exclude the rare case who may turn out to have a non-malignant cause for their clinical presentation. An adequate tissue sample is required and this can rarely be achieved by a fine needle aspirate. The strategy is to confirm the diagnosis of metastatic cancer before attempting to identify by investigating the primary tumor site. For example, in patients who present with clinical and radiographic evidence of liver metastasis without an obvious primary tumor site, a liver biopsy is the appropriate initial investigation and in one series 30% proved to have specific histological variants, e.g. small cell carcinoma or carcinoid thereby dictating the sequence of subsequent investigations which may be appropriate.

Once the histological subtype of metastatic disease has been determined by appropriate biopsy with attention to relevant immunocytochemical, hormone receptor and other simple characterization, it is appropriate to retake the clinical history etc. in order to explore symptomatology which may indicate the likely primary tumor site. A complete physical examination including a pelvic examination is an essential part of the assessment, as well as a chest X-ray. In patients with cervical lymphadenopathy and particularly a squamous morphology, formal ENT examination of the oropharynx and nasopharynx is appropriate and many advocate blind biopsies of these mucosae in these patients.

LABORATORY AND RADIOGRAPHIC INVESTIGATIONS IN PARTICULAR SUBSETS OF PATIENTS PRESENTING WITH CARCINOMA FROM AN UNKNOWN PRIMARY

Tumor markers

The case for measuring routinely blood Beta HCG, α-fetoprotein and PSA (the latter in men) is based largely on the importance of not overlooking an undifferentiated cancer with germ cell features which may respond dramatically to cisplatin-based therapy, but also on the sensitivity and modest specificity of PSA as a screening test for prostatic cancer. Some believe that CEA and CA125 should also be measured in patients with abdominal disease although the sensitivity, specificity and likely influence of these test results on treatment strategy and outcome is modest.

Routine blood tests

It is conventional to perform a full blood count and a biochemical screen but rarely will the results of these investigations be valuable in detecting the primary tumor site. The finding of hypercalcemia, and of metabolic derangement characteristic of "ectopic" hormone production may in some circumstances influence the probability of primary lung tumors, etc., but more commonly the results of these tests will signify only the extent of metastatic disease.

Radiographic investigations

In some clinical settings, radiographs may be a simple means of confirming a clinical suspicion of a likely primary tumor site. For example in patients who present with evidence of metastatic brain disease, a chest X-ray may sometimes identify an obvious but clinically occult primary lung cancer. In some cases, skeletal X-rays which demonstrate bony metastases with sclerotic or lytic characteristics may help to confirm the likely primary

Table 26.2. Radiographic investigation of patients with unknown primary cancer.

	Barium meal	Barium enema	IVP	Mammogram
Total patients tested	497	449	438	59
Positive	53	42	41	6
True-positive	28	22	15	6
False-positive	25	20	26	0

Data from Didolkar, Osteen, Nystrom and Stewart

tumor site in patients with other known metastatic disease. The status of abdominal CT-scan as part of the routine work-up of patients with metastatic cancer from an unknown primary site is arguable. A recent report of the diagnostic yield of this investigation and the likely impact on patient management and disease outcome has noted that although abdominal CT-scan in up to 20% of patients may identify the likely primary tumor site, in only very occasional patients has this investigation led to useful interventions or particular treatments which have impacted favorably on patient outcomes. My view is that abdominal CT-scan should not be considered part of the routine investigation of patients with CUP, but in those patients who have specific abdominal symptoms – backache suggestive of retroperitoneal lymphadenopathy, etc., this investigation may sometimes clarify the cause of the symptoms and thereby assist in the selection of effective treatments. Mammography may be a useful investigation in woman who present with axillary lymphadenopathy or in those who have bony metastases from an unknown primary tumor site.

The role of isotopic imaging in patients with metastatic cancer from an unknown primary is rarely to assist in the identification of the primary tumor site except very occasionally in patients with neuroendocrine tumors where an MIBG study may rarely identify the primary tumor.

Table 26.2 summarizes the status of specific radiographic investigations in patients with metastatic cancer from an unknown primary site, and indicates the limited value of these approaches to identify the primary tumor.

Endoscopy

Apart from patients with cervical lymphadenopathy with squamous metastasis, endoscopy is rarely of great value in patients with cancer from an unknown primary. On the other hand, in patients with

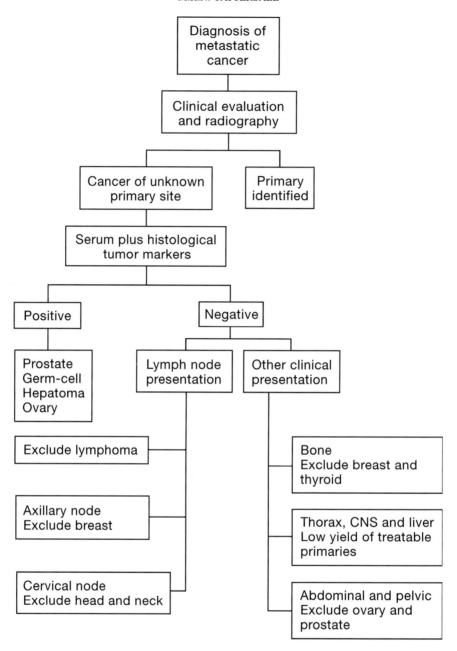

Figure 26.1. Identification of treatable cancer of unknown primary site.

obvious symptoms, e.g. hematuria, rectal bleeding, hemoptysis, and metastatic disease from an unknown primary, endoscopy may identify the source of bleeding and confirm a primary tumor site. However, rarely will this information be of major assistance in determining treatment although local treatment to bleeding sites may sometimes have a major place in symptom control.

A DIAGNOSTIC STRATEGY IN PATIENTS PRESENTING WITH CARCINOMA FROM AN UNKNOWN PRIMARY SITE

Figure 26.1 identifies a practical diagnostic approach which minimizes patient inconvenience and costs and is likely to identify all patients with "treatable" cancers.

Treatment

In patients in whom the above diagnostic strategy does not identify a specifically "treatable" metastatic tumor, the case for empirical therapy is not well made. While efforts should be directed at treating specific metastatic disease sites which are symptomatic, e.g. palliative radiotherapy to symptomatic bone metastases, etc., the impact of empirical systemic chemotherapy is rarely impressive. Some investigators have utilized tamoxifen as a semi-placebo treatment for relatively asymptomatic patients with metastatic cancer from an unknown primary, and have reserved trials of toxic chemotherapy for the younger than average patient with rapidly advancing disease. Few randomized trials in this setting have been reported, but platinum-based therapy, doxorubicin-based therapy and regimens including fluorouracil and folinic acid have all been advocated and have reported tumor response rates in about 20% of patients. Since the average survival of patients with CUP is about three months, the status of empirical therapy is questionable, but when a patient presents with features suggestive of a chemosensitive disease even though this has not been proven, a case for empirical chemotherapy directed at the presumed primary tumor can be justified so long as its effectiveness is assessed and the morbidity is not excessive.

References

1. Alberts, A.S., Falkson, G., Falkson, H.C. and Van der Merwe, M.P. (1989). Treatment and prognosis of metastatic carcinoma of unknown primary site: analysis of 100 patients. *Med. Ped. Oncol.*, **17**, 188–192.

2. Altman, E. and Cadman, E. (1986). An analyses of 1539 patients with cancer of unknown primary site. *Cancer*, **57**, 120–124.

3. Dalrymple, J.C., Bannatyne, P., Russell, P., Solomon, H.J., Tattersall, M.H.N., Atkinson, K.A., *et al.* (1989). Extraovarian (peritoneal) serous papillary carcinoma; a clinicopathological study of 31 cases. *Cancer*, **64**, 110–115.

4. Didolkar, M.S., Fanous, N., Elias, E.G. and Moore, R.H. (1977). Metastatic carcinomas from occult primary tumors. *Annals of Surgery*, **186**, 625–630.

5. Kirsten, F., Chi, C.H., Leary, J.A., Ng, A.B.P., Hedley, D.W. and Tattersall, M.H.N. (1987). Metastatic adeno or undifferentiated carcinoma from an unknown primary site: natural history, and guidelines for identification of treatable subsets. *Quart. J. Med.*, **62**, 143–161.

6. Nystrom, J.S., Weiner, J.M., Wolf, R.M., Bateman, J.R. and Viola, M.V. (1979). Identifying the primary site in metastatic cancer of unknown primary origins, inadequacy of roentgenographic procedures. *J.A.M.A.*, **241**, 381–383.

7. Osteen, R T., Kopf, G. and Wilson R.E. (1978). In pursuit of the unknown primary. *Am. J. Surg.*, **135**, 494–498.

8. Stewart, J.F., Tattersall M.H.N., Woods, R.C. and Fox, R.M. (1979). Unknown primary adenocarcinoma, incidence of overinvestigation and natural history. *Brit. Med. J.*, **1**, 1530–1533.

27. Childhood Cancer

MICHAEL BURGESS and MARTIN MOTT

Bristol Royal Hospital for Sick Children, St. Michael's Hill, Bristol, UK

Childhood cancer is rare and accounts for about 1% of all malignancies. It is, however, the second commonest cause of death in children between 1 and 14 years of age (16% of all deaths in this age group).[1] Although pediatric malignancies are rare, they must be included in the differential diagnosis for many different clinical presentations since delay in diagnosis may adversely effect outcome.

The management of children with malignant disease differs in many respects from that of adults and should take place wherever possible in a child-orientated environment. Most adult tumors are carcinomas and are usually classified by their site of origin; pediatric tumors arise from a variety of different tissues and are therefore classified by histological type. Tumor types common to both adults and children, such as lymphoma and leukemia, differ in their biology, behaviour and prognosis and hence demand different treatment. Some embryonal tumors presenting in infancy undergo spontaneous remission or maturation.

The optimal management of children with cancer is achieved by close interaction between medical, nursing, social and educational services together with the active co-operation of the parents. The medical needs of the child must be delivered in an environment which can respond to the differing needs of each age group. Periods of hospitalization should be kept to a minimum during which time efforts should be made to continue education and development. The child should be encouraged to return to a normal family routine and to school as soon as is feasible. Adolescents are a special group in which the growing need for independence may be threatened by extrinsic forces (disease, treatment regimens, hospital routines). Alopecia, sickness and even mutilation consequent on treatment may adversely affect body image. Support too for the parents and siblings is essential. Family facilities within the hospital are a fundamental part of helping them to continue to function as an effective unit.

EPIDEMIOLOGY

The annual incidence of pediatric malignancy in the South-West Region of the UK is 111/million children under 15 years of age (Table 27.1). This figure agrees closely with those found in other regions of the UK and in the USA. The age at presentation shows a bimodal distribution, with one peak between 2 and 4 years and another between 12 and 14 years of age.[2]

Table 27.1. The relative incidence of pediatric malignancy by tumor type in South-West England (1976–1985).

Tumor type	Relative incidence
Acute lymphoblastic leukemia	29.6%
Brain tumors	24.0%
Lymphoma	8.3%
Wilms' tumor	6.8%
Acute non-lymphoblastic leukemia	6.7%
Rhabdomyosarcoma	4.7%
Bone tumor	4.1%
Neuroblastoma	3.7%
Others	12.7%

Many childhood malignancies are more common in boys. There are worldwide variations in the incidence of certain types of tumors, which may have etiological implications. For example, in the USA, Ewing's sarcoma is seldom seen in African Americans and the incidence of leukemia in this group is also far lower than in Caucasians. The concept that the incidence of nephroblastoma (Wilms' tumor) is relatively consistent worldwide is now being challenged.

ETIOLOGY

In most cases the cause of childhood malignancy remains unknown and some of the most favored hypotheses are currently the subject of a national study. In a small number of cases an etiological agent, such as viruses, drugs or radiation, may be identified (e.g. Epstein-Barr virus and lymphoma, Hepatitis B and hepatocellular carcinoma and transplacental diethylstilboestrol and clear-cell sarcoma of the vagina).

Currently the contribution played by the genetic constitution is under considerable scrutiny. Nonrandom cytogenetic abnormalities occur not uncommonly in tumor cells (e.g. deletion at chromosome 11p in Wilms' tumor and at 13q in retinoblastoma, translocation between chromosomes 11 and 22 in Ewing's tumor and 8 and 14 in lymphoma). Over 200 single gene disorders are associated with an increased incidence of neoplasia. These include cutaneous syndromes (e.g. neurofibromatosis), defects of DNA repair (e.g. Xeroderma Pigmentosum) and immune deficiency (e.g. Wiskott Aldrich syndrome and Bruton's Agammaglobulinaemia). Importantly a further genetic mechanism of neoplasia is the loss of function of tumor suppressor genes e.g. loss of WTI function in Wilms' tumor and p53 function in the family cancer syndrome (Li-Fraumeni syndrome). An increasing proportion of childhood malignancies are best defined by specific genetic abnormalities rather than by conventional pathological techniques.

INVESTIGATIONS

If there are reasonable grounds to suspect a malignancy, appropriate investigations must be undertaken urgently. Radiological examination will depend on the nature of the suspected lesion and the facilities available. Taking this into consideration, appropriate advice should be sought from the regional paediatric oncology unit. Biopsy should ideally, only be performed in regional specialist centers where the necessary support services are available (e.g. molecular biology services) and once radiological examination of the lesion is complete. Biopsy sites must be within potential radiation fields, as malignant cells may seed along the biopsy track. Staging investigations may be performed following biopsy. Biological markers should be obtained prior to surgery, e.g. urinary catecholeamines for neuroblastoma, lactate dehydrogenase in lymphoma and α-fetoprotein in germ cell tumors.

STAGING

Once the diagnosis has been confirmed, the extent of the tumor must be established:

- The staging of the disease directs the treatment given and should help to avoid excessive therapy; in easily curable conditions, excessive therapy is known to put the child at increased risk of adverse late effects of treatment.
- The stage of the disease also tends to reflect the prognosis and, consequently, aids the counseling of both child and parents.
- Staging systems generally progress from localized disease (stage 1) to widespread disease (stage 4) and are based on results obtained from clinical examination, radiodiagnosis and pathology.

TREATMENT

Surgery, radiotherapy and chemotherapy are the primary modalities used in the treatment of childhood malignancy. The treatment regimen employed depends on the pathology and the stage of the disease. Most treatment schedules involve cyclical chemotherapy together with individually tailored courses of radiotherapy and surgical intervention. This cyclical approach to therapy is designed to reduce the emergence of resistant clones of malignant cells.

Radiotherapy is associated with specific problems. It requires that the child remain motionless in isolation while the dose is administered. In the treatment of brain tumors in particular, there is the additional constraint of a mask. (A clear plastic mask is constructed from a plaster mold of the child's head. This is attached to the radiotherapy table and the child then lies on the table with either his face or head in the mask. This allows accurate and precise application of the radiotherapy field.) Skilled play leaders and considerable patience can often avoid the need for repeated sedation or general anesthetic. Radiation damage to immature organ systems gives rise to significant treatment morbidity. Radiation should be avoided altogether where possible in children under the age of 2 years.

Bone marrow toxicity has in the past limited the dose of chemotherapeutic agents which can be administered. For solid tumors of poor prognosis, with standard treatment regimens, high dose single or multiple agent chemotherapy can be administered with the support of rescue procedures such as cytokine (e.g. G-CSF) administration, autologous or allogeneic bone marrow transplant or more recently peripheral blood stem cell transplantation. These regimens remain experimental at present.

Competent care for the child must include care of the whole family. Parents and siblings are often also fearful of the disease, its treatment and its prognosis. Feelings of guilt, anger and hopelessness are common and need to be managed actively.

PROGNOSIS

The prognosis for many childhood malignancies has improved dramatically over the past 30 years. The five-year survival rate for all childhood malignancies was 68% for children treated at this center in the decade 1980–89 (Table 27.2). The cure rate

Table 27.3. Factors adversely affected by treatment for childhood malignancy.

- Growth
- Thyroid function (radiation)
- Secondary sexual development
- Fertility (radiation and cyclophosphamide)
- Pregnancy outcome (radiotherapy may affect uterine size and vascular supply, and both surgery and radiotherapy may affect the bones of the pelvis)
- Intelligence (cranial radiation — dose related)
- Education (time out of school)
- Hearing (cisplatin, aminoglycosides)
- Peripheral neural function
- Musculoskeletal development (selective radiation)
- Cardiac function (myopathy from anthracyclines)
- Pulmonary function (fibrosis from bleomycin, methotrexate)
- Renal function (radiation, cisplatin, methotrexate)
- DNA repair leading to secondary tumors (alkylating agents, radiation)

for Wilms' tumor stage I is 98%, the five-year survival rate for childhood lymphoblastic leukemia or lymphoma, which was once universally fatal, is about 75% in some centers and an increasing proportion of many other solid tumors can be cured. However, the prognosis for patients presenting with widespread metastatic disease, especially those with neuroblastoma, rhabdomyosarcoma and Ewing's sarcoma, remains relatively poor.

LATE EFFECTS OF TREATMENT

Although the majority of children can nowadays be cured of their cancer treatment continues to exact a toll. In addition to the acute effects of chemotherapy and radiotherapy there are significant long-term sequelae of the treatments on growing and developing organ systems.

Emphasis is thus increasingly being focused on the morbidity following treatment. Many areas of concern have been identified and strategies have been devised to reduce the impact of many of these problems (Table 27.3). These are important public health issues, as 1 in 1000 young people entering adult life is now a survivor of childhood cancer.

Table 27.2. A comparison of the overall five-year survival (%) for all malignancies and that defined by tumor type for the decades 1970–79 and 1980–89.

Diagnosis	1970–79	1980–89
All malignancies	53	68
ALL	60	76
ANLL	7	44
Non-Hodgkin's lymphoma	52	74
Wilms'tumor	85	91
Neuroblastoma	24	43
Rhabdomyosarcoma	48	68
Bone tumors	35	56

LEUKEMIA

Acute lymphoblastic leukemia (ALL)[3] is the commonest malignancy of childhood. It accounts for

75% of all leukemias in this age group. Acute myeloid leukemia (AML) occurs less frequently. Chronic myeloid leukemia (CML), both adult type with a t(9;22) translocation and juvenile type with an elevated HbF, occur rarely.

Acute lymphoblastic leukemia

The prevalence is approximately 1 in 3000. In the UK the peak incidence of ALL is among 3–4-year-olds. It is more common in boys in whom the prognosis is worse. ALL is rare under the age of 1 year and is then often associated with a particular chromosomal translocation, t(4;11)(q21;q23), which confers a poorer prognosis. There is an increased prevalence in siblings (1 in 720) and with certain genetic and DNA fragility syndromes (Down syndrome 1 in 95 and Bloom's syndrome 1 in 8). Leukemia clusters around power lines and nuclear installations have been widely reported in the press, but there is no proven causal association.

A variety of karyotypic and cytogenetic abnormalities have been described in ALL. Ploidy (chromosome number) has been shown to be a prognostic indicator. Children with greater than 50 chromosomes have the best prognosis and those with near-haploidy the worst. The translocations t(8;14), t(4;11), t(l;19) and t(9;22) have high rates of early treatment failure while a translocation between chromosomes 12 and 21 which is present in 16% of childhood B-lineage ALL defines a good prognostic group.

Cell surface markers are used to characterize the cell of origin and stage of differentiation.[4] Subclasses of ALL recognized by immunophenotyping include Common ALL, which is the most prevalent and has the best prognosis, T-cell ALL, which presents with a mediastinal mass and often a high white cell count, B-cell ALL, which may be similar to B-cell lymphoma in presentation and treatment and null ALL which has the worst.[4]

Thus, for example, the best prognosis is for girls aged between 2 and 10 years, with a presenting white cell count less than 50×10^9 cells/1, common immunophenotype, hyperdiploidy and with clearance of bone marrow blasts by Day 14 of treatment.

Clinical presentation

Children present with the consequences of marrow and tissue infiltration with immature blasts. Normal hemopoesis is severely compromised and thus pallor, infection and bleeding or bruising are common. General malaise, weight loss and anorexia often accompany signs of bone marrow failure. Joint and bone pain are not uncommon. Infiltration and enlargement of lymph nodes and liver and/or spleen may be apparent on examination.

In half the patients the white cell count will be less than 10×10^9 cells/l and in a quarter it will be over 100×10^9 cells/l. The diagnosis is confirmed by bone marrow aspirate. Samples must be sent for cytology, immunophenotyping and cytogenetics.

Treatment

Over 70% of children with ALL can expect to be cured with modern chemotherapy. This improved state of affairs has come about because of the treatment trials that have taken place over the past 30 years. Currently therapy lasts two years and consists of induction, intensification and maintenance phases. The vast majority of this will be administered at home by parents. Hospitalization is required only for the initial induction and intensification. It has previously been shown that two blocks of intensification treatment with vincristine, prednisolone, daunorubicin, cytosine, etoposide and thioguanine were more effective than either one block or none. The current trial is examining whether three blocks may be better still. Obviously any potential advantage has to be balanced with the increased risk of adverse toxic events so randomized trials are the only way to proceed.[5]

In the majority of cases remission will be achieved in the first four weeks but these patients will nonetheless still have a considerable leukemic burden. Premature cessation of treatment is associated with early relapse. A period of continuation chemotherapy is required to eradicate residual leukemia. Experience suggests that this should be approximately two years. This treatment consists of daily 6-mercaptopurine, weekly oral methotrexate, monthly vincristine and prednisolone and three-monthly intrathecal methotrexate in those not having cranial irradiation. Treatment is adjusted to maintain a total white cell count between 2.5 and 3.5×10^9 cells/l with at least 0.5×10^9 granulocytes/l.

The blood brain barrier provides a sanctuary for leukemic cells within the CNS and without attention to this site over half of patients will relapse there. Radiotherapy in combination with intrathecal methotrexate has been the mainstay of CNS directed treatment. The dose of cranial radiation initially used was effective; however, side effects in a minority such as mild learning defects and poor growth from hypothalamic-pituitary damage proved unacceptable. The dose of radiation has therefore been decreased from 24 Gy to 18 Gy and in the current protocol for low count patients it has been superseded by continuing intrathecal methotrexate with or without high dose intravenous methotrexate.

Another sanctuary site, in boys, is the testis which must be carefully examined at presentation, during and after treatment.

For patients who relapse or who have poor prognosis disease on standard therapy a bone marrow transplant may be a suitable treatment. There is controversy about the use of autologous transplantation for childhood ALL, but allogeneic transplantation either from a relative or a volunteer has proved efficacious in some circumstances.

In the first few days of induction therapy tumor lysis may cause significant problems. Serum uric acid is often elevated at diagnosis. Alkalinized fluids and allopurinol are given to reduce this serum level and protect against urate nephropathy. Rarely dialysis is required. Blood and platelet support as well as intravenous antibiotics for fever associated with neutropenia are required throughout treatment. Infection continues to be a major cause of treatment-associated mortality. Patients should report to hospital with significant fever during times of neutropenia. Any contact with chicken pox and measles should also be reported. Live vaccines should not be given until six months off treatment when immunosuppression has largely reversed.

Other leukemias

In general the other leukemias are no different to their adult counterparts in terms of disease characteristics or treatment. The clinical presentation for AML is the same as for ALL. The survival for patients with AML treated with chemotherapy alone is approximately 50%. Treatment consists of blocks of intensive chemotherapy over a six-month period. Radiotherapy is only used as part of transplant conditioning. The role of autologous BMT is currently being studied while allogeneic BMT is an acceptable treatment for relapsed or resistant AML and for CML.

LYMPHOMA

Non-Hodgkin's Lymphoma (NHL)

Non-Hodgkin's lymphoma is more common in childhood than Hodgkin's disease (62% vs. 38% in our unit 1980–1995) and is the third most common childhood malignancy after leukemia and brain tumors. NHL forms a completely distinct group of diseases to those found in adults. The disease tends to be more widespread at diagnosis with a greater propensity for dissemination to the bone marrow and CNS and less nodal disease.

NHL is rare under the age 2, but the incidence increases with increasing age. There is considerable geographical variation. In Africa, for example, NHL accounts for 50% of all malignancy because of the high incidence of Burkitt's lymphoma. In this case there is a clear association with Epstein-Barr virus, which is not so readily apparent with sporadic Burkitt's lymphoma in the West. The etiology of sporadic cases is less clear. Important understanding has come from the discovery of particular translocations present in some Burkitt's (small cell) NHL. In 1976 a translocation between chromosome 8 and 14 was described which brings the c-myc oncogene under the influence of the promoter for the immunoglobulin heavy chain gene resulting in the aberrant expression of c-myc driving the cell to excessive proliferation. Subsequently two other translocations t(8;22) and t(2;8) were found less frequently which bring c-myc under the influence of Kappa and Lambda light chain genes. Many other translocations specific for childhood malignancies have since been found, often with less frequent variants which drive aberrant oncogene expression.

The histological classifications appropriate for adults have very little relevance in children. The classification and staging in adults is confused and confusing. In childhood the most useful classification brings together the clinical features, histopathology and surface immunophenotype to indicate T-cell, B-cell or undifferentiated lineage. Follicular lymphomas are rare in childhood, almost all cases having diffuse morphology.

Clinical presentation

The site of presentation of NHL often corresponds to the cell type. Mediastinal disease tends to be

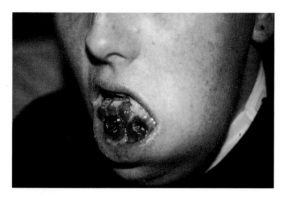

Figure 27.1. A large fungating anaplastic lymphoma of the mouth. Not surprisingly this tumor interfered with speech and eating.

T-cell in lineage and presents with dyspnoea, stridor, cough, pleuritic pain and swelling in the neck and face secondary to superior vena cava obstruction. It tends to grow and spread rapidly and malignant T-cell lymphoblasts are often present in bone marrow. By convention if there is greater than 25% involvement of the marrow then this is classified as T-cell lymphoblastic leukemia. Abdominal disease presents with pain swelling and intestinal obstruction and is B-cell in lineage. NHL is a rare, but important cause of intussuseption. Large cell anaplastic disease frequently presents similarly to B-cell disease, but may present in unusual sites, e.g. bone, skin (Figure 27.1).

In addition to the site-specific symptoms described above patients may also have generalized features such as fever, anorexia, weight loss and fatigue. There may be generalized or local lymphadenopathy.

Investigation

Bone marrow aspirate and/or biopsy is essential and offers a quick and easy method for diagnosis which if positive negates the need for formal lymph node biopsy. Staging investigations may include computed tomography (CT) scans of the head, chest, abdomen and pelvis. Radio-isotope bone scan will indicate any bone involvement. Examination of the CSF must always be included to exclude meningeal involvement.

Treatment

The mainstay of treatment is intensive combination chemotherapy. In B-cell and anaplastic disease treat-

ment can be limited to six months, but for T-cell disease treatment with maintenance therapy usually continues for two years (as for ALL). In both cases CNS prophylaxis with intrathecal drugs are used. Massive tumor lysis frequently follows the start of treatment so great care to minimize nephropathy must be taken. Adequate hydration and allopurinol or uricozyme reduce the likelihood of renal failure. The use of steroids to treat stridor or croup in childhood may have catastrophic consequences if the stridor is due to lymphoma and is not recognized.

Urgent treatment is indicated for airway or renal obstruction. Steroids or low dose radiotherapy can often eliminate the need for intubation and ventilation in mediastinal disease and relieve any obstructive nephropathy in abdominal disease. Abdominal obstruction with the exception of intussusception may be treated conservatively. Tumor shrinkage in response to chemotherapy should restore intestinal continuity.

Hodgkin's disease

This disease was originally described in 1832 by Thomas Hodgkin. There are approximately 50 new childhood cases in the UK each year. There is a definite bimodal age distribution with an early peak in adolescence and a later peak in adulthood. It is more common in boys. The etiology is unknown, but it appears to be more common in immunodeficiency syndromes (e.g. ataxia telangiectasia, Wiskott-Aldrich syndrome).[6]

Hodgkin's disease is characterized histologically by the Reed-Sternberg cell although this cell has been found in other conditions e.g. infectious mononucleosis. There are four main subtypes: lymphocytic predominant, lymphocytic depleted, mixed cellularity and nodular sclerosing; the last two are the most common in childhood. Lymphocyte depleted is extremely rare in children.

Clinical presentation

The usual clinical presentation is one of painless lymphadenopathy. This most commonly involves nodes in the cervical area or supraclavicular fossa. The spleen is more likely to be involved than the liver and extranodal primary site disease is rare. Systemic ("B") symptoms of fever, night sweats, anorexia, weight loss, malaise and indeed alcohol intolerance occur in 20% of children. Mediastinal involvement is common and chest X-ray is imperative in all individuals in whom this diagnosis is suspected.

Investigation and staging

The investigation of Hodgkin's disease is the same as that for NHL. The Ann Arbor staging classification is used in Hodgkin's disease. About 30% of children will be stage IIA at presentation and 20% each IA or IIIA.

Treatment

The overall prognosis for Hodgkin's disease is excellent (91% five-year survival for all stages; 97% for stage I and 70% for stage IV).

In the UK clinical stage I disease has been treated with radiotherapy alone. For cervical lymph nodes the radiation field is applied bilaterally to minimize later skeletal deformity. Chemotherapy is the treatment of choice for stage II–IV disease. In the past regimens have produced unacceptably high male infertility rates and alkylating agents are also associated with the induction of second malignancy. The current treatment regimen is ChlVPP (chlorambucil, vincristine, procarbazine and prednisolone) and ABVD (adriamycin, bleomycin, vincristine and DTIC) is given if there is no response or disease progression. For refractory or relapsed disease very high dose chemotherapy and transplantation have been successful in controlling resistant disease.

It is worth noting that patients with Hodgkin's disease are immunosuppressed and are at risk of transfusion-associated graft-versus-host disease and should only receive irradiated blood and blood products.

TUMORS OF THE CENTRAL NERVOUS SYSTEM

CNS tumors account for 25% of all paediatric malignancy and unlike adults 50% occur infratentorially. The relative incidence of central nervous system tumors is shown in Table 27.4.

The etiology of childhood brain tumors is largely unknown. Hereditary associations are known with Li-Fraumeni families and also with neurofibromatosis. Environmental factors may play a role. There is an increased incidence of CNS tumors in survivors of childhood ALL which may relate to

Table 27.4. The relative occurrence of tumors of the Central Nervous System in the South-West of England (1985–1994).

Tumor	Relative incidence
Medulloblastoma	23.2%
Supra tentorial astrocytoma	17.1%
Cerebellar astrocytoma	14.0%
Brain stem glioma	16.5%
Ependymoma	10.4%
Optic glioma	6.7%
Craniopharyngioma	4.3%
Pineal tumors	1.8%
Other	6.1%

prophylactic cranial irradiation. The incidence of medulloblastoma appears to have declined over the past decade coincident with the increasing use of folic acid in early pregnancy to prevent neural tube defects.

Clinical presentation

The clinical presentation of a child with a CNS tumor is varied and this reflects the age of presentation and the site of the lesion. A common mode of presentation is raised intracranial pressure produced by obstruction to the normal efflux of CSF through the third and fourth ventricles. Typically the child presents with headache which is worse in the morning and on rising. There is associated nausea and vomiting and if left untreated consciousness will eventually be impaired. Importantly papilloedema may not be present. Rapid progression of symptoms suggests a rapidly growing lesion or sudden expansion secondary to tumor hemorrhage. More commonly the tumor expands more slowly and the presentation of raised intracranial pressure is more insidious. In young children failure to thrive, irritability and developmental delay often occur prior to acute presentation. Increasing head circumference with expansion of the cranial sutures and bulging of the fontanelle is seen in infants. Occasionally a squint develops due to cranial nerve compression. Sunsetting of the eyes is rarely seen nowadays. In school age children the deteriorating school performance, change in personality and vague headache over weeks can occur before the diagnosis is obvious.

The signs and symptoms of neurological impairment are determined by the relationship to the structures involved. Infratentorial lesions present with truncal and gait ataxia and cranial nerve palsies. Unilateral facial weakness, squint and disturbances of speech and swallowing often with dribbling imply compression or destruction of the brain stem. In contrast lesions in the supratentorial region are varied and often non-specific and non-localizing. Convulsions are an uncommon presentation, but are more likely to occur in slow growing low grade astrocytomas. Upper motor neurone signs such as hemiparesis and hyperreflexia accompanied on occasion by sensory loss may present in a child with a frontoparietal lesion. Visual disturbance, anorexia, disorders of puberty, growth retardation and diabetes insipidus all occur in pituitary or hypothalamic tumors.

In addition to the clinical features outlined above some CNS tumors (e.g. Primitive neuroectodermal tumor (PNET), medulloblastoma) disseminate down the spinal cord. Children may thus present with back or radicular pain, bladder or bowel dysfunction or long tract signs.

Imaging

There is little place for plain skull X-rays in the diagnosis of intracranial tumors. Radiological signs of raised intracranial pressure and the calcification seen with teratomas, craniopharyngiomas, and pineal tumors can all be seen clearly on computed tomography (CT) scans. Furthermore a CT scan with or without contrast provides additional information about the site of the lesion and hence of the obstruction. Magnetic resonance imaging (MRI) provides additional advantages over CT. The anatomical detail on a MRI scan aids the planning of surgery. Lesions, especially in the posterior fossa, or slow growing infiltrative lesions are often evident on MRI before CT. The spinal cord can be examined for metastases where appropriate at the same session. Gadolinium-DPTA enhancement has improved the resolution of such scans. MRI, however, is more sensitive to movement artefact and the scan acquisition times tend to be longer, compounding the problem. During scanning the individual is completely enclosed within the scanner and many people find this confinement disturbing. It is seldom possible to perform MRI on a young child without sedation. Indeed in many instances a general anesthetic is required for which special equipment is necessary because of the high magnetic field. New MRI scanners have faster acquisition times and open scanners are becoming available.

Thus far positron emission tomography has not been extensively explored in children, but is likely to prove useful in the future.

Treatment

The distribution of paediatric neurosurgical services within the United Kingdom means that most children will present to hospitals without such a facility. In many cases transfer can be arranged for the following day; however, the mode of presentation in some means that urgent treatment of raised intracranial pressure is required. A combination of steroids, dexamethasone (0.5–1 mg/kg initially and 0.25–0.5 mg/kg/day divided six hourly subsequently), mannitol and if necessary intubation and hyperventilation are the treatments of choice. Urgent neurosurgical referral for CSF shunt or stenting should then be arranged. Brain stem tumors effecting the lower cranial nerves produce airway compromise and may necessitate intubation to protect the airway prior to transfer.

Surgery

Ideally complete surgical removal is the treatment of choice. Unfortunately the location and infiltrating nature of many tumors prevents achievement of this goal despite the use of modern computer-guided equipment. Partial resection or biopsy alone are the only alternatives. Treatment with radiotherapy or chemotherapy can permit a complete resection at second look surgery. Indeed this approach has been more successful in the treatment of ependymoma than initial heroic surgery. Insertion of a Ventriculo-Peritoneal or Ventriculo-Atrial shunt will be required if the normal circulation of CSF cannot be re-established.

Radiotherapy

Radiotherapy plays a major role in the treatment of CNS tumors in children. Megavoltage radiation from a linear accelerator should be used. A mask for immobilizing the child in an accurate and reproducible position is essential. In general, adequately prepared children tolerate both the mask and the radiotherapy well. Radiotherapy is used to treat the entire CNS in tumor known to disseminate through the CSF, wide margins of apparently normal tissue infiltrating tumors and with limited volumes and small margins to normal tissue in circumscribed tumors. The dose of radiation varies according to the age of the child and the tumor type.

Although most children tolerate radiotherapy remarkably well, regular clinical review is essential. Acute tumor swelling in response to treatment can be ameliorated with steroids, but this has to be differentiated from progressive disease. Temporary alopecia is seldom troubling, but a hat and sun barrier creams must be used to protect sensitive skin from sun burn. Radiation of particularly the whole neuroaxis is associated with marrow suppression which may necessitate transfusion of blood and or platelets or a temporary cessation in treatment. Profound lethargy, anorexia and headache, "somnolence syndrome", may occur 4–8 weeks after treatment. Long-term complications result from injury to normal tissues. Radiation necrosis occurs in less than 1% of patients. Second malignancies, including a variety of soft tissue sarcomas, are increasingly being reported in long-term survivors.

Chemotherapy

A plethora of drugs have been shown to have a temporary beneficial effect on many CNS tumors. Drugs are normally administered intravenously. In theory the blood brain barrier should limit the concentration of drug achievable in the brain and CSF. However, it is likely that in the area of the tumor the blood brain barrier is disrupted. There is no advantage, therefore, in administering drug directly into the CSF. In addition the drug is required not in the CSF but in the substance of the brain. The most widely used agents are vincristine, methotrexate, etoposide, CCNU and DTIC. Increasingly high dose carboplatin, cyclophosphamide and thiotepa are being studied in clinical trials. Very high dose chemotherapy and autologous bone marrow or peripheral blood stem cell rescue have been explored for poor prognosis disease (e.g. high grade astrocytoma, medulloblastoma), but results so far have been disappointing.

WILMS' TUMOR (NEPHROBLASTOMA)

Nephroblastoma is an embryonal tumor and is the most common renal tumor of childhood. Approximately 1 in 10,000 children per-year will develop

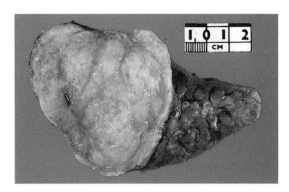

Figure 27.2. A resection specimen of an upper pole Wilms' tumor from a patient with aniridia and an 11p deletion.

a Wilms' tumor. The incidence is 2–3 times greater for blacks in Africa and in the United States compared to that of East Asians. Caucasians have an intermediate incidence. The sex ratio is equal as is the laterality. The peak age of diagnosis is 2–3 years, earlier in boys than girls and earlier for bilateral disease. In the National Wilms' Tumor Study (NWTS), 1969–1985, the median age of presentation with a unilateral tumor was 36 months for boys and 43 months for girls. In contrast the median age was 23 months for boys and 30 months for girls in individuals with bilateral disease.

Wilms' tumors associated with a range of congenital abnormalities; particularly aniridia, Beckwith-Wiedemann syndrome, hemihypertrophy and genitourinary abnormalities (Drash Syndrome). A constitutional chromosomal deletion of chromosome 11 (11p13) is seen in patients with aniridia in which there is a 30% risk of developing nephroblastoma. (Figure 27.2) A tumor suppressor gene, WTI, has been identified at this site. Another gene implicated in the genesis of Wilms' tumor is WT2 which is located at 11p15 and identified from studies of Beckwith-Wiedemann syndrome. Loss of heterozygosity for chromosome 16 has been identified as conferring a poorer prognosis.[7]

Pathology

Nephroblastoma arises from the mesonephros and is usually unilateral (95%). Surrounding renal tissue is compressed and displaced. The tumor may extend in to the renal pelvis and via the renal veins into the vena cava. Local and regional lymph nodes may be infiltrated. The cut surface is pale gray and yellow. Hemorrhage, necrosis and cysts may all be present.

Histological examination may differ from one part of the tumor to another. The classical pattern is triphasic, including blastema, epithelial and stroma elements indicative of disordered embryogenesis. Areas of nephroblastomatosis are often recognized. There is increasing evidence that nephroblastomatosis is a premalignant condition although the process of malignant transformation remains unknown. The presence of anaplasia confers a poorer prognosis. In the first NWTS anaplasia was noted in 11% of all cases, but in 52% of the deaths. Anaplasia is recognized by the presence of hyperdiploid mitotic figures, three-fold or greater nuclear enlargement and nuclear hyperchromasia. Not all Wilms' tumors are of the classical pattern and this occasionally may give rise to diagnostic confusion.

In infancy Wilms' tumor should be differentiated from congenital mesoblastic nephroma and rhabdoid tumor both of which have a very different treatment and prognosis. Congenital mesoblastic nephroma is curative with surgery alone and associated with an excellent prognosis. In contrast rhabdoid tumor is associated with bone metastases, hypercalcemia and chemoresistance. The prognosis is poor with mortality rate in excess of 80%. Clear cell carcinoma of the kidney presents identically to Wilms' tumor, but is distinct histologically and has a much higher relapse rate. Renal cell carcinoma occasionally presents in childhood and is usually fatal.

Clinical presentation

The usual presentation is a well child with a combination of an abdominal mass, abdominal discomfort (1/3 of cases) or hematuria (less than 1/4). Hypertension and features of the congenital syndromes discussed above may be noted on examination.

Imaging studies can often be confined to ultrasound examination of the abdomen, characteristically demonstrating a mass displacing and distorting normal kidney and a chest X-ray to exclude pulmonary metastasis. CT scan, intravenous pyelography and arteriography may be useful if there is diagnostic doubt or to plan surgery.

Staging

The extent of the disease has important implications for treatment and prognosis. The prognosis

for stage 5 disease equates to that of the individual tumors.

Stage	Classification
Stage 1	Tumor localized to the kidney and completely resected.
Stage 2	Tumor extends beyond the kidney, but is completely excised.
Stage 3	Residual tumor confined to the abdomen e.g. macro or microscopic tumor beyond resection margins, lymph node disease.
Stage 4	Distant metastasis.
Stage 5	Bilateral disease.

Treatment

Wilms' tumor is the most curable of all childhood malignancy. The current multimodal approach is associated with an overall 80% survival. Treatment strategies for low stage favorable histology tumors are therefore aimed at reducing sequelae while continuing to preserve the efficacy of treatments

Surgery

Current controversy surrounds the timing of surgery and the role of biopsy. Surgical resection is the initial treatment of choice in most cases in the USA. Tumors judged unresectable may be shrunk with pre-operative chemotherapy and radiotherapy. In Europe pre-operative chemotherapy, with or without biopsy, is the routine. In theory a biopsy will convert a hitherto stage 1 tumor to stage 2 and gives rise to the possibility of recurrence in the biopsy tract. The current UK Wilms' tumor study aims to address the timing of surgery by examining initial surgery against biopsy and pre-treatment with surgery following after three courses of chemotherapy. Subsequent treatment is then based on the stage of the resected specimen.

Chemotherapy

Studies have identified three drugs, vincristine, actinomycin D and doxorubicin, which used either singly or in combination have proven useful in the treatment of Wilms' tumor. The addition of cyclophosphamide increased side effects and did not enhance survival. Cyclophosphamide is therefore used almost exclusively in relapsed or non-responsive tumors. Current treatment strategies range from weekly vincristine alone for 10 weeks to triple therapy with vincristine, actinomycin D and doxorubicin for one year.

Radiotherapy

Post operative radiotherapy is indicated for all stage 2 unfavorable histology and above tumors. The aim is to eradicate residual tumor. Anterior and posterior fields are applied to the tumor bed and the fields are extended across the midline so as to minimize later skeletal malformation. Lung metastases visible on chest X-ray, not those on CT scan alone, are treated with radiation to the whole chest.

Prognosis and follow-up

Overall the prognosis for Wilms' tumor is excellent. Low treatment-associated morbidity is now the aim for most stages. Anthracycline cardiotoxicity, actinomycin D induced hepatic failure and skeletal malformation following unilateral radiotherapy are important adverse consequences of treatment. Follow-up should be at least monthly for the first six months, two-monthly in the second year and three-monthly in the third and sixth monthly thereafter. At each visit blood pressure should be measured and periodically a chest X-ray examined.

NEUROBLASTOMA

Neuroblastoma is derived from primitive neural crest cells which generate the normal sympathetic nervous system. The variation in location, presentation and degree of differentiation reflects this. In contrast to other childhood tumors progress in the treatment of neuroblastoma has been painfully slow. The prognosis for localized disease remains excellent, but that of advanced disease, with the exception of stage 4S disease, is dismal.

The prevalence is approximately 1 in 8000 live births. As with Wilms' tumor it is mainly a disease of pre-school children, 75% occurring under five years of age. Some studies have shown a biphasic trend with an initial peak incidence under a year of age and a second peak at 2–4 years of age. There is a slight male excess (1.2:1). There is a suggestion of a genetic predisposition to neuroblastoma, but in general there are no associations with congenital anomalies. Rare associations with neurofibromatosis and colonic aganglionosis have been reported.[8]

Pathology

Neuroblastoma is one of the "small round blue cell" family of tumors. These tumors can present anywhere along the craniospinal axis and may differ considerably in their differentiation and hence malignant potential. In contrast to Wilms' tumor, neuroblastomas are often infiltrating, becoming friable with areas of calcification and hemorrhage. Histologically neuroblastoma is densely cellular, the cells containing dense hyperchromatic nuclei and scant cytoplasm. The presence of neuritic process or neuropil is a pathognomonic feature. Some tumors are composed entirely of mature ganglion, neuropil and schwann cells. These ganglioneuromas are benign and form well-encapsulated masses which do not metastasize. Ganglioneuroblastoma is a term used to reflect an intermediate histology in which there is focal or diffuse maturation within a neuroblastoma.

It is essential to distinguish neuroblastoma from other small round blue cell tumors. This is best accomplished by a combination of immunohistochemistry and electron microscopy. In addition, neuroblastoma may be differentiated cytogenetically by the presence of homogenous staining regions or double minutes. These are areas of amplification of the n-myc oncogene, the number of repeat copies of which is associated with prognosis. Also of prognostic significance is deletion of lp, which is often associated with high repeat number n-myc amplification, and expression of the TRK-A nerve growth factor receptor.

Clinical presentation

Presenting features depend upon the site of the lesion, but unlike Wilms' tumor these children often appear unwell. Approximately 60% occur in the abdomen and pelvis and thus present with an abdominal mass. Airway compromise, superior vena caval obstruction and Horner's syndrome are features of cervical/thoracic disease. Limb paralysis and pain are features of compression of the spinal cord by a "dumb-bell" tumor infiltrating through the intervertebral foramen. Primary intracranial sites are rare.

Symptoms from metastatic disease are common. In addition to general malaise, fever, irritability, weight loss and bone pain there are a number of classical signs associated with neuroblastoma. The predilection of this tumor for the skull and retro-

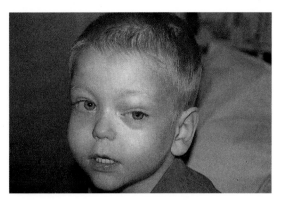

Figure 27.3. Proptosis in 4-year-old boy with disseminated neuroblastoma. This subsequently resolved with chemotherapy.

orbital tissues results in proptosis and periorbital ecchymosis (Figure 27.3). Opsomyoclonus, dancing eye syndrome, and ataxia are examples of paraneoplastic phenomena. Skin involvement, manifest as subcutaneous nodules with a bluish hue are seen exclusively in stage 4S disease. Finally symptoms of excessive catecholeamine production e.g. hypertension tachycardia and perspiration, can be seen.

Investigation

Anemia and thrombocytopenia are indicative of bone marrow involvement. In this circumstance bone marrow aspirate and trephine will show clumps of neuroblastoma cells arranged in pseudorosettes. Biochemically the diagnosis is suggested by elevated urinary catecholeamine metabolite levels. Elevated vanillylmandelic acid (VMA) and homovanillic acid (HVA) are seen in 75% of cases. The levels fall with treatment and hence can be used serially to monitor treatment and subsequently to detect subclinical relapse.

Imaging studies are important both in terms of defining the primary lesion and as a means of assessing distant spread. A plain X-ray may show mass effect and calcification. Abdominal ultrasound is often useful to examine the adrenal glands. CT or MRI scanning are the most useful modalities particularly if there is brain or spinal cord involvement. Bone involvement can be identified by radionucleotide bone scan. In addition [131]Iodine-labelled MIBG (metaiodobenzylguanidine) which is taken up by catecholeamine secreting tissue may be used

both to determine the extent of disease and intraoperatively to aid resection.

Staging

The staging of neuroblastoma has varied over time. Below is shown the current neuroblastoma staging system.

Stage	Classification
Stage 1	Tumor confined to the organ or structure of origin; complete gross excision with or without microscopic residual disease; lymph nodes (ipsitateral and contralateral) negative microscopically.
Stage 2a	Unilateral tumor with incomplete gross excision. Lymph nodes (ipsitateral and contralateral) negative microscopically.
Stage 2b	Unilateral tumor completely or incompletely excised with positive ipsilateral and microscopically negative contralateral lymph nodes.
Stage 3	Tumor infiltrating across the midline with or without regional or bilateral lymph node involvement or unilateral disease with contralateral node involvements.
Stage 4	Disseminated disease.
Stage 4S	Tumor as for stages 1 and 2 with dissemination to liver, skin and/or bone marrow.

Treatment

The management of airwav compromise, with intubation and ventilation, and central nervous system manifestations if present must be a priority. Steroids should be used to treat spinal cord compression. Emergency radiotherapy is useful at controlling both pain and central nervous system disease prior to starting dedicated treatment.

For stage I and 2 disease surgical excision is often curative. Outside of this, biopsy only is necessary initially; definitive surgery being delayed until the bulk of the tumor is reduced with chemotherapy or radiation. Open biopsy is preferred as it is often necessary to obtain a large sample for histology, immunohistochemistry and molecular diagnostic procedures. Laminectomy has also been used in the past to overcome spinal cord compression although the later development of scoliosis, which can be severe, is not an uncommon consequence.

Chemotherapy is the main modality of treatment. A number of effective drugs either singly or in combination have been identified. Most therapeutic protocols employ a multidrug approach. Modifications are made based on the age of the child and the stage of the disease. There is currently little evidence to support the use of aggressive chemotherapy and bone marrow transplantation in children with stage 4 disease. In contrast to the appalling prognosis for stage 4 neuroblastoma, stage 4S disease may undergo spontaneous regression. Consequently its treatment is limited to surgical resection and minimal chemotherapy or radiation. Life threatening respiratory compromise as a result of massive abdominal organomegaly is a particular risk in this group.

Radiotherapy is useful as adjuvant therapy in combination with surgery and chemotherapy. It is particularly efficacious at controlling pain and hence has a very valuable role in the palliative care. Radionucleotide therapy with high dose ^{131}I-MIBG has been used in an attempt to cure aggressive or recurrent disease with limited success, although it does produce excellent palliation.

Prognosis, sequelae and follow-up

In a now historical series the prognosis is indicated by the age, stage and molecular pathology of the tumor. The overall two-year disease-free survival for children under 1 was 75% compared to 12% for those over 2 years. The two-year disease-free survival for stage 1 was 85%, stage 4S was 77%, stage 2 was 63%, stage 3 was 37% and stage 4 was 6%.[9]

Deformities, neurological deficits and second malignancies are all important complications of the disease and its treatment. Neurosurgical procedures and unilateral radiotherapy exact a price on the growing skeleton which can impact severely on the needs and demands of a growing child. Loss of neurological function as a consequence of disease does not always improve with treatment. Physiotherapy and specialist aids may be required. Other malignancies have been reported with increased frequency in survivors.

Long-term surveillance is essential. Relapse is common and may occur some years after the original presentation. Regular follow-up and the intermittent measurement of urinary VMA and HVA is advised. Follow-up also allows for the assessment of ongoing orthopaedic, physiotherapy and emotional problems.

RHABDOMYOSARCOMA

Rhabdomyosarcoma (RMS) is the most common tumor of connective tissue in childhood. Most patients present before 5 years of age. The tumor arises from mesenchymal tissue that mimics striated muscle. Any site can be involved, but the most common are:

- head and neck — 40% (including parameningeal 20% and orbit 10%)
- genitourinary tract — 20%
- extremities — 20%

Rhabdomyosarcomas have been reported in association with neurofibromatosis, Rubenstein-Taybi syndrome and fetal alcohol syndrome. Some occur in Li-Fraumeni cancer families where close relatives have premenopausal breast cancer and soft tissue sarcomas. Many patients with this syndrome inherit a germline mutation in the p53 tumor suppressor gene. Cytogenetic anomalies have been identified in this and other of the soft tissue sarcomas. Translocations of chromosome 2 and 13 (t(2;13) PAX3-FKHR gene fusion) and chromosomes one and 13 (t(1;13) PAX7-FKHR gene fusion) have been reported in alveolar rhabdomyosarcoma. Other translocations occur infrequently in this and other soft tissue sarcomas.[10]

Pathology

Rhabdomyosarcomas are characterized by rapid growth and widespread local infiltration. Spread by hematogenous and lymphatic routes is common and bone marrow involvement is seen in 20% of cases.

Rhabdomyosarcomas are poorly differentiated and varied histological appearances may be present within the same tumor making the diagnosis extremely difficult. The feature most often sought by light microscopy is cross striation mimicking striated muscle. Immunocytochemistry using specific skeletal antibodies is extremely useful.

Four main categories are described: embryonal, alveolar, pleomorphic and mixed. Embryonal tumors constitute 50% of all RMS and occur primarily in the head, neck and genitourinary tract. Furthermore a subtype sarcoma botryoides occurs in the bladder vagina and nasopharynx and these have the best prognosis. In contrast the alveolar subtype which can be differentiated from other RMS by the translocations described above and histologically by any alveolar pattern occurs on the extremities and trunk and has a poor prognosis. Pleomorphic RMS is extremely rare in childhood.

Clinical presentation

The mode of presentation varies depending on the site. Orbital disease may present with proptosis, diplopia and chemosis. Nasopharyngeal tumors present with nasal discharge which may be blood stained, airway compromise and a protruding mass. Tumors of the abdomen present with a mass, pain, hematuria or testicular swelling (paratesticular RMS) and of the extremities present as discrete lumps. Bloody vaginal discharge and urinary obstruction occur with genitourinary disease.

Investigation

A biopsy is essential for diagnosis. Staging investigations should also be complete prior to starting treatment. Plain X-rays are not helpful. MRI scan is the best imaging modality for the primary lesion. CT scans of the chest and radionucteotide bone scans are required because of the high incidence of pulmonary and bone metastases. Bone marrow aspirate and trephine will exclude marrow invasion. CSF cytology is indicated in parameningeal disease.

Staging

The stage of the tumor is based on the site of origin and its clinical behavior.

Stage	Classification
Stage 1	Localized disease, completely resected in a favorable site, i.e. orbit, paratestis and genitourinary tract.
Stage 2	Non-favorable sites; tumor < 5 cm; regional nodes not involved.
Stage 3	Non-favorable sites; tumor > 5 cm; and/or regional lymph nodes involved.
Stage 4	Distant disease.

Treatment

Complete removal of the tumor is the ideal. The frequent presence of micrometastasis at diagnosis means, however, that chemotherapy is used in all cases. Pre-operative chemotherapy reduces the need

for mutilating surgery in many instances. The exact role of surgery will depend upon the site, size and extent of tumor. Where complete excision cannot be achieved biopsy is required.

The current European treatment study, MMT95, aims to reduce the amount of chemotherapy given to stage 1 and 2 tumors, but to intensify treatment for higher stage disease which continues to have a poor prognosis. Thus for stage 1 paratesticular disease following surgical excision treatment continues for six months with vincristine and actinomycin D. In contrast stage 4 disease requires treatment with a six-drug regimen administered over four courses initially followed by high dose etoposide, cyclophosphamide and finally carboplatin with autologous bone marrow or peripheral blood stem cell rescue.

Radiotherapy is needed in many patients to enhance the chances of local control. Careful planning is required particularly with orbital and parameningeal primaries. Radiation is again useful for symptom control as part of palliative care.

Follow-up

Local relapse and pulmonary metastasis may become evident some time after the end of treatment. Regular chest X-ray and clinical examination is therefore required. Skeletal malformations can be particularly troublesome and can require surgical intervention. Overall 65% of patients should be cured.

OSTEOSARCOMA

Osteosarcoma is the most common primary malignant bone tumor in childhood (60%) and is derived from primitive bone forming mesenchyme. The peak incidence is in the second decade during the adolescent growth spurt. The etiology of osteosarcoma is unknown although a familial incidence has been described. The strongest genetic association is with retinoblastoma. There is an increased risk of nonocular osteosarcoma in patients with retinoblastoma. Indeed there appears to be partial deletion, loss of heterozygosity or altered expression of the paternal RB gene in some osteosarcomas. The majority have normal RB alleles and expression. Li-Fraumeni families also have an increased incidence. Radiation is implicated as an etiological agent. This was first described in association with orthovoltage therapeutic radiation, but there is increasing recognition of these tumors following treatment with megavoltage radiotherapy. Alkylating agents have also been linked to the subsequent development of osteosarcoma. Approximately 2% of patients with Paget's disease develop osteosarcoma.

Pathology

Osteosarcoma is characterized by the production of osteoid associated with malignant sarcomatous stroma and bone. There is variation in the proportion of each of these present within an individual tumor. Fibrosarcoma and chondrosarcoma are differentiated from osteosarcoma by the lack of osteoid. Approximately 50% of cases have abundant osteoid and are designated osteoblastic osteosarcoma. In 25% differentiation is towards cartilage and these are known as chondroblastic osteosarcoma. Other minor subclassifications are described.

Clinical presentation

Pain and swelling is the commonest mode of presentation. Often there is a history of trivial trauma some weeks previously. The infiltration of local nerves gives rise to severe pain and paraesthesia. Fracture through the tumor may perchance initiate medical contact. The lower femoral and upper tibial metaphyses are the predominant sites affected followed by the upper humerus and pelvis, but any bone can be involved.

Metastatic disease is present in 10–20% of patients at diagnosis. Although most will be pulmonary and clinically silent bone metastases also occur. The presence of multifocal bone disease raises the question of multiple primary lesions. Synchronous and metachronous tumors are well described.

Imaging

An incidental plain X-ray occasionally gives the first clue to the presence of tumor. Characteristically there is destruction of the normal traebecular pattern without expansion of the bone shaft. Intense periosteal new bone formation and the extension of bone spicules into the tumor mass gives a sun-ray appearance. MRI provides more detailed information and extension into the marrow cavity is more easily defined. Metastatic disease is evaluated by

CT scans of the chest (more sensitive than MRI) and radioisotope bone scan.

Treatment and prognosis

This depends upon the site of the tumor and the presence of distant disease. Osteosarcomas are not radiosensitive. Primary surgery is usually limited to biopsy. Limb salvage surgery using endoprostheses, bone grafting or in some cases simple resection (fibula) is deferred until chemotherapy has achieved tumor shrinkage. Amputation should be avoided if possible, but failure to gain local control or disease progression with appropriate chemotherapy may necessitate this. Isolated pulmonary metastases can be surgically removed.

Adjuvant chemotherapy has reduced the number of patients who relapse with metastatic disease from 80% to 30%. Chemotherapy is based on an intensive multidrug regimen. Renal and cardiac toxicity may limit treatment; there may also be an unacceptable degree of nausea and bone marrow suppression.[11] The current regimen in this unit is based on five cycles of ifosfamide vincristine and actinomycin D (IVA) alternating three weekly with carboplatin, etoposide, epirubicin and vincristine (CEEV). Disease-free survival is 75% (median follow-up is 24 months) without significant renal and cardiac toxicity. Other drugs, notably methotrexate, likewise have a role to play particularly in the treatment of relapse.

Since this is a disease of the adolescent years and the treatment regimen is long and arduous conflict with health-care staff and parental desires can occasionally arise. Psychological support is often required. Regular follow-up must be maintained. Discomfort in a limb stump can necessitate revision. Continued skeletal growth may obligate revision of the endoprosthesis or a change of artificial limb.

EWING'S TUMOR

Ewing's sarcoma is the second most common malignant tumor of bone. Unlike osteosarcoma it principally affects the axial skeleton and is not of endothelial origin and consequently may also occur in soft tissues. The cell of origin is probably neural. Ewing's sarcoma of bone shares many characteristics with extraosseous Ewing's sarcoma (Askin tumor), primitive neuro-ectodermal tumors (PNET) and possibly desmoplastic small round cell tumor of the abdomen.

The Ewing's sarcoma family of tumors most commonly presents in the second decade (64%), but is not uncommon in the first (27%) and can present in adulthood. There is a slight excess of boys (1.4:1). Ewing's sarcomas are rare in races other than white Caucasians. Associations with congenital and skeletal abnormalities are not infrequently reported. A consistent cytogenetic abnormality is identified in Ewing's sarcoma and links the members of the family together.[12] It consists of a reciprocal translocation t(11;22) which can be found in the majority of Ewing's tumors of bone and also in extraosseous disease, in Askin tumor and in PNET. The translocation brings together the EWS gene on chromosome 22 with FLI-1 gene on chromosome 11 or a number of variants. In addition in desmoplastic small round cell tumor of the abdomen the EWS gene is fused with WT1 gene at 11p13.

Pathology

As might be expected there is considerable variation in the light microscopic appearances of these tumors. Typical Ewing's tumor of bone is composed of sheets of small round blue cells with scant cytoplasm which stains positive for glycogen. Immunocytochemistry is invaluable to differentiate this tumor from the other small round blue cell tumors. Neurone specific enolase is consistently positive.

Clinical presentation

Symptoms and signs are related to the site. Pain, mass and fracture are again the commonest modes of presentation. In addition constitutional upset with fever and weight loss is not unusual. Since the axial skeleton is the most common site, symptoms and signs of spinal cord compression are another method of presentation. Metastatic disease occurs in a third of patients at presentation. Bone deposits may be palpable and pain from multiple deposits can be debilitating.

Investigation

Serum lactate dehydrogenase (LDH) is elevated. Anemia and thrombocytopenia may indicate mar-

row involvement which would be evident on bone marrow biopsy. Although plain X-ray may show erosion of the cortex and spread into soft tissues accompanied by periosteal reaction ("onion peel") MRI is the optimal imaging modality. STIR sequences define soft tissue involvement and readily show compression of the spinal cord.

Treatment

No formal staging system exists. Most are disseminated at presentation. The treatment of cord compression is an emergency (see neuroblastoma). All too often surgery can only offer biopsy. Local control can be achieved with a combination of radiotherapy and local surgery, particularly for lesions of the extremities. However, with this approach most will recur: chemotherapy is therefore, essential. Different drug regimens have been tried and many are useful in treating localized disease. This combined approach has resulted in a significant cure rate for patients presenting with localized disease. Unfortunately the outlook for disseminated Ewing's sarcoma is mediocre. High dose treatment regimens with autologous or allogeneic bone marrow or PBSC transplantation has not improved the ultimate survival in most series. Better understanding of the biology of this disease may permit the design of more novel treatment strategies.

GERM CELL TUMORS

Germ cell tumors are benign or malignant growths derived from primordial germ cells. Any or all extraembryonal or embryonal elements can be found in any one tumor. Germ cell tumors account for 3% of malignant disease in children. Most germ cell tumors are found outside the gonads and must therefore be considered in the differential diagnosis of a mass arising in the sacrococcygeal region, abdomen, mediastinum and pineal gland. The tumor markers α-fetoprotein, produced if yolk-sac elements are present, and βHCG, produced if trophoblastic elements are present, may aid diagnosis and permit monitoring of treatment and in exclusion of relapse. (It should be noted that α-fetoprotein is normally raised after birth and decreases over the first 3–6 months of life. Moreover α-fetoprotein is raised in other condition, e.g. hepatoblastoma, tyrosinaemia.)

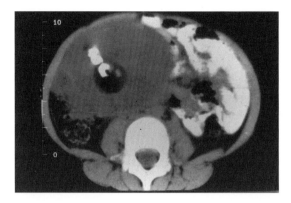

Figure 27.4a. CT scan of the abdomen in 12-year-old girl with abdominal enlargement. Note the presence of a soft tissue mass in which teeth can clearly be seen.

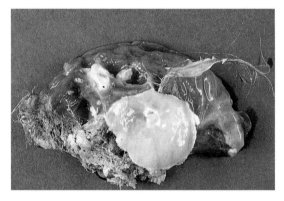

Figure 27.4b. The cut surface of this teratoma in which teeth, hair and fat can be seen.

The most common site for germ cell tumors is the sacrococcyx. Approximately 40% of all germ cell tumors are sacrococcygeal teratomas and 70% of these occur in girls. Over half present in neonates and although they may be very large they tend to be benign. Malignant potential increases with increasing age of presentation. Many of the symptoms and signs of these tumors relate principally to their physical size (Figure 27.4).

For benign tumors surgical resection is the treatment of choice. Large tumors in neonates present a considerable surgical challenge. All malignant tumors with the exception of localized testicular disease (orchidoblastoma) will require additional chemotherapy. The prognosis of the group as a whole has become excellent with modern treatment.

Intracranial tumors present with headache and paralysis of upward gaze (Parinaud's syndrome) and may be of any germ cell type. It is advisable

to measure (α-fetoprotein and βHCG both in the serum and the CSF. Treatment comprises surgery and chemotherapy for secreting tumors. Radiotherapy alone is effective in the treatment of intracranial germinomas and may be used in combination with other modalities in the treatment of intracranial disease, but is of limited value outside the CNS.

RARITIES

Langerhans' Cell Histiocytosis[13]

This disorder accounts for 2% of all paediatric malignancy. It is more common in boys and usually presents under the age of 2 years. There is a spectrum of disease from benign through to highly malignant. There are three defined syndromes:

1. Eosinophilic granuloma which presents as a solitary painless swelling often on the skull. X-ray demonstrates a lytic lesion with well-defined borders. Granulomata may also occur in the soft tissues. These may undergo spontaneous healing, but are curable by curettage or low-dose radiotherapy.
2. Hand-Schuller-Christian disease in which granulomata result in the classical triad of bone lesion, exophthalmos and diabetes insipidus.
3. Letterer-Siwe syndrome which is the more disseminated form.

The last two require systemic treatment with steroids, vincristine, cyclophosphamide, etoposide and methotrexate either singly or in combination.

Other forms of histiocytoses include familial erthrophagocytic lymphohistiocytosis (FEL) and its sporadic counterpart virus associated haemophagocytic syndrome. Treatment of these may involve chemotherapy and bone marrow transplantation.

Retinoblastoma

Approximately 40 new cases present each year in the UK of which about a third are bilateral. The genetics of retinoblastoma led Knudson to postulate his two-hit hypothesis for the etiology of cancer. About 40% are inherited and these are diagnosed earlier, may be either bilateral or unilateral and have a germline mutation in the retinoblastoma

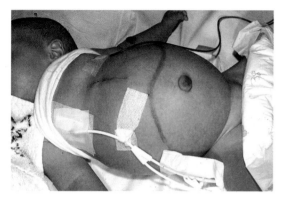

Figure 27.5. Massive hepatomegaly compromising respiration in a 4-month-old girl with hepatoblastoma. In addition, there was marked thrombocytosis and osteoporosis.

tumor suppressor gene (Rb). In contrast the remaining 60% arise spontaneously and present later and are always unilateral. These patients do not carry a germline mutation in the Rb gene and consequently require two post-zygotic events rather than one in the inherited form to inactivate the gene. Patients present with leukocoria, strabismus or orbital inflammation. Treatment should be at a national referral center and consists of enucleation and radiotherapy. Chemotherapy is of limited value in selected patients.

Hepatoblastoma

Hepatoblastoma presents with a large abdominal mass, thrombocytosis (tumor produces thrombopoetin) and osteopenia. α-Fetoprotein is greatly elevated. Treatment is with chemotherapy and surgery. Liver transplant has proven successful in treating central otherwise irresectable tumours (Figure 27.5).

Others

There are a number of tumors both embryonal (orchidoblastoma) and adult (carcinoma of the colon, squamous carcinoma) that occur extremely rarely. Management of the adult tumors in childhood is essentially that for the individual tumor occurring in adulthood; it is important, however, to explore the possibility of a cancer-predisposition (e.g. Li-Fraumeni, Familial Polyposis Coli). The rare embryonal tumors are best treated using international protocols.

References

1. Botting, B. (1996). The Health of our children. Decennial Supplement. Office of Population Censuses and Surveys.
2. Ries, L.A. Hankey, B.F. and Miller, B.A. (1991). Cancer Statistics Review 1973–1988. NIH Publication No. 91–2789.
3. Cortes, I.E. and Kantarjian, H.M. (1995). Acute Lymphoblastic Leukaemia. A Comprehensive Review with Emphasis on Biology and Therapy. *Cancer* **76**, 2393–2417.
4. General Haematology Task Force of BCSH, (1994). Immunophenotyping in the diagnosis of acute leukaemias. *J. Clin. Pathol.*, **47**, 777–781.
5. MRC UKALL XI Randomised clinical trial for the treatment of childhood acute lymphoblastic leukaemia.
6. Gatti, R.A. and Good, R.A. (1971). Occurrence of malignancy in immunodeficiency disease: A literature review. *Cancer*, **28**, 89–98.
7. Mott, M.G. (1995). The Molecular genetic basis of childhood neoplasia. *Clinical Oncology*, **7**, 279–286.
8. Brodeur, G.M. (1991). Neuroblastoma and other peripheral neuroectodermal tumours. In *Clinical Paediatric Oncology*, edited by D.I. Fernbach and T.I. Vietti, 4th edn. St Louis: Mosby Year Book.
9. Philip, T. (1992). Overveiw of current treatment of neuroblastoma. *Am. J. Paed. Haem./Oncol.*, **14**, 97–102.
10. Cooper, C.S. (1996). Translocations in solid tumours. *Current Opinion in Genetics and Development*, **6**, 71–75.
11. Pratt, C.B., Champion, J.E. and Fleming, I. (1990). Adjuvant chemotherapy for osteosarcoma of the extremity. Long-term results of two consecutive prospective protocol studies. *Cancer*, **65**, 439–445.
12. Donaldson, S., Shuster, J. and Andreozzi, C. (1989). The Paediatric Oncology Group (POG) experience in Ewing's sarcoma of bone. *Med. Pediatr. Oncol.*, **17**, 2834.
13. The French Langerhans' Cell Histocytosis Study Group (1996). A multicentre retrospective survey of Langerhans' cell histiocytosis: 348 cases observed between 1983 and 1993. *Archives of Disease in Childhood*, **75**, 17–24.

General Reading

Pizzo, P.A. and Poplack, D.G. (1997). *Principles and Practice of Pediatric Oncology*. 3rd Edition. Philadelphia: J.B. Lippincott.
Pinkerton, R. and Plowman P.N. (1996). P*aediatric Oncology; Clinical Practice & Controversies*. 3rd edn. London: Chapman and Hall Medical.

Frequency of childhood cancers
USA, SEER, 1973–82

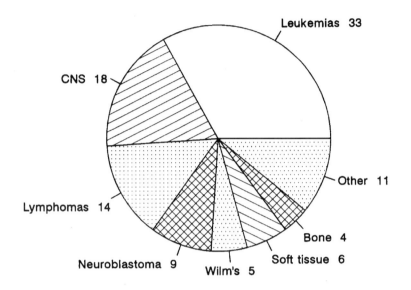

Males

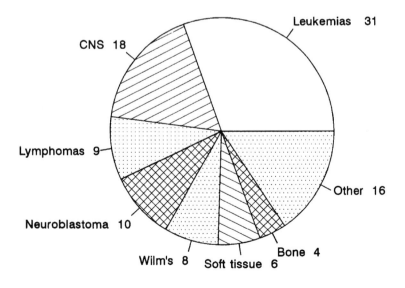

Females

28. HIV Associated Malignancies

DAVID GOLDSTEIN

Prince of Wales Hospital, Randwick, Sydney, Australia

HIV infection is associated with gradual deterioration in immune function, which can be quantified by measuring the number and proportion of T-cells expressing the CD4 cell surface marker. The decrease in T-cell count is accompanied by the occurrence of opportunistic infections and malignancies, increasing in severity over time and associated with mortality. Although HIV-related neoplasia is associated with decreasing immunity, the relationship is less clear than for the major opportunistic infections such as atypical mycobacterium.

One in six HIV positive individuals ultimately develops a neoplasm. Some of the neoplasms associated with HIV may be characterized as "opportunistic" in that viral agents other than HIV appear to be involved in their pathogenesis. The best examples of these are:

- Non-Hodgkin's lymphomas of which about 50% are positive for Epstein-Barr virus
- Genital papillomas
- Anal and Cervical intra-epithelial neoplasia
- There is also some evidence that Kaposis sarcoma has an infectious origin.

All of the HIV associated neoplasms are complicated by co-existence of opportunistic infections and a poor response to standard therapy.

A clear parallel can be established between the HIV associated malignancies and the transplantation associated malignancies, which were first described in the late sixties once patients had started to be followed for extended periods following renal transplantation. An increased incidence of Non-Hodgkin's lymphoma, Kaposi's sarcoma, renal cell carcinoma, vulval and perineal squamous cell carcinomas have now been described in these patients.

In the HIV setting Non-Hodgkin's Lymphoma, Kaposi's Sarcoma and cervical carcinoma are all accepted as AIDS-defining conditions and are discussed below. An increased incidence and severity of Hodgkin's Disease has been documented but is not yet accepted as an AIDS defining illness.

NON-HODGKIN'S LYMPHOMA

Approximately 3% per year of AIDS-defining illnesses are NHL; the overall incidence in advanced HIV disease being 9% per year. The probability of developing NHL increases dramatically with time following AIDS diagnosis. In one series, it was estimated to be 29% in AIDS patients who had been on AZT for longer than 36 months.

Non-Hodgkin's lymphoma (NHL) has very clearly been shown to have an increased incidence in immunosuppressive states. The incidence of NHL

Correspondence: Current Address — Department of Medical Oncology, Institute of Oncology, Prince of Wales Hospital, Randwick 2031. E-Mail:D.Goldstein*unsw.edu.au

in transplant recipients has been estimated to be between 30 and 40 times that of the general population. NHL in HIV disease is estimated to occur as much as sixty times more frequently than in the general population.

AIDS associated NHL is characterized by aggressive histological subtypes with the majority of tumors being high grade, either large cell immunoblastic or small non-cleaved (Burkitt-like), and the rest being intermediate grade (see Chapter 24 on lymphoma). Those of large cell immunoblastic histology are generally EBV positive, polymorphic, associated with a low CD4 count and are found in the gastrointestinal tract, brain and the oral mucosa. Its incidence increases with increasing age. The small non-cleaved histology are EBV negative and associated with genetic changes such as c-myc deregulation and P53 inactivation, occur at higher CD4 counts and have a distribution involving lymph nodes and bone marrow. Its incidence peaks in the under 20 age group. A possible model for NHL pathogenesis involves chronic antigenic stimulation of lymphocytes resulting in excessive production of factors that stimulate resting B-cells to proliferate. Cells co-infected with the EBV virus

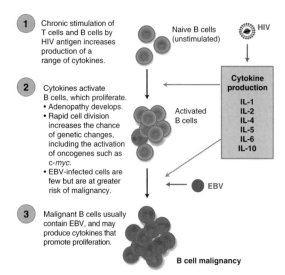

1. Chronic stimulation of T cells and B cells by HIV antigen increases production of a range of cytokines.

2. Cytokines activate B cells, which proliferate.
   • Adenopathy develops.
   • Rapid cell division increases the chance of genetic changes, including the activation of oncogenes such as c-*myc*.
   • EBV-infected cells are few but are at greater risk of malignancy.

3. Malignant B cells usually contain EBV, and may produce cytokines that promote proliferation.

Naive B cells (unstimulated)

HIV

Cytokine production

IL-1
IL-2
IL-4
IL-5
IL-6
IL-10

Activated B cells

EBV

B cell malignancy

In the setting of HIV infection, antigen is not cleared, cytokine production remains disordered, HIV replication continues and cells in the early stages of malignant conversion are not deleted by host immunoregulatory mechanisms

EBV = Epstein–Barr virus; IL = interleukin.

Figure 28.1. How HIV leads to lymphoma (a model based on current knowledge). Source: Millar, J.L., Goldstein, D. and Gelmon, K.A. (1996). "HIV and Kaposi's Sarcoma". *MJA*, **164**, 539–542. © Copyright 1996 *The Medical Journal of Australia* — reproduced with permission".

have a proliferative advantage. Ultimately the hyper-proliferative B-cells transform into a malignant clone. These clones may then establish an autocrine growth factor loop, most likely with the cytokine Interleukin 6 (see Figure 28.1).

The most common presentations of HIV associated NHL are with mass lesions and B-symptoms, and in contrast to Non-HIV lymphoma, there is a preponderance of extra-nodal disease (up to 80% of patients). Over a quarter of patients have involvement of their bone marrow at diagnosis and a similar proportion have involvement of the gastrointestinal tract with features such as rectal and anal abscesses. Central nervous system involvement occurs in over 30% of peripheral lymphomas, hepatic involvement in over 15% and nearly 20% will have positive CSF cytology.

As with all lymphomas appropriate staging includes chest and abdomino-pelvic CT scans, bone marrow aspirate and trephine and CSF fluid cytology to assess extent of disease and other sites, e.g. endoscopy of the gastrointestinal tract as indicated, serum levels of lactate dehydrogenase and total body gallium scans.

Favorable prognostic factors include performance status, the absence of extra-nodal disease, the absence of bulky disease, a CD4 count greater than 100, absence of a previous AIDS-defining illness, absence of CNS involvement and treatment with relatively lower doses of Cyclophosphamide than is standard in the non-HIV setting.

Most of the combination chemotherapy regimens used in non-HIV associated NHL have been tried and it seems clear that the response rates are consistently lower, in the order of 50–60%, with remission durations varying from 5–15 months.

A high incidence of opportunistic infections and poor tolerance of bone marrow suppression has led to the use of chemotherapy regimens with marked reductions in dose. Levine and colleagues showed that a regimen of MBACOD (combination chemotherapy with Methotrexate, Bleomycin, Adriamcyin, Cyclophosphamide, Vincristine, Dexamethasone) at 50% of standard doses achieved a response rate similar to that seen at higher doses. Their response rate was 50% with a median survival of five months. About half the responders achieved a complete response, with a median survival of 15 months. Levine also showed that at least 50% of the deaths in the group who were complete responders could be attributed to non-malignant causes. This has since been confirmed in a large randomized trial of low dose versus standard dose MBACOD at least for the more immunocompromised patients.

In Australia we have used a CHOP-like (Cyclophosphamide, Adriamycin, Vincristine, Prednisone) regimen with Adriamycin replaced by Epirubicin – CEOP. Treatment is generally commenced at 50% of standard doses and escalated according to hematological tolerance. In the first 18 patients treated in this manner, the response rate was over 80% with a median duration of 14 months. This regimen was well tolerated and could be delivered entirely in the outpatient setting. We and others have subsequently demonstrated that antiviral therapy can be safely given with chemotherapy which may decrease the incidence of deaths from opportunistic infections. In addition novel schedules such as infusional chemotherapy and biological agents including interleukin-2 and monoclonal antibodies as consolidation therapy hold promise for further improvement in durable responses.

Although lymphoma remains a major cause of mortality in AIDS, there is reason for guarded optimism in the ability of cytotoxics to provide good palliation and potentially extended survival.

PRIMARY CNS LYMPHOMA

By contrast to the encouraging results for systemic presentations, in terms of response and tolerance to chemotherapy, primary central nervous system lymphoma has a much poorer prognosis. It is almost always EBV positive and is associated with very low CD4 counts, typically under 50 cells per microlitre. The majority of cases present with central nervous system symptoms. It has a characteristic appearance on CT-scan with hyperattenuated lesions and subependymal spread. However, because it is frequently difficult to exclude toxoplasmosis, treatment with sulphadiazine and pyrimethamine is recommended. Stereotactic biopsy may be required for definitive diagnosis. Treatment is generally palliative, i.e. whole brain irradiation which gives symptomatic improvement in approximately 50% of patients, The median survival is 4–5 months.

KAPOSI'S SARCOMA

Kaposi's sarcoma (KS) was first reported by the Hungarian dermatologist, Kaposi, in 1872. He described a disease with a slow and benign progress requiring little in the way of intervention and therapy. This remained a rare condition more recently described in transplant recipients where it was shown that withdrawal of immunosuppressive treatment would often result in spontaneous regression. In the early 1980's an increase of KS in young homosexual men was noted and was the earliest manifestation of the AIDS epidemic. The proportion of patients presenting with KS as their AIDS-defining illness has decreased over the past decade. Nevertheless, the overall prevalence of the disease remains relatively unchanged. Furthermore, with increasing control and prevention of opportunistic infections, the role of KS as a cause of morbidity and mortality is, if anything, increasing. In Australia about 14% of primary AIDS-defining diagnoses are KS and overall risk is estimated to be 30% within three years. The percentage of AIDS patients with KS is greatest between the ages of 20–49. A fall in incidence in parallel with that of AIDS strongly supports a sexual transmission etiology. Recent Australian data suggests a life time risk of 35% of contracting KS and when confounding factors are taken into account show no difference in prognosis between initial and later presentation as an AIDS-related condition.

A new herpes virus, HHV-8, was first described in 1994 as being associated with KS. It has subsequently been identified in KS tumors from HIV and non-HIV-affected individuals. Serologic data shows an increased presence in high risk groups as opposed to the general population in western countries but a much higher incidence in African countries where KS is seen in the non-HIV-affected population. Definitive evidence of direct causation and mechanism is yet to be elucidated.

The current most favored etiological model is that exposure to HIV, together with another putative infectious agent, possibly a novel herpetic virus, results in both activation of the immune system and dysregulation with inappropriate release of a variety of cytokines, many of which cause mesenchymal cell/target cell proliferation. Multiple cells of endothelial and smooth muscle origin then tend to proliferate and form tumors in the presence of other activators, such as one of the proteins of the HIV virus, the tat protein. It is this relatively benign stage that is likely to be manifested as the limited cutaneous disease of initial presentation. Ongoing proliferation may then increase the likelihood of

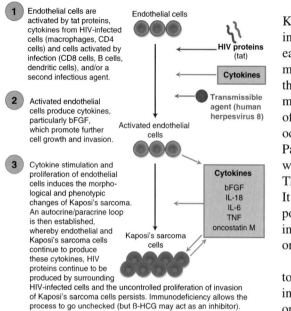

1 Endothelial cells are activated by tat proteins, cytokines from HIV-infected cells (macrophages, CD4 cells) and cells activated by infection (CD8 cells, B cells, dendritic cells), and/or a second infectious agent.

2 Activated endothelial cells produce cytokines, particularly bFGF, which promote further cell growth and invasion.

3 Cytokine stimulation and proliferation of endothelial cells induces the morphological and phenotypic changes of Kaposi's sarcoma. An autocrine/paracrine loop is then established, whereby endothelial and Kaposi's sarcoma cells continue to produce these cytokines, HIV proteins continue to be produced by surrounding HIV-infected cells and the uncontrolled proliferation of invasion of Kaposi's sarcoma cells persists. Immunodeficiency allows the process to go unchecked (but ß-HCG may act as an inhibitor).

bFGF = basic fibroblast growth factor; ß-HCG = ß human chorionic gonadotrophin; IL = interleukin; TNF = tumour necrosis factor.

Figure 28.2. How HIV leads to Kaposi's sarcoma (a model based on current knowledge). Source: Boyle, M.J., Goldstein, D.A., Frazer, I.H. and Sculley, T.B. (1996). "How HIV promotes malignancies". *MJA*, **164**, 230–232. © Copyright 1996 *The Medical Journal of Australia* — reproduced with permission".

malignant transformation manifested by the development of autocrine growth factor production, most particularly the fibroblast growth factors and IL-6 with its manifestation as a true sarcoma with the capacity to metastasize (Figure 28.2).

The cell of origin is controversial, but may well be a combination of mesenchymal cell types, rather than any one type. The histological features include vascular proliferation leading to slit-like vascular channels and the development of a spindle cell population, associated with extravasated erythrocytes.

It is characterized by violaceous, raised nodules. Three characteristic stages are recognized, a patch stage with pigmented macules in the dermis containing small bands of spindle cells, a plaque stage with palpable lesions containing spindle cells associated with reticular and collagen fibres and a nodular stage with sheets of spindle cells and trapped erythrocytes and larger vascular networks leading to more defined tumor masses.

Unlike many other of the AIDS-defining illnesses, KS often occurs at a much higher CD4 count, and in many cases is restricted to cutaneous-only disease for the duration of life. The cutaneous form may be quite indolent or it may progress to involve the entire body, becoming almost confluent. The macular lesions are usually small, faint in color often on the soles, hard palate or nose. Oral lesions occur in up to 45% of those with cutaneous disease. Papular lesions are more commonly on the trunk with larger plaques found on the elbows and knees. The plaques can be associated with painful oedema. It may be quite debilitating, either from a cosmetic point of view or because of pain from weight bearing areas such as the soles of the feet, or pressure on peripheral nerves.

KS in HIV infection may also result in asymptomatic visceral disease particularly of the gastrointestinal tract but may also present with blood loss or abdominal pain. Approximately 10% of patients present with pulmonary or hepatic disease, commonly involving the lung parenchyma with resulting dyspnoea and a widespread nodular infiltrate on chest X-ray.

As with NHL, conventional approaches to the management of KS in HIV infection have not met with great success. A staging system based on involvement of multiple sites and or other organs did not appear to correlate very well with outcome. More recently, a TNM-like system (TNM — International staging system combining size of tumor, presence of lymph nodes and metastases to assess extent of disease) has been used in which the principal features used are:

- the spread of the tumor, restriction to the skin and/or lymph nodes indicating a lower risk of progression than a tumor associated with oedema and/or visceral involvement;
- the degree of immunosuppression, the cut-off point being a CD4 count greater than 200;
- the presence or absence of systemic illness or prior opportunistic infection.

Investigations should be guided by presentation; for indolent limited disease (<10 lesions), careful review of the trunk and limbs and a CXR are all that are required. Those with extensive skin disease should also have an abdomino-pelvic CT scan to assess liver and nodal involvement and endoscopy if clinically indicated prior to initiation of treatment.

Since in the majority of patients with IUV associated KS the disease is indolent for extended periods of time, the initial treatment is watchful observation. Liquid nitrogen cryotherapy is an effective treatment for small lesions; complete recurrences are frequent but edge recurrence is a problem in larger lesions. Intralesional chemotherapy can be used for somewhat larger lesions. For problems of disfiguring or incapacitating lesions, the best approach is radiation therapy with a response rate in the order of 60–70%. A variety of radiation schedules and doses have been used, ranging from single doses of 8 gray up to 20 fractions for a total of 36–40 gray. The major toxicities seen are hyperpigmentation of the site of irradiation and blister formation in thick lesions and on the sole of the foot. In sites involving mucosa such as anorectal and oral disease, quite marked and brisk mucosal reactions occur which are often severe. Radiation is most effective for relief of bleeding up to 80% complete response and least effective for oedema — 30% complete response.

For patients with widespread progressive cutaneous disease, radio-resistant or symptomatic visceral disease, systemic chemotherapy is the remaining therapeutic option. The main agents which have shown responses are Etoposide, Vinca Alkaloids, Adriamycin and Bleomycin. Response rates vary between 50 and 75%, with the anthracyclines, Bleomycin and Etoposide all apparently equivalent in efficacy. Duration of response is relatively short, varying between three and nine months. Combination chemotherapy was initially tried, but caused considerable morbidity and mortality due to the high incidence of associated opportunistic infections and myelosuppression. Morerecently the use of lower doses of chemotherapy has resulted in much better tolerance. For patients with extensive cutaneous disease but no evidence of active visceral involvement, the combination of Bleomycin and Vincristine is well tolerated, principally because of its more limited hematological toxicity. The response rate is in the order of 60% when given at two- to four-weekly intervals. Another commonly used regimen is the combination of Adriamycin, Bleomycin, and Vincristine, given at two-weekly intervals at doses lower than those used in conventional chemotherapy. When compared to a regimen using a conventional dose of Adriamycin there was a lower incidence of opportunistic infections but a similar tumor response rate. However, the increased hematological toxicity of this regimen means its use should be restricted to patients with visceral involvement, most importantly in the lung. The use of G-CSF may improve tolerance but is not recommended as standard therapy.

More recently a liposomal formulation of anthracycline (both doxorubicin and daunorubicin) has shown comparable or better efficacy with markedly reduced toxicity, and is now the treatment of choice as first-line chemotherapy.

The Australian experience with a liposome encapsulated doxorubicin (Doxil) suggests a response rate of 30–40% in advanced disease, but with a marked reduction in toxicity compared to standard chemotherapy. Interferons are not commonly used but in the small group of patients with CD4 counts > 200/ul and no prior opportunistic infections, responses of nearly 50% are described.

Overall median survival is about 15 months; it varies according to TIS (KS-TNM stage), the most favorable group being 2.5–3 years, 1.5 years for intermediate prognosis and nine months for the least favorable.

Novel drug approaches include taxol and possibly antiangiogenesis agents, topical retinoids and possibly in the future antiviral agents against HHV-8.

ANO-GENITAL MALIGNANCIES

Other important HIV associated malignancies are anal neoplasms in gay men and cervical neoplasia in women. A number of studies in gay men have demonstrated much higher incidence of anal intraepithelial neoplasia in HIV positive versus HIV negative men. Anogenital neoplasia appears to be linked to HPV subtypes 16 and 18 which are detected in up to 30% of patients. In women invasive cervical carcinoma has recently been adopted as an AIDS-defining condition. Recent meta-analysis of a number of studies shows an odds ratio of 4.9 for cervical intraepithelial neoplasia (CIN) in HIV positive women. There is an increased incidence in areas with the highest rate of heterosexually acquired HIV infection. The relatively low incidence of anal and cervical carcinoma may well be related to deaths from other opportunistic infections, before sufficient time has elapsed to allow progression to invasive cancer. So far treatment has been the same as the non-HIV setting. In the future, however, the improvement in control of other opportunistic infections may result in an increasing incidence of invasive carcinoma. The poor outcome of conventional therapy suggests that more novel approaches as used in NHL may be needed. Aggressive screening, with cervical screening at six-monthly intervals and early colposcopy if CIN is reported is recommended and treatment of intra-epithelial disease is also required because of the very poor prognosis in this population of men and women.

CONCLUSION

Major strides have been made in improving both the efficacy and tolerability of treatments both for HIV associated Non-Hodgkin's lymphoma and KS. An increase in the effectiveness of new highly active antiretroviral therapy is likely to lead to improved survival in HIV-infected individuals. Accompanying this phenomenon may well be an increase in the prevalence of HIV-related malignancies. This increases the need to identify better treatment strategies. The ultimate goal, however, has to be prevention of the underlying etiological factor for HIV associated malignancies, which is HIV itself. Only by increasing education and awareness of strategies to prevent exposure and acquisition of the HIV virus can the incidence of the HIV associated malignancies be drastically reduced and ultimately eliminated.

References

1. Crowe, S.M., Carlin, J.B., Stewal, K.I. *et al.* (1991). Predictive value of lymphocyte-CD4 numbers for the development of opportunistic infections and malignancies in HIV infected persons. *J. Acquir. Immune Defic. Syndr.*, **4**, 770–776.

2. Reynolds, P., Saunders, L.D., Layefsky, M.E. and Lemp, G.F. (1993). The spectrum of acquired immunodeficiency syndrome (AIDS) — associated malignancies in San Francisco 1980–1987. *Am. J. Epidemiol.*, **137**, 19–30.

3. Herndier, B.G., Kaplan, L.D., McGrath, M.S. *et al.* (1994). Pathogenesis of AIDS Lymphomas. *AIDS*, **8**, 1025–1049.

4. Levine, A. (1992). Acquired Immunodeficiency Syndrome-Related Lymphoma. *Blood*, **80**, 8–20.

5. Kaplanb, L.D., Straus, D.J., Testa, M.A., *et al.* (19??). Low-dose compared with standard-dose m-BACOD chemotherapy for Non-Hodgkin's lymphoma associated with human immunodeficiency virus infection. *The New England J. Med.*, **336**(23), 164.

6. Sparano, J.A., Wiernik, P.H. and Hu, Z. (1996). Pilot trial of unfusional Cyclophosphamide, Doxorubicin and Etoposide plus Didanosine and Filgrastim in patients with human immunodeficiency virus-associated Non-Hodgkin's lymphoma. *Clin. Oncol.*, **14**(11), 3026–3035.

7. Remick, S.C., Diamond, C., Migliozzi, J.A. *et al.* (1990). Primary central nervous system lymphoma in patients with and without the acquired immune deficiency syndrome: A retrospective analysis and review of the literature. *Medicine*, **69**, 345–360.

8. Peters, B.S., Beck, E.J., Coleman D.G. *et al.* (1991). Chan disease patterns in patients with AIDS in a referral centre in the United Kingdom: the changing face of AIDS. *BMJ*, **302**, 203–206.

9. Padiglione, A., Goldstein, D., Law, M.G, *et al.* (19??). Prognosis of Kaposi's Sarcoma as an initial and later AIDS associated illness. *Ann Oncol* (in Press).

10. Chang, Y., Cesarman, E., Pessin, M.S. *et al.* (1994). Identification of Herpes-like DNA sequences in AIDS associated Kaposi's sarcoma. *Science*, **226**, 1865–1869.

11. Kedes, D.H., Operskalski, E., Busch, M., *et al.* (1996). The seroepidemiology of human herpesvirus 8 (Kaposi's sarcoma-associated herpesvirus): Distribution of infection in KS risk groups and evidence for sexual transmission. *Nature Med*, **2**, 918–24.

12. Ensoli, B., Gendelman, R., Maiham, P. *et al.* (1994). Synergy between basic fibroblast growth factor and HIV-1 tat protein in induction of Kaposi's Sarcoma. *Nature*, **371**, 674–680.

13. Krown, S.E., Metroka C., Wernz, J.C. *et al.* (1989). Kaposi's sarcoma in the acquired immune deficiency syndrome. *J. Clin. Oncol.*, **7**, 1201–1207.

14. Chang, L.L., Reddy, S. and Shidnia, H. (1992). Comparison of radiation therapy of classic and epidemic Kaposi's sarcoma. *Am. J. Clin. Oncol.*, **15**, 200–206.

15. Gill, P.S., Rarick, M., McCutchan, J.A. *et al.* (1991). Systemic treatment of AIDS-related Kaposi's sarcoma: results of a randomised trial. *Am. J. Med.*, **90**, 427–433.

16. Goebel, F.-D., Goldstein, D., Goos, M., *et al.* (1996). Efficacy and Safety of Stealth Liposomal Doxorubicin in AIDS related Kaposi's sarcoma. *Bri Cancer*, **73**, 989–994.

17. Gill, P.S., Wernz, J., and Scadden, D.T. (1996). Randomised Phase III trial of Liposomal Daunorubicin versus Doxorubicin, Bleomycin and Vincristine in AIDS related Kaposi's Sarcoma. *J Clin Oncol*, **14**(8), Aug., 2353–2364.

18. Palefsky, J.M., Holly, E.A., Gonzales, J. *et al.* (1992). Natural history of anal cytologic abnormalities and papillomavirus infection among homosexual men with group IV HIV disease. *J. Acquir. Immune Def. Syndr.*, **5**, 1258–1265.

19. Mandelblatt, J.S., Fahs, M., Garibaidi, K. *et al.* (1992). Association between HIV infection and cervical neoplasia: implications for clinical care of women at risk for both conditions. *AIDS*, **6**, 173–8.

29. Pancreatic Cancer

J. JORGENSEN[1] and C.W. IMRIE[2]

[1] *St. George Private Medical Centre, Kogarah, Australia*
[2] *PancreatoBiliary Surgery Unit, Royal Infirmary, Glasgow, Scotland*

INTRODUCTION

Pancreatic cancer is one of the more common causes of cancer-related death in the western world. Improved survival has been defined in early cases. However, most patients present with advanced disease due to the absence of early symptoms and lack of effective screening programs. Surgery for cure occurs in the minority of cases with most patients requiring some form of palliation. This chapter discusses recent advances in diagnosis, staging, curative surgery, palliation and adjuvant therapy for pancreatic carcinoma.

INCIDENCE

In western and industrialized countries pancreatic cancer is the fourth leading cause of cancer-related death in men and the fifth in women. The incidence of pancreatic carcinoma rose three-fold in the western world from the 1920s and stabilized in the late 1970s. This increase in incidence is believed genuine and not simply a consequence of improved diagnostics. Ecologic studies have documented an increase in dietary protein and fats, and cigarette smoking over the same time period.

SEX

There is a higher incidence in men (1.5–1) with the gender bias lessening with advancing age.

AGE

Incidence increases with age. Cases under the age of 40 years are rare. More than 80% of cases occur between the ages of 60 and 80 years.

PREDISPOSING AND RISK FACTORS

Genetic

Black Americans appear to have the highest incidence of pancreatic carcinoma. Other ethnic groups with a high incidence are New Zealand Maoris, Korean Americans and native female Hawaiians. However, environmental factors also play an important role as evidenced by the increased incidence of pancreatic carcinoma in American Blacks over African Blacks and American Japanese migrants compared to resident Japanese.

Pancreatic cancer has been associated with following genetic syndromes: Lynch II, Ataxia-telangiectasis, familial atypical mole-malignant melanoma and hereditary pancreatitis. There is some evidence of a weak familial predisposition to pancreatic carcinoma.

Chromosomal abnormalities associated with pancreatic carcinoma have recently been defined. Most pancreatic carcinomas (90%) have the K-ras mutation at codon 12. Mutations of the p53 suppressor gene occurs in around 70% of cases. There is reduced expression of the DCC gene in 50% of cases and deletions of other tumor suppressor genes have been defined but are less common.

Environmental

Case-control and cohort studies have linked cigarette smoking to an increased risk of developing pancreatic cancer. The relative risk (odds ratio) in most reports range from 1.5 to 3.0. Some work has demonstrated a dose-dependent increase in risk. The increase in pancreatic carcinoma from the 1920s to late 1970s correlates well with an increase in tobacco use over that time. Nitrosamines produced by smoking have been shown to be carcinogenic to the pancreas in animal models. Smokers have been documented to have cytological changes of the pancreatic duct epithelium at autopsy.

There would seem to be an increased risk with diets rich in meat which has been attributed to the protein content. Diets rich in saturated fats and cholesterol have also been linked to an increased risk of pancreatic carcinoma. Both protein and fat stimulate cholecystokinin release. This gut hormone is trophic to pancreatic duct mucosa resulting in increased cell proliferation. Fiber, raw fruit, vegetables and vitamin C have been shown to have a negative risk effect.

Data on alcohol and coffee are conflicting. At this time no convincing evidence exists for alcohol and little if any for coffee as promoters of pancreatic carcinoma.

Association with other disease

Diabetes mellitus has been associated with an increased risk of pancreatic carcinoma in many studies. If recent onset diabetes (i.e. those cases that may have been caused by the cancer) is excluded, the link between the two conditions weakens considerably. Recent work has shown that pancreatic cancer results in increased insulin resistance due to a change in the levels of somatostatin, glucagon and islet associated amyloid polypeptide. This may explain the link between recent diabetes and pancreatic cancer. However, there probably still remains a small association between diabetes mellitus and carcinoma of the pancreas.

Similar problems of cause and effect exist for non-hereditary chronic pancreatitis and pancreatic carcinoma. The observed association may be only reflecting pancreatitis as a symptom of the pancreatic malignancy. If any link exists between the two conditions it is thought to be weak.

PROTECTIVE FACTORS

The consumption of raw fruit and vegetables and vitamin C has been shown to have a negative impact on the development of pancreatic carcinoma. Tonsillectomy has been linked with a lower risk of pancreatic carcinoma. Also, allergy associated conditions such as asthma and eczema have been correlated with a reduced pancreatic carcinoma risk. These findings suggest a role of the immune system in the pathogenesis of pancreatic carcinoma.

PATHOLOGY

A number of tumors arise from the exocrine pancreas. The lesion commonly termed "pancreatic carcinoma", accounts for more than 90% of pancreatic tumors and is a malignant neoplasm arising from ductal epithelial cells. Other tumors are more rare but are of importance as their biologic behavior is often more favorable, having significant implications for therapy as well as prognosis. With lesions that are confined to the pancreas (i.e. no metastases) it is crucial that all histological subtypes have been considered (with or without biopsy) before decisions about treatment and prognosis are made.

Peri-ampullary tumors are often discussed in the context of pancreatic carcinoma as they have the common feature of arising within close proximity of the ampulla of Vater. Peri-ampullary tumors include lesions arising from the pancreatic duct, lower common bile duct, ampulla and the duodenum. The prognosis of the latter three are much better than that for pancreatic carcinoma and this is why all patients with a pancreatic head lesion who are fit for pancreaticoduodenectomy should be referred for expert surgical consultation.

TUMOR TYPE

Classification of primary pancreatic exocrine tumors according to biological behavior are as follows.

Benign
Microcystic serous adenoma

Uncertain biological behavior
Mucinous cystic tumor
Solid-Cystic tumor

Malignant

Microcystic serous adenocarcinoma
Mucinous cystadenocarcinoma
Adenocarcinoma
Acinar cell carcinoma
Pancreaticoblastoma
Small cell carcinoma
Anaplastic tumor

MACROSCOPIC AND MICROSCOPIC FEATURES

Pancreatic carcinoma arises in different areas of the gland as follows: head (70%), body (15%), tail (10%) and multifocal (5%). Macroscopically, the tumors are white or gray and of a hard consistency. There may be central necrosis of the lesion with haemorrhage. A surrounding halo of pancreatitis is usually present secondary to an obstructed pancreatic duct. This makes accurate intra-operative size estimation difficult. The most common histological appearance is of a well-differentiated adenocarcinoma with formation of ducts and a characteristic desmoplastic reaction. Ducts are not normally arranged and individual cells show atypia. There are many descriptive histological variants. On flow cytometry, 20% are aneuploid and this confers a poorer prognosis to the patient. Up to 80% of pancreatic cancers can be shown to have peri-neural invasion on careful histological examination.

MODES OF SPREAD

Pancreatic carcinoma spreads directly, peri-neurally, via lymphatics or the blood stream (portal venous), and finally trans-peritoneal. Within the pancreas, the tumor spreads along inter lobular septa and, when the capsule of the gland is reached, invasion of surrounding tissues occur and the patient effectively becomes incurable. This is much more common for body and tail lesions, as the size of these lesions tends to be greater at presentation.

Common bile duct obstruction, and the resultant jaundice, alerts the patient and the medical profession to the presence of a pancreatic head lesion at a smaller size. The normal anteroposterior diameter of the pancreatic head is between 3–4 cm, hence, only a small lesion can be accommodated in the pancreatic parenchyma before extra pancreatic invasion occurs. Pancreatic head lesions tend to invade into the common bile duct, retroperitoneum, portal vein, duodenum and the root of the transverse mesocolon. Lesions in the tail invade the splenic vessels, the left kidney and adrenal, and the stomach. Peri-neural spread is a feature of pancreatic carcinoma and its presence infers a poor prognosis. This is likely to be due to incomplete excision of the cancer at surgery as the standard Whipple resection does not include a para-aortic and coeliac neurectomy. Lymphatic dissemination is early and occurs even in small lesions. Fifty percent of pancreatic head lesions of < 2 cm have positive lymph node involvement and the incidence of nodal metastases increases with the size of the lesion. The presence of carcinomatous lymphadenopathy is an independent poor prognostic factor. Liver metastases are common and increase with the size of the lesion. Transperitoneal spread is common with advanced disease. However, even in disease thought to be localized to the pancreas on CT, peritoneal lavage will reveal positive cytology in up to 20% of cases. Systemic metastases rarely occur without extensive intra-abdominal disease. After resection disease recurrence occurs equally in the pancreatic bed and the liver. Again systemic metastases are rare in the absence of intra-abdominal disease.

SCREENING

The few 5 year survivors of pancreatic carcinoma attest to the fact that most patients present too late for cure. Screening offers the hope of increasing the number of early cases that present a potential for surgical cure. The problem, at present, is that no high risk population has been defined and imaging modalities such as CT scanning and ERCP are expensive, invasive and have trouble diagnosing very early cases (< 2 cm). Endoscopic ultrasound has been shown to be superior in detecting small lesions but it is not freely available and is very operator dependent. Current serum tumor markers lack the sensitivity and specificity to be useful for screening with the sensitivity of CA 19-9 being 70%, CEA 60% and CA 125 30%. Recently, genetic markers of pancreatic carcinoma have been sought. K-ras mutations have been detected in duodenal juice obtained at endoscopy after secretin stimulation. The test was positive in 60% of patients with pancreatic carcinoma. Ductal hyperplasia has recently been defined as a potential precursor or premalignant lesion. Twelve K-ras mutations are associated with some of these types of hyperplasia. The utility of genetic testing awaits further study but points to possible molecular biology strategies for screening. Invasive imaging may then be selectively used on people defined by genetic testing.

CLINICAL PRESENTATION

Lesions of the pancreatic head present differently to those arising in the body and tail. Most patients (> 90%) with pancreatic head lesions will become jaundiced. The jaundice tends to get progressively worse in most cases; however, it may fluctuate in up to 10%. It usually results from tumor compression of the intra-pancreatic common bile duct. Depending on how close the original lesion is to the common bile duct (CBD) the cancer may be relatively early or advanced by the time jaundice appears. For example, lesions arising in the region of the ampulla tend to present early, whereas jaundice from a lesion arising in the uncinate process usually reflects advanced disease. These patients are classically said to have painless jaundice; however, most do have abdominal pain (although it is true most of them do not suffer severe acute attacks of pain characteristic of biliary colic). The pain is usually upper abdominal and constant and thought to be caused by stretching of the pancreatic capsule. Another source of pain is obstruction of the pancreatic duct with resultant pancreatitis. Discomfort is often exacerbated by intake of food, which increases the pressure in the obstructed pancreatic ductal system. Back pain may reflect retro-peritoneal neural invasion or obstructive pancreatitis. Weight loss is an early and common symptom and is not always due to advanced disease. Recent onset diabetes in an elderly patient should raise the suspicion of an underlying carcinoma. Migrating thrombophlebitis is a sign of advanced pancreatic or other malignancy. Physical examination may be normal or diagnostic depending on the stage of the disease. A palpable gallbladder in the presence of jaundice is said to exclude choledocholithiasis as the cause, but the sign is not reliable. A palpable mass or nodular hepatomegaly signifies advanced disease, as do ascites, supraclavicular lymphadenopathy and a peri-umbilical mass.

Tumors of the body and tail have usually grown to a large size by the time of presentation. Symptoms are usually secondary to advanced disease. Jaundice in these patients often reflects hepatic metastases or common hepatic duct obstruction by metastatic nodes in the liver hilum. Pain is due to pancreatic capsular stretching and invasion into the extra pancreatic tissues. Splenic vein invasion and subsequent thrombosis can lead to left sided portal hypertension and bleeding from fundal varices. Physical examination in these patients often reveals the signs of advanced disease discussed above.

INVESTIGATIONS

The first aim of investigations is to secure a diagnosis. Staging the malignancy may or may not be appropriate, depending on the individual patient and the therapy contemplated.

DIAGNOSIS

Most patients present with obstructive jaundice, and an ultrasound (US) is an excellent initial test. Reliable information will be obtained about the size of the CBD and the presence of gallstones. Pancreatic morphology is not always reliably defined by US. A dilated pancreatic duct (> 4 mm) can often be seen but imaging of the body and tail is usually unsatisfactory secondary to intestinal gas. In good hands a sensitivity and specificity of 90% and 80% have been reported. After US the clinician will have a good idea if the patient truly has obstructive jaundice (i.e. dilated CBD > 5 mm), if there are gallstones or liver secondaries, the presence of ascites and finally any abnormalities of the pancreatic head.

In most patients, where a suspicion of pancreatic carcinoma remains after US, a high resolution dynamic contrast-enhanced CT of the abdomen will be indicated. The radiologist should be shown the US and specifically asked to address the differential diagnosis posed. Lesions of 1 cm and above can be detected with accuracy. A false positive rate of 10% for a mass results from focal pancreatitis, lymphoma and anatomical variation. Secondary signs of pancreatic carcinoma are dilatation of the CBD and main pancreatic duct (MPD) (the double duct sign), invasion of surrounding structures, liver secondaries, lymphadenopathy (if > 2 cm) and ascites. Lesions of the tail and body are accurately defined by the CT and rarely present diagnostic problems.

ERCP is often the next step in the diagnostic process and has the highest sensitivity of all tests for pancreatic carcinoma (> 95%). False negatives occur with small lesions in the uncinate and acinar cell tumors. Diagnostic ERCP comes with a morbidity (5%) and mortality (< 0.5%), and injection of dye into an obstructed biliary tree has a significant risk of converting sterile obstructive jaundice into cholangitis. The test should be performed only after careful consideration of previous non-invasive imaging. Reasons for ERCP are: visualization of the ampulla to diagnose duodenal or ampullary carcinomas, definition of pancreatic and biliary duct morphology to aid diagnosis, brush cytology of strictures and, finally, stenting for palliation of jaundice where indicated.

Clinical, US, CT and ERCP findings combine to give a confident clinicoradiological diagnosis of carcinoma of the pancreas in most patients.

Of the many tumor markers studied in the context of pancreatic cancer CA19-9 has been the most thoroughly evaluated. With a specificity of only < 75% it is clearly not useful for diagnosis. New methods for detection of genetic abnormalities, such as the K-ras mutation, may make genetic testing valuable in the future.

Final diagnosis depends on cytological or histological confirmation. Tissue can be obtained at ERCP with cytology of pancreatic secretions and brush cytology of strictures. These endoscopic maneuvers require some skill and only produce positive results in < 70% of cases. However, they are relatively safe with no risk of tumor dissemination. Fine needle aspiration biopsy (FNAB) and core biopsy can be performed under radiological guidance. False negatives occur, especially with small lesions, and reflect sampling error, but a diagnosis can be achieved in more than 80% of cases. Complications increase with the number of passes and include pancreatitis, pancreatic fistula and bleeding. Seeding of the tract has not been reported, but it is known that pre-operative biopsy increases the rate of positive peritoneal washings. For the above reasons, radiological biopsy should be reserved for patients in whom surgery is not planned. It is important to note that FNAB cannot always distinguish between carcinoma, cystic tumors and neuroendocrine lesions. Those patients proceeding to laparotomy can undergo intra-operative biopsy under optimal conditions. It is the small < 2 cm lesion that often defies all attempts at histological diagnosis. This is the very case where surgery is indicated as the patient has a real chance of cure with surgical excision. Excision will be required in some of these cases without histological proof, highlighting the importance of careful pre-operative clinical, CT and ERCP assessment.

STAGING

Once a diagnosis of pancreatic carcinoma has been arrived at, the patient should be considered for staging. Those deemed unfit for major surgery will need no futher investigations but simply histological confirmation of the diagnosis and appropriate palliation.

Patients who are surgical candidates should undergo US, CT and laparoscopy, in the above order, to define the extent of disease, so that appropriate therapy can be offered. The US and CT will detect signs of advanced disease such as liver metastases and ascites. CT will more accurately define locoregional spread such as invasion or encasement of the portal vein and superior mesenteric artery. Lymphadenopathy may be seen but, on its own, should not preclude exploration unless FNAB is positive for carcinoma. Endoscopic ultrasound has recently been developed to provide further information about local spread. For lesions in the head of the pancreas the relationship to the major vessels can be accurately defined and biopsy of suspicious lymph nodes has been reported. In the future, endoscopic ultrasound may become an important staging tool. Laparoscopy is, finally, done to identify patients with small peritoneal and liver nodules (< 5 mm). These are beyond the resolution of current imaging. Fit patients with disease confined to the pancreas after the above staging are then explored at laparotomy. This is the final arbitrator and only patients judged to have potentially curable disease undergo pancreaticoduodenectomy.

STAGING SYSTEM

The TNM staging system for pancreatic carcinoma is as follows.

Stage 1	T1–T2	N0	M0
Stage 2	T3	N0	M0
Stage 3	any T	N1	M0
Stage 4	any T	any N	M1

T1	No direct extension of tumor
T1 a/b	</> 2 cm in size
T2	Limited direct extension into duodenum, CBD, or peri-pancreatic tissue
T3	Advanced direct extension into adjacent tissues (unresectable)
N0	No lymph node metastases
N1	Lymph node metastases
M0	No distant metastases
M1	Distant metastases

PROGNOSTIC FACTORS

After a curative pancreaticoduodenectomy for carcinoma of the head of the pancreas the following factors have been defined as independent prognostic factors: tumor size, lymph node metastases, positive surgical excision margins and DNA content of the lesion.

Pancreatic carcinomas of < 2 cm are thought to represent "early" disease. The prognostic significance of size has been confirmed in many series with median survival of 20 months for small lesions versus 10 months for large lesions. It is important to note that size is measured from pathological specimens. Pre-operative or intra-operative size estimations are fraught with inaccuracy, due to the halo of pancreatitis that often surrounds pancreatic carcinomas. Patients should not be excluded from surgery pre-operatively on grounds of size alone.

Positive lymph nodes significantly impact on long-term survival. Median survival is reduced from 28 months to 12 months in the presence of lymph node metastases. At this time, there exists no evidence that a more radical operation with a wider lymphadenectomy improves survival. As for breast cancer, positive nodes indicate, in the majority of cases, disseminated disease not curable by surgery alone.

Incomplete excision with resultant positive margins results in a poorer prognosis. Median survival falls from 18 months to 10 months. The 10-month survival is not different to that achieved by surgical biliary bypass, hence there seems little justification for palliative pancreaticoduodenectomy.

The DNA content of the tumor has a strong influence on outcome. Patients with aneuploid tumors have a median survival of 11-months compared to 24 months with diploid tumors.

TREATMENT

Surgery offers the patient with pancreatic carcinoma the only chance of cure. The mortality of pancreaticoduodenectomy has fallen to around 5% in most specialist pancreatic surgical centers. Accompanying this fall in operative mortality have been reports of improved five-year survivals of 15–20%. These improved survival statistics have been scrutinized and cannot be simply dismissed on grounds of better case selection, lead time bias or inclusion of favorable histology tumors. Therefore, indiscriminate "stenting" of patients with disease localized to the pancreatic head cannot be supported. As well, a pre-operative diagnosis of pancreatic carcinoma is sometimes wrong, with the patient having a better prognosis tumor. For these reasons, all patients with non-disseminated disease, who are fit for surgery, should have a surgical consultation. Those patients who, after staging, are thought to have potentially curable disease should undergo a laparotomy. This will account for < 15% of all patients, with the vast majority requiring some form of palliative treatment.

CURATIVE TREATMENT

For lesions in the pancreatic head, a standard pancreaticoduodenectomy remains the operation of choice. This includes resection of all of the duodenum with a short segment of jejunum, the pancreatic head, cholecystectomy and excision of the CBD and a distal gastrectomy. Reconstruction is by way of a hepatico-jejunostomy, gastrojejunostomy and usually a pancreaticojejunostomy. Anastomosis of the pancreas is the Achilles heel of the operation and many different methods of anastomosis have been developed all with their advocates. Total pancreatectomy performed to avoid the risk of pancreatic fistula has not been shown to be safer or oncologically superior; post-operative problems with blood sugar control have been considerable with mortalities directly related to diabetic coma. Pylorus-preserving resection has been shown to have comparable outcome to the standard pancreatico-duodenectomy. The procedure offers some benefits to the patient with regards to post-operative nutrition and reduced post-gastrectomy symptoms. Where the tumor is located in the upper portion of the head, and margins may be compromised by a pylorus-preserving resection a standard resection may be safest. Recently there have been some reports of improved survival with a more radical resection that incorporates an extensive retro-peritoneal and para-aortic lymphadenectomy and neurectomy. To date, no controlled data exist to support such an approach which is accompanied by a higher perioperative morbidity and mortality.

Mortality of pancreaticoduodenectomy has fallen over recent years to around 5% and there are many reasons for this. Care of these patients has tended to be concentrated in expert surgical centers, resulting in increased experience and skill in pre-, intra- and post-operative care. Also, the patients are much better selected with modern staging modalities, thereby improving the case mix.

The morbidity of the procedure remains high at 30–40%. Common post-operative complications are: delayed gastric emptying (20–30%), pancreatic fistula (10–15%), intra-abdominal abscess (10%), hemorrhage, wound infection (5%) and respiratory problems. Delayed gastric emptying usually resolves with conservative measures. It is important to exclude peri-gastric sepsis as a cause and to ensure there is no mechanical obstruction to gastric outflow. Otherwise, prolonged nasogastric suction will usually resolve the situation. Occasionally prokinetic agents such as cisapride suppositories are used in an attempt to hasten resolution. The most common serious post-operative problem is the development of a pancreatic fistula although this can also usually be managed conservatively with prolonged intra-abdominal drainage. CT scanning and sinogram studies will define the fistula anatomy and radiologically placed drains can be employed to secure optimal drainage of fistula fluid. Rarely (< 10%) surgical reintervention is needed to control sepsis from a leaking pancreatic anastomosis. A completion pancreatectomy or drainage of the pancreas into an isolated Roux-loop is usually undertaken. The use of perioperative somatostatin, to suppress pancreatic secretions, has been shown to reduce pancreatic fistula rates, and most surgeons now use it routinely. Intra-abdominal abscess cavities are related to pancreatic fistulas in more than 50% of cases. Leaks from the other two anastomoses are rare. Treatment is adequate drainage either radiological or surgical, depending on the anatomy.

Radiological drainage is preferred, if it can be performed safely and effectively, with surgery reserved for radiological failures. Early hemorrhage reflects inadequate intra-operative hemostasis and is best managed by prompt reoperation. Delayed hemorrhage usually reflects intra-abdominal sepsis and re exploration will be required. Angiography may have a role to play with bleeding that occurs in the context of known intra-abdominal abscess.

Five-year survival figures are in the order of 5–20%. The best results are achieved in diploid lesions that are < 2 cm with negative lymph nodes and clear surgical margins, with five-year survival figures of > 30%. Most resected patients will, however, die from their disease with median survivals of 18-months. Recurrence tends to be loco-regional in the pancreatic bed or hepatic. Systemic metastases are rare in the absence of intra-abdominal disease. For context, duodenal, ampullary and CBD lesions have five-year survivals of 40%, 30% and 20% respectively.

PALLIATIVE TREATMENT

Palliative treatment is concerned with three main problems: jaundice, gastric outlet obstruction and pain.

Jaundice

Jaundice can be palliated effectively (> 90% success) with percutaneous, endoscopic or surgical means. Many trials have been performed to try to define the optimal mode of jaundice palliation but some controversy still exists and the "goal-posts of best practise" are continually shifting with the development of new technology such as expandable metallic stents and laparoscopic surgery. Trans-hepatic drainage was the initial non-operative mode of jaundice palliation. Results were hampered by the discomfort, inconvenience and electrolyte loss of having a permanent external biliary fistula. The development of internal–external drains improved the situation a little from an electrolyte point of view but patients still had an uncomfortable external reminder of their disease. Fully internalized endoprostheses were developed but needed 12–14Fr delivery systems which were associated with significant problems such as bleeding and bile peritonitis. When endoscopic stenting became available, it was shown to be as effective as percutaneous techniques but with lower morbidity. For these reasons, ERCP became the minimally invasive technique of choice for bile duct stenting. The development of expandable metallic stents, which can be effectively delivered via 7Fr tracts transhepatically, have now improved what can be offered radiologically. As most clinicians use ERCP as the procedure of choice for a diagnostic cholangiogram, it is logical to use ERCP as therapeutic tool at the same time. Stenting at ERCP will be successful in over 90% of cases. Percutaneous techniques are reserved for ERCP failures, where either a combined procedure can be done or if appropriate a metal stent placed from above. In summary, ERCP, with occasional help from radiology, can successfully palliate jaundice in most patients. This comes with a low morbidity (< 10%) and low mortality (< 1%). Thirty day mortality remains high, at 10–20% due to the nature of the patient cohort. The problem with endoscopic stenting remains stent occlusion. The median patency of stents for CBD strictures is 4–6 months. As the median survival of patients stented is six months, many will not need a further procedure. But, up to 30% will need repeat stent exchanges for stent occlusion with cholangitis. Surgical bypass is known to have a much lower recurrent jaundice rate (< 10%). ERCP has been compared to open surgical by-pass in prospective randomized trials. In summary, data indicates a reduced initial mortality for endoscopic stenting but this advantage is lost with time as stent occlusion and gastric outlet obstruction occurs. Thirty-day mortality and overall survival are similar. Therefore, it would seem sensible to stent the elderly and infirm and those patients with an expected survival of < six months (the current plastic stent patency). Surgical by-pass should be reserved for fit patients who are predicted to outlive stent patency. Selection of this group of patients should reduce operative mortality to well below 5%. Apart from a more secure long term solution to jaundice, a surgical approach offers the patient the opportunity to undergo gastric by-pass as prophylaxis against gastric outlet obstruction which occurs in 10–15% of patients. Pain can also be effectively reduced by intra-operative chemical splanchnicectomy with 50% alcohol. Also, it should be remembered that, if any doubt exists about the diagnosis or potential for cure, surgical exploration is indicated. Patients found to be non-resectable can then undergo surgical palliation. The contribution of metal stents and laparoscopic biliary by-pass surgery is not known at this time, but considerable potential exists to further improve the quality of palliation with these techniques.

Gastric outlet obstruction

Gastric outlet obstruction occurs in 10–15% of patients. Occasionally, this reflects terminal disease with gastroparesis secondary to neural invasion. These patients are best treated with supportive care only, as surgical by-pass will not relieve their problem. In most patients, however, the gastric outlet obstruction is secondary to malignant duodenal stenosis which should be confirmed by radiology and endoscopy. A gastrojejunostomy will solve the problem in most patients. If the patient is adequately stented and, therefore, no biliary by-pass is required, a laparoscopic gastroenterostomy can be performed. To avoid having to operate on patients at an advanced stage of their illness, most surgeons favor a prophylactic gastroenterostomy at the time of biliary by-pass surgery. Reports of endoscopically placed expandable metallic stents are interesting, and this approach may be valuable in the frail patient.

Pain

Pain will become problematic in most patients. Management by an experienced pain team optimizes their palliation. Most patients' pain can be controlled on regular oral opiates. Anti-emetics are given for nausea and careful attention is needed to prevent constipation. If patients are undergoing surgical palliation, intra-operative chemical splanchnicectomy may be performed. Results of this have been reported to be good, with little in the way of side effects. Thoracoscopic splanchnic nerve division is another operative option for patients who are poorly palliated with narcotics. Percutaneous coeliac axis blocks are also effective with significant pain relief obtained by 80% of patients. External beam radiotherapy has been used effectively in some patients. In patients with pain following a meal, presumably due to main pancreatic duct (MPD) obstruction, stenting of the MPD has resulted in good pain relief, in the small numbers so treated.

PALLIATIVE CHEMORADIOTHERAPY

Combined modality therapy with 5-FU and radiotherapy has been shown to prolong survival in patients with unresectable pancreatic carcinoma. The increase in survival is modest (3–4 months) and this gain needs to be balanced against toxicity and increased hospitalization. Response rates have been instructive for the development of adjuvant chemo-radiation regimes.

ADJUVANT THERAPY

The motivation for using adjuvant therapy, after a curative resection for pancreatic carcinoma, is the predictable low cure rate and the high loco-regional recurrence rate. Combined modality therapy with 5-FU and radiotherapy is currently used and there is some evidence of increased survival with such an approach. Recruitment of suitable patients into prospective randomized trials is crucial, so that the role of adjuvant therapy can be further defined. The European Study of Pancreatic Cancer (ESPAC 1) is an important trial currently under way and should help define the role of adjuvant threrapy. Future advances in the treatment of pancreatic carcinoma are likely to come from better adjuvant therapy.

FOLLOW-UP

From an oncological point of view there is little justification for an intensive follow-up program after a curative resection. Patients presenting with recurrence are deemed incurable and an early diagnosis of recurrence does not improve the outlook. Follow-up, however, is important in the context of audit, research and importantly patient confidence.

References

1. Haddock, G. and Carter, D.C. (1990). Aetiology of pancreatic cancer. *Br J Surg*, **77**, 1159–66.
2. Warshaw, A.L., Gu, Z.Y., Wittenberg, J. and Waltman, A.C. (1990). Preoperative Staging and Assessment of Resectability of Pancreatic Cancer. *Arch Surg*, **125**, 230–233.
3. Trede, M., Schwall, G. and Saeger, H. (1990). Survival After Pancreatoduodenectomy. *Ann Surg*, **211**, 447–458.
4. Cameron, J.L., Pitt, H.A., Yeo, M.D., *et al.* (1993). One Hundred and Forty-five Consecutive Pancreaticoduodenectomies Without Mortality. *Ann Surg*, **217**, 430–438.
5. Geer, J.R. and Brennan, M.F. (1993). Prognostic Indicators for Survival After Resection of Pancreatic Adenocarcinoma. *Am J Surg*, **165**, 68–73.
6. Nitecki, S.S., Saar, M.G., Colby, T.V., *et al.* (1995). Long-term Survival After Resection For Ductal Adenocarcinoma of the Pancreas. Is it Really Improving? *Ann Surg*, **221**, 59–66.
7. Smith, A.C., Dowsett, J.F., Russell, R.C.G., *et al.* (1994). Randomized trial of endoscopic stenting versus surgical bypass in malignant bile duct obstruction. *Lancet*, **344**, 1655–1660.
8. Lillemore, K.D., Sauter, P., Pitt, H.A., *et al.* (1993). Current status of surgical palliation of periampullary carcinoma. *Surg Gynaecol Obstet*, **176**, 1–10.
9. Moertel, C.G., Frytak, S., Hahn, R.G., *et al.* (1991). Therapy of Locally Unresectable Pancreatic Carcinoma: A Randomized Comparison of High Dose (6000 Rads) Radiation Alone, Moderate Dose Radiation (4000Rads + 5-Fluorouracil), and High Dose Radiation + 5-Fluorouracil. *Cancer*, **48**, 1705–1710.
10. Kaleser, M.H. and Ellenberg, S.S. (1985). Pancreatic Cancer. Adjuvant Combined Radiation and Chemotherapy Following Curative Resection. *Arch Surg*, **120**, 899–903.
11. Gastrointestinal Tumor Study Group (1987). Further Evidence of Effective Adjuvant Combined Radiation and Chemotherapy Following Curative Resection of Pancreatic Cancer. *Cancer*, **59**, 2006–2010.

Pancreatic Cancer

Worldwide: 15th most common
             More common in developed countries

Lifetime risk
in USA whites:
  M   1 in 90
  F   1 in 80

Relative five-year survival in 1983–87
in USA whites:
  M   2.3 %
  F   3.6 %

Risk factors
Tobacco
Dietary factors suspected

Geographical variation in 1983–87
Highest rate
M: 13.7 per 100,000 in USA, Alameda, black
F: 11.9 per 100,000 in USA, Alameda, black
Lowest rate
M: 0.7 per 100,000 in India, Ahmedabad
F: 0.2 per 100,000 in India, Ahmedabad

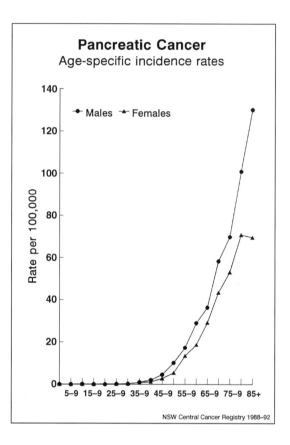

Pancreatic Cancer
Age-specific incidence rates

NSW Central Cancer Registry 1988–92

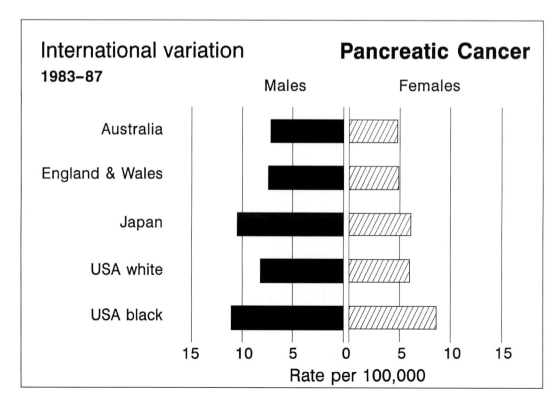

International variation
1983–87

Pancreatic Cancer

Males   Females

Rate per 100,000

30. Management of Metastatic Cancer

WILLIAM B. ROSS and JOHN KEARSLEY

The St. George Hospital, Kogarah, Australia

INTRODUCTION

There can be little doubt that the patient with metastatic disease poses one of the most challenging problems for the oncologist. It has been estimated that approximately 30% of all newly diagnosed cancer patients will have detectable metastases at the time of first diagnosis, and 60–70% of patients will develop metastatic disease at some time prior to death.

As a general rule, the advent of metastatic disease implies incurability, and the primary focus of treatment becomes the maintenance of a good quality of life for as long as possible. Therefore, almost all patients with metastatic disease will require palliative and supportive care, and the oncologist must be ever vigilant to ensure that active intervention promotes a good quality of life rather than causes harm. Skilled management of patients with metastatic disease requires careful thought as to the most appropriate treatments for individual patients; for some patients with relatively slowly growing metastases, aggressive interventions, e.g. radical surgical resections and high dose chemotherapy, may be totally appropriate. In other cases where metastatic disease runs an aggressive course, symptomatic measures alone may suffice. The therapeutic approach must be individualized and will vary according to the extent of tumor burden, the presence of troublesome symptoms, a patient's performance status and the time interval between clinical diagnosis of cancer and the diagnosis of metastatic disease.

LIVER

Of the many tumors which metastasize to the liver, the most common arise from primary lesions within the gastrointestinal tract, pancreas, lung and breast. The prognosis for patients with extensive liver metastases is poor in most cases and symptoms include right upper quadrant discomfort, anorexia, nausea, fevers, malaise and weight loss. A CT scan of the abdomen is the method of choice for detection of hepatic metastases and the evaluation of a potential primary site within the remainder of the abdomen or pelvis. In most cases, serum alkaline phosphatase and gamma glutamyl transpeptidase (GGT) levels will be raised.

Less advanced metastatic disease may be found coincidentally on ultrasound or CT scanning, or may be diagnosed following the detection of a rising CEA level in patients with a past history of colorectal malignancy. A small proportion of colorectal patients are found to have a solitary hepatic metastasis, and surgical resection can offer a five-year survival rate of 35% in selective patients. More extensive involvement of a single lobe may also be resected in certain cases with good palliation. Prolonged survival after resection of hepatic metastases in the absence of extra hepatic disease is better if the number of metastases is small, the disease-free interval long or tumor marker levels not unduly raised. Radiation therapy can relieve pain due to localized symptomatic liver deposits although the limiting factor in treating hepatic metastases with radiotherapy is the restricted tolerance of normal liver. Regional hemoperfusion with 5-FU or FUDR may offer a survival advantage in patients with unresectable colorectal cancer liver metastases. In the presence of rapidly developing extra hepatic metastases, symptomatic treatment alone usually suffices in allaying distressing symptoms.

LUNG

The lung is a very common site for metastatic spread from many cancers, particularly cancers of the breast, kidney, melanoma, sarcomas and many GI cancers. Whereas some lung metastases may be large, e.g. sarcomas, germ cell tumors, renal cell carcinoma, other lung metastases are characteristically small, e.g. thyroid cancer.

Most lung metastases are detected on routine radiology during follow-up of treated malignancy. Patients with lung metastases may be asymptomatic, yet others may complain of shortness of breath on exertion, a dry hacking cough and pleuritic chest pain. At the time of detection, most patients will have metastases at other sites and active intervention is often based on the use of systemic chemotherapy appropriate to the primary tumor. Surgery can remove solitary lung metastases for diagnosis or therapeutic purposes, particularly if there has been a long disease-free interval. Long-term survival may be possible following resection of selected patients with lung metastases, e.g. osteosarcoma. Radiotherapy can relieve occasional symptoms of haemoptysis, bronchial obstruction or pain and small fields with abbreviated treatment regimens will be used. However, radiotherapy for lung metastases is limited by the radiosensitivity of normal lung tissue. In several radiosensitive childhood malignancies, whole lung irradiation may be possible with good long-term survival.

Chemotherapy can be curative in sensitive tumors such as germ cell malignancy, chorio carcinoma and Hodgkin's disease. In other patients with lung metastases from breast cancer or colonic malignancy, worthwhile palliation using chemotherapy can be achieved.

BRAIN

The most common causes of brain metastases are primary cancers of the breast, lung, kidney and melanoma. Symptoms of brain metastases include headaches, nausea, vomiting, incoordination, disordered gait, seizures and localized sensory symptoms. A CT or MRI scan will be the investigation of choice. The conventional treatment of patients with brain metastases is radiotherapy, commonly to a dose of 30 Gy delivered over a two-week period. Dexamethasone is also used in conjunction with radiotherapy although dexamethasone dosage should be reduced promptly following completion of radiotherapy in order to prevent distressing corticosteroid-induced side effects. Brain metastases from melanoma usually respond poorly to radiotherapy.

The surgical excision of brain metastases is rarely indicated. Urgent relief of raised intracranial pressure by surgical intervention may be indicated in selected patients who do not respond to high dose corticosteroids. Optimal treatment for patients with single brain metastases includes surgical excision followed by post-operative radiotherapy. Most recently, stereotactic radiosurgery has been used in several centers for the treatment of small solitary radiographically-defined brain metastases.

Chemotherapy has been given by the intrathecal route, but is limited to only a few sensitive cancers, e.g. small cell lung cancer, breast cancer, testicular cancer and lymphoma.

BONE

Pain is a major symptom for many patients with metastatic cancer. The major cause of severe pain is metastatic bone disease. Apart from producing pain bone metastases cause pathological fractures.

The vast majority of bone metastases are caused by cancer of the lung, breast and prostate. In metastases from the solid organ cancers management is aimed at palliation rather than cure.

The principal symptom is of course pain. A radioisotope bone scan will detect lesions at an earlier stage than plain X-rays. It should be noted that in renal cell carcinoma and thyroid carcinoma lytic bone lesions are often not associated with bone regeneration and may not be detected on isotope scans.

In the limb local treatment is directed at preventing pathological fractures. Radiotherapy is the treatment of choice; internal fixation may also be required.

In the spine, metastatic tumors can cause compression of the cord or spinal nerve roots. MR or myelographic CT scans are considered the most useful investigations in a patient suspected of cord compression. Suspected cord compression is a medical emergency requiring rapid investigation and surgical decompression and/or radiotherapy may be required to avoid devastating neurological sequelae. Substantial metastatic damage may cause instability of the spine which may require internal fixation.

The majority of bone metastases are multifocal and systemic treatment of the primary cancer may be considered. Breast cancer responds well to treatment with hormones or chemotherapy. Similarly, hormone treatment in patients with prostate cancer can achieve good palliation. Myeloma will often respond well to chemotherapy. Patients with bony cancer, on the other hand, have a very limited prospect of survival in the presence of bony metastases and chemotherapy may be of little benefit.

Treatment with biphosphonates may relieve pain in patients with osteolytic lesions. Osteoblastic lesions caused by prostate cancer may respond well with relief of pain to radioactive strontium.

Widespread bony metastases may cause hypercalcemia (discussed later).

MALIGNANT ASCITES

Malignant ascites is caused by involvement of the peritoneal cavity by the malignant process. Other causes of ascites such as cirrhosis and heart failure should be excluded. Tumors which are the usual causes of ascites include ovarian, endometrial, breast, pancreatic and gastric cancer. Increasing abdominal distension causes discomfort and may affect respiration.

Peritoneal paracentesis for cytology may assist diagnosis. If the tumor is sensitive to chemotherapy, e.g. breast or ovarian, then systemic therapy may help the ascites. For others installation of chemotherapeutic agents into the peritoneal cavity has variable results. Peritoneal ascites can be shifted to the venous system by placement of a peritoneal venous shunt. Circulatory overload can cause congestive heart failure. Disseminated intravascular coagulation is another important complication. Subsequently, the shunts may block or thrombose.

In contrast to cirrhotic ascites, dietary salt restriction and diuretic drugs have only limited success in the management of malignant ascites.

Repeated paracentesis seems to gain little while causing great distress to the patient. It can be complicated by protein depletion, and damage to intra-abdominal organs.

Intraperitoneal instillation of chemotherapeutic agents is attracting interest and may be of use in the future in colon cancer. Good results have been described in mucinous cancers of the appendix.

PERICARDIAL EFFUSION

Most cases of neoplastic cardiac tamponade result from metastatic invasion of the pericardium. Fluid accumulates in the pericardial sac which prevents filling of the cardiac chambers. Cancers with the greatest risk for causing this complication include breast and lung cancer, lymphoma, leukemia and melanoma. Non-malignant causes of pericardial effusion such as radiation induced pericarditis and infections are important and should be considered in a cancer patient. Many patients with pericardial effusions are asymptomatic. Patients present often with non-specific symptoms of weakness and lethargy caused by the poor cardiac output. Other signs of cardiac failure may also be present by chest pain, peripheral oedema, dyspnoea. The diagnosis is usually confirmed by echocardiography or CT scan.

Cardiac tamponade requires urgent treatment by emergency paracentesis. Examination of the aspirated fluid will determine the cause, be it malignant or infectious.

The definitive management of malignant pericardial effusion has not been fully clarified. Treatment options include systemic chemotherapy, pericardial radiotherapy, pericardial drainage or surgery to make a pericardial pleural window. The type of management will be influenced by the primary tumor and by the prognosis of the patient.

MALIGNANT PLEURAL EFFUSION

Malignant pleural effusions may be caused by increased capillary permeability due to inflammation or disruption of the capillary epithelium or by malignant obstruction of lymphatic drainage. Malignant effusions are therefore generally exudative with a high protein content.

Malignancies which commonly cause pleural effusions include those arising in breast, lung, ovary, gastrointestinal tract and also lymphomas. As with pericardial effusions, only half of pleural effusions in cancer patients are due to a malignant process. Again, diagnosis is a key step in management. Congestive heart failure and infection are two common causes of pleural effusion. Aspiration and pathological examination of pleural fluid should be done at an early stage. However, only 50% of malignant pleural effusions will have positive cytology at this stage. Pleural biopsy may be required to confirm the diagnosis.

The treatment of the pleural effusion will depend on the tumor type. Malignant effusions caused by breast cancer, small cell lung cancer and lymphoma may be sensitive to chemotherapy or hormones unless there has been a substantial prior treatment.

Other treatments are available. Thoracocentesis alone gives temporary relief of symptoms only. Tube thoracotomy combined with pleural sclerosis with bleomycin or tetracycline (doxycline) will have success in two-thirds of cases. Thorascopic insufflation of sclerosing agents is more successful. Pleural stripping is the most effective treatment but has very high morbidity.

A pleuro peritoneal shunt can also be inserted surgically but this procedure has a 25% risk of shunt occlusion.

SPINAL CORD COMPRESSION

The bones of the vertebral column represent the most common site of metastatic disease, and compression of the spinal cord or cauda equina is not infrequently seen in patients with advanced cancer, particularly from primary tumors of the lung, breast, prostate and melanoma. Spinal cord compression is an oncologic emergency, and delay in treatment will result in irreversible paralysis and sphincteric incontinence.

Although many patients will present with back or chest wall radicular pain, the first sign in many patients may involve heaviness of the lower limbs or incoordination. The vertebra may be tender to palpation at the involved level, but once sensory, motor or autonomic symptoms develop, progression to irreversible paraplegia is often rapid.

Should spinal cord compression be suspected, then corticosteroid therapy is instituted immediately and the diagnosis is made by CT or MRI scanning.

Treatment is aimed at preserving neural function, control of locally advanced malignancy, stabilization of the vertebral column and the relief of pain. Both

radiotherapy and surgery (decompression laminectomy) alone or combined can achieve these goals. However, the presence of paraplegia at the time of diagnosis is associated with a very poor prognosis. Clinical trials have not determined the superiority of a particular treatment regimen although surgery is usually favored when the onset of paraparesis is rapid or when a tissue diagnosis is lacking.

SUPERIOR VENA CAVAL SYNDROME

Nearly all cases of superior vena caval (SVC) syndrome are caused by malignancy. Most common primary tumors include lung, lymphoma, and rarely germ cell tumors. The clinical features of SVC syndrome include suffusion and swelling of the subcutaneous tissues of the head and neck, a raised jugular venous pressure, headaches, distended upper chest wall veins, visual disturbances and plethora/oedema of the upper extremities.

The diagnosis is based on the characteristic clinical signs and symptoms and a chest X-ray will reveal a mass lesion adjacent to the superior vena cava in the majority of cases. CT and MRI scans may reveal more detailed information.

Treatment is aimed at the relief of symptoms, usually by a combination of corticosteroids and local field irradiation. In some patients with chemosensitive malignancies, e.g. small cell lung cancer, chemotherapy may be combined with radiotherapy. The syndrome improves in more than 70% of patients and death from the syndrome is unusual unless there is a complicating factor such as cerebral metastasis or tracheal obstruction.

HYPERCALCEMIA

Hypercalcemia is a frequent complication in certain types of cancer. It has life threatening potential and can have an insidious onset which delays recognition of the problem.

Breast and lung cancer are important causes as are lymphoma, leukemia and multiple myeloma. With breast cancer hypercalcemia may occur in up to one third of patients with metastatic disease. It should be noted that hypercalcemia can occur in the absence of bony metastases.

The symptoms of hypercalcemia include anxiety, fatigue, weakness, anorexia, nausea, abdominal pain, polydipsia, constipation and mental disturbances. On examination there may be evidence of muscle weakness and decreased reflexes. Mental changes include restlessness, difficulty in concentrating, depression, apathy, lethargy, confusion, acute psychoses and ultimately decreased consciousness leading to coma.

Treatment of hypercalcemia in a patient with advanced cancer should follow the principles of palliative care — in particular to maintain quality of life.

Intravenous fluid (isotonic saline) in large volumes is given in the acute case. Immobilization increases resorption of calcium from bone and should be avoided. Dialysis may be appropriate for patients with renal failure who have a relatively good prognosis with their cancer. A high dietary calcium intake is contraindicated.

Drugs which are known to precipitate hypercalcemia should be withdrawn. These include estrogens, antiestrogens and thiazide diuretics. Chemotherapy directed at the underlying malignancy may produce remission. In breast cancer the initial use of hormonal therapy may actually aggravate hypercalcemia, e.g. tamoxifen.

Hypercalcemia can be reversed in most cases if recognized and treated aggressively. Increasing severity of the initial hypercalcemia worsens the prognosis.

Biphosphonates inhibit bone resorption of calcium and are an effective treatment. Pamidronate is effective in 80% of cases. Etidromate is less effective while clodromate is more effective but takes longer to achieve the effect. Phosphate therapy and calcitonin have limited roles.

The drug of first choice in the treatment of tumor induced hypercalcemia is disodium pamidronate. The recommended dose is 30–90 mg as a single dose or 15–30 mg/day for 2–3 days. The drug is given as a slow intravenous infusion.

31. Paraneoplastic Syndromes, Emergencies and Neuroendocrine Cancer

DAVID L. MORRIS

UNSW Department of Surgery, The St. George Hospital, Kogarah, Sydney, Australia

PARANEOPLASTIC SYNDROMES

While both primary and secondary tumors can produce symptoms due to the mechanical effects of the tumor they can also present with symptoms and signs produced at a remote site, and these are called paraneoplastic syndromes. The mechanism may involve a hormone, e.g. ACTH or PTH, or a growth factor.

Common examples include Cushing's syndrome from lung cancer, inappropriate ADH secretion (lung cancer), hypercalcemia (small cell cancer), acromegaly (carcinoid, pancreatic cancer). Gynecomastia, precocious puberty and menstrual disturbance can be due to gonadotrophic secretion by cancers (pituitary, gestational trophoblastic tumors including hydatiform mole and choriocarcinoma, testicular and ovarian germ cell tumors, and occasional lung cancers).

Neurological paraneoplastic syndromes

CNS paraneoplastic syndromes are less common than brain mets or embolism but include subacute cerebellar degeneration, dementia, optic neuritis and spinal cord and peripheral nerve syndromes.

Hematology Paraneoplastic Syndromes

Polycythemia (hypernephroma, hepatoma due to erythropoietin). Anemia due to blood loss, bone marrow invasion but also due to bone marrow damage from radiotherapy or chemotherapy.

Hemolytic syndromes can also be seen in cancer. Thrombocythemia (>400,000/µl) is common in cancer patients and contributes to their increased risk of DVT. Thrombocytopenia in cancer is usually related to marrow injury from chemotherapy or radiotherapy. An ITP-like syndrome can be seen in cancer. Migratory thrombophlebitis (Trousseau's syndrome) is particularly associated with mucus secreting adenocarcinomas (especially pancreas).

Disseminated intravascular coagulation (DIC) is not common in cancer but can be associated with leukemia, lung, pancreas and prostate cancer.

Fever can be regarded as a paraneoplastic syndrome; it is especially seen in lymphoma, hypernephroma, osteogenic sarcoma and liver tumors.

Gastrointestinal paraneoplastic syndromes

The commonest syndromes are those due to hormone secretion, including the Zollinger Ellison (gastrin), carcinoid syndrome (5HT). These and other less common neuroendocrine tumors are covered later in the chapter.

ONCOLOGICAL EMERGENCIES

Superior vena cava compression syndrome

Patients can present with dyspnoea, facial swelling, oedema and cyanosis, cough, arm swelling, venous distension. Frequent cancer causes include primary lung cancer and lymphoma. Urgent treatment by chemotherapy or radiotherapy is indicated.

Spinal cord compression

This is covered in Chapter 12.

Metabolic

Hypercalcemia is the commonest of the metabolic emergencies and is most commonly seen in myeloma and breast cancer but can be seen in many other cancers. It is due to excess bone resorption and may be seen in the presence or absence of bone metastases. It is often due to a PTH-related protein but prostaglandins and growth factors can also be involved. Patients can present with:

GI	Anorexia, nausea, vomiting, constipation
CNS	Fatigue, depression, psychosis
Renal	Thirst, polyuria, polydypsia

Treatment is with IV isotonic saline, perhaps 400 ml/hour for 3-4 hours then re-check electrolytes (K^+ and Mg^{2+} will fall). Corticosteroids produce short-term inhibition of osteoclast activity and reduce GI absorption, calcitonin has a modest but rapid effect increasing renal excretion and reducing bone resorption.

Bisphosphonates — these are absorbed into the hydroxyapatite and inhibit resorption.
Mithromycin — this kills osteoclasts but can have significant renal, hepatic and coagulation side effects. Dialysis may be considered if there is marked renal insufficiency.

Hyperuricemia

Renal insufficiency can occur when the urine is supersaturated with urate. It can be seen in leukemia and lymphoma. It is treated with IV hydration, alkalinization of urine and a diuretic to maintain urine output. Allopurinol can be used because it inhibits xanthene oxidase and xanthine is more soluble than uric acid.

Tumor lysis syndrome

Rapid release of intracellular constituents causing hyperuricemia, hyperkalemia, hypocalcemia, hyperphosphatemia, cardiac arrhythmia and acute renal failure may result. It is most frequently seen in lymphoma/leukemia; we produce a similar syndrome with large volume hepatic cryotherapy.

Hypoglycemia

This is mainly due to insulinoma but can also be seen in hepatoma and with sarcomas.

Lactic acidosis

This is usually seen in lymphoma and leukemia. It results in hyperventilation, hypotension and tachycardia. It may be treated with IV bicarbonate and treatment of the underlying malignancy. It has a poor prognosis.

Adrenal insufficiency

Due to destruction of adrenals by tumor, produces weight loss, weakness, anorexia, hyperpigmentation and postural hypotension. Collapse and shock are not common. Treat with parenteral corticosteroid.

Surgical emergencies

The common complications of GI neoplasms are those of hemorrhage, obstruction and perforation (or bleed, block and bust). Surgery may be required for perforation of gut following chemotherapy where intestinal neoplasm, commonly lymphoma, has been lysed during treatment.

Hepatic artery catheters

Hemorrhage from arterial access devices, especially hepatic artery catheters, either into the GI tract or peritoneum, can be a life threatening but relatively easily remediable complication. Any patient with pain during arterial chemo should be urgently investigated for this complication (UGI scope, portacathogram).

Airway

Thyroid neoplasms can produce life threatening airway compression which may be very difficult to manage — tracheostomy through a large vascular tumor can be a most difficult and dangerous procedure. Whenever possible the situation should be avoided by urgent treatment of the thyroid neoplasm, usually by radiotherapy.

Urology

Bladder hemorrhage can be due to tumor or a complication of chemotherapy/radiotherapy. Clot retention may require bladder washout under anesthesia and/or an irrigating catheter. While a conservative approach is usually appropriate when the bleeding is a complication of treatment, specific anti-tumor treatment endoscopic resection/diathermy is usually required for bladder tumors if they cannot be removed. Obstruction of the urinary tract by tumor can occur at several levels, ureteric compression by retroperitoneal cancer is not uncommonly seen in advanced disease, endoscopically placed stents may palliate the obstruction. It is commonly held that uraemia is a pleasant way to die and that malignant ureteric obstruction should not be treated but this will depend on the type of tumor, possibility of response to further therapy and the patient's wishes.

Priapism is a pathological engorgement and sustained erection of the penis due to thrombosis of the corpora cavernosa. It is seen in leukemia. Spinal anesthesia, anti-coagulation or washouts of the corpora may be of value and a communication between the unengorged glans and the corpora cavernosa may be created surgically or with a trucut biopsy needle. An anastamosis between the saphenous vein and corpora can also be used.

NEUROENDOCRINE CANCERS

Carcinoid tumor

These tumors arise from neuroectodermal cells characterized by argentaffin staining. They commonly affect the appendix and small bowel but stomach, rectal and bronchial carcinoids are seen. Malignancy varies with the tumor site — characteristically, those of the appendix are quite benign and those of the rectum more malignant. Excess serotonin secretion by liver metastases may lead to the carcinoid syndrome of flushing, diarrhea and bronchospasm. Hypertension, valve lesions and telangiectasis can also occur. Carcinoid syndrome is not seen with primary carcinoid tumor because the liver metabolizes the serotonin. Investigations include measurement of 5HIAA in the urine and serotonin in the blood. Treatment is resection of the primary tumor, and liver metastases should be resected or treated by cryotherapy. Prolonged palliation for inoperable liver disease can be achieved by hepatic artery embolization. Specific chemotherapy with streptozotocin can be useful. Long-acting somatostatin analogs are useful in controlling symptoms but also can sometimes produce tumor regression. Many carcinoid tumors do not secrete 5HT.

Multiple Endocrine Neoplasia (MEN)

The cells involved are called APUD (Amino Precursor Uptake Decarboxylase) cells and are derived from neuroectoderms.

MEN 1   Parathyroids, pancreatic islets, pituitary, adrenal cortex
Often presents with peptic ulcer from gastrinoma

MEN 2   Parathyroid hyperplasia, phaeochromocytoma, medullary thyroid carcinoma. (High calcitonin).

Gastrinoma (Zollinger Ellison Syndrome)

An adenoma or carcinoma producing gastrin of variable malignancy. Typically presents with peptic ulceration and can affect not only duodenum but oesophagus or jejunum. Measure serum gastrin, treat ulceration with omeprazole, assess pancreatic tumor for resectability, often slowly growing and worth resecting primary and nodes/liver metastases.

Insulinoma

This produces hypoglycaemia, alteration in mood, neurologic disturbance, 70% are single benign tumor, 10% are multiple, 10% malignant. CT scan, angiography and selective venous sampling are used to localize tumors. Resection is the preferred treatment.

VIPOMAS

Excess secretion of vasoactive intestinal peptide results in watery diarrhea, hypokalaemia and achlorhydria (WDHA) or pancreatic cholera.

Index